ANIMAL
BEHAVIOUR

ANIMAL BEHAVIOUR

For
B.Sc. and M.Sc. students of Universities of India and abroad.
Candidates preparing for Civil Services (Mains) conducted by UPSC.
Aspirants of National Eligibility Test (NET) for lectureship conducted by UGC.
Students preparing for Junior Research Fellowship (JRF) conducted by CSIR.
Selection Test for Lectureship (SLET) conducted by different States.
Persons interested in wildlife and pet animals.

S. PRASAD M.Sc., Ph.D., FAZ
Professor & Head, Deptt. of Zoology
M.G. College, Gaya (Bihar) 823001

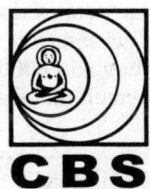

CBS

CBS Publishers & Distributors Pvt. Ltd.

New Delhi • Bengaluru • Chennai • Kochi • Kolkata • Mumbai
Hyderabad • Nagpur • Patna • Pune • Vijayawada

ISBN: 979-81-239-1066-5 (PB)
ISBN: 81-239-1131-9 (HB)

First Edition: 2004
Reprint: 2007, 2011, 2018

Published by **Satish Kumar Jain** and produced by **Varun Jain** for
CBS Publishers & Distributors Pvt. Ltd.,
4819/XI Prahlad Street, 24 Ansari Road, Daryaganj, New Delhi - 110002
delhi@cbspd.com, cbspubs@airtelmail.in • www.cbspd.com
Ph.: 23289259, 23266861, 23266867 • Fax: 011-23243014

Corporate Office: 204 FIE, Industrial Area, Patparganj, Delhi - 110 092
Ph: 49344934 • Fax: 011-49344935
E-mail: publishing@cbspd.com • publicity@cbspd.com

Branches:
• *Bengaluru:* 2975, 17th Cross, K.R. Road, Bansankari 2nd Stage,
  Bengaluru - 70 • Ph: +91-80-26771678/79 • Fax: +91-80-26771680
  E-mail: cbsbng@gmail.com, bangalore@cbspd.com
• *Chennai:* No. 7, Subbaraya Street, Shenoy Nagar, Chennai - 600030
  Ph: +91-44-26681266, 26680620 • Fax: +91-44-42032115
  E-mail: chennai@cbspd.com
• *Kochi:* Ashana House, 39/1904, A.M. Thomas Road, Valanjambalam,
  Ernakulum, Kochi • Ph: +91-484-4059061-65
  Fax: +91-484-4059065 • E-mail: cochin@cbspd.com
• *Kolkata:* 6-B, Ground Floor, Rameshwar Shaw Road, Kolkata - 700014
  Ph: +91-33-22891126/7/8 • E-mail: kolkata@cbspd.com
• *Mumbai:* 83-C, Dr. E. Moses Road, Worli, Mumbai - 400018
  Ph: +91-9833017933, 022-24902340/41 • E-mail: mumbai@cbspd.com

Representatives:

• Hyderabad: 0-9885175004	• Nagpur: 0-9021734563
• Patna: 0-9334159340	• Pune: 0-9623451994
• Jharkhand: 0-9811541605	• Uttarakhand: 0-9716462459

Printed at:
India Binding House, Noida, UP (India)

Dr. Hari Mohan Prasad

Professor & Head, Deptt. of English,
Dean, Faculty of Humanities,
Magadh University, Bodh-Gaya,
Vice-Chairman, J.S.S. Gaya
Est. Under Ministry of HRD
Govt. of India, New Delhi,
Editor − Orbit.

Aastha,
M-74, Housing Colony,
Gaya, Bihar.
Tel. : 420868
E-mail − Harimohanpd.@yahoo.com.in.

FOREWORD

Centuries ago, the great English Romantic poet Wordsworth warned us that mankind would face extinction if man did not maintain a mutually nourishing reciprocal relationship with Nature that is environment. What was his poetic creed then has become scientific truth now. We have sullied our rivers, ransacked our woods, mutilated our hills and, above all, we have played havoc with the wildlife, which is the prime centre of ecological balance. We have killed them for our pleasure and pastime, for our cuisine and commercial gains. The need of the hour is to protect and preserve them.

Dr. Prasad's book "Animal Behaviour" is a sensitive response to awaken in human beings a keen interest in the world of fauna. In a lucid, easy-to-understand language with attractive visuals, Mr. Prasad has unfolded the fascinating world of animals. Their behaviours surprise us, excite us, enthral us and sometimes baffle us. The book is not only a rich treasure of information but also an enchantingly readable narrative. All those enlightened people who watch National Geographic channel or Discovery channel or Animal Planet avidly will find an equivalent counterpart in black and white in this book. The book is relevant for each of us if we are sensitive to the world around us.

Hari Mohan Prasad

PREFACE

Konrad Lorenz's remark that *"people mostly deal only with lifeless artificial objects in their daily work, with objects that are not particularly beautiful and that are by no means appropriate to inspire awe. That is why most people have forgotten how to live with living creatures"* is no longer truism.

In fact, the scenario is changing fast in the 21st century. The popularity of cartoon films featuring Mickey and Minnie Mouse, Donald Duck, Tom and Jerry etc. reflect the imaginative expression of keen human interest in animals. Now-a-days Discovery channel and National Geographic channel are most popular channels for TV viewers because they mostly exhibit episodes of animal behaviour. Now, almost all universities of India have introduced *"Animal Behaviour"* as a subject of study at undergraduate and postgraduate levels.

The study of animal behaviour is known as "ethology". This element of life science is both intriguing and fascinating, but surprisingly enough both foreign and Indian authors have overlooked to present the subject in a systematic manner. A new empirical approach is thus the cry of the hour.

This book is the first serious attempt to arrange scattered materials on 'Animal Behaviour' in a systematic and coherent manner intending to build a cogent perspective on the topic. Self-developed relevant diagrams along with charts and tables in required numbers have been given to impart clarity to concepts and their implications. It has been taken care that the language of the book remains simple and direct throughout.

I am greatly indebted to my colleagues for their valuable suggestions. I am obliged to my friend Dr. Hari Mohan Prasad, Professor and Head, P.G. Department of English, Magadh University, Gaya, for correcting the text carefully.

I am thankful to my artist Mr. R.K. Samaiyar who made illustrations with utmost care, clarity and accuracy. I highly appreciate the alround cooperation of Mr. Satish Kumar Jain, Managing Director; Mr. Vinod Jain, Production Director; Mr. H.S. Poplai, General Manager; Mr. S.K. Verma, Marketing Manager of CBS Publishers & Distributors for publishing and releasing this book.

Finally, I solicit sincere and honest suggestions from all corners so that the book is improved in next edition.

Sept. 2003

S. Prasad

CONTENTS

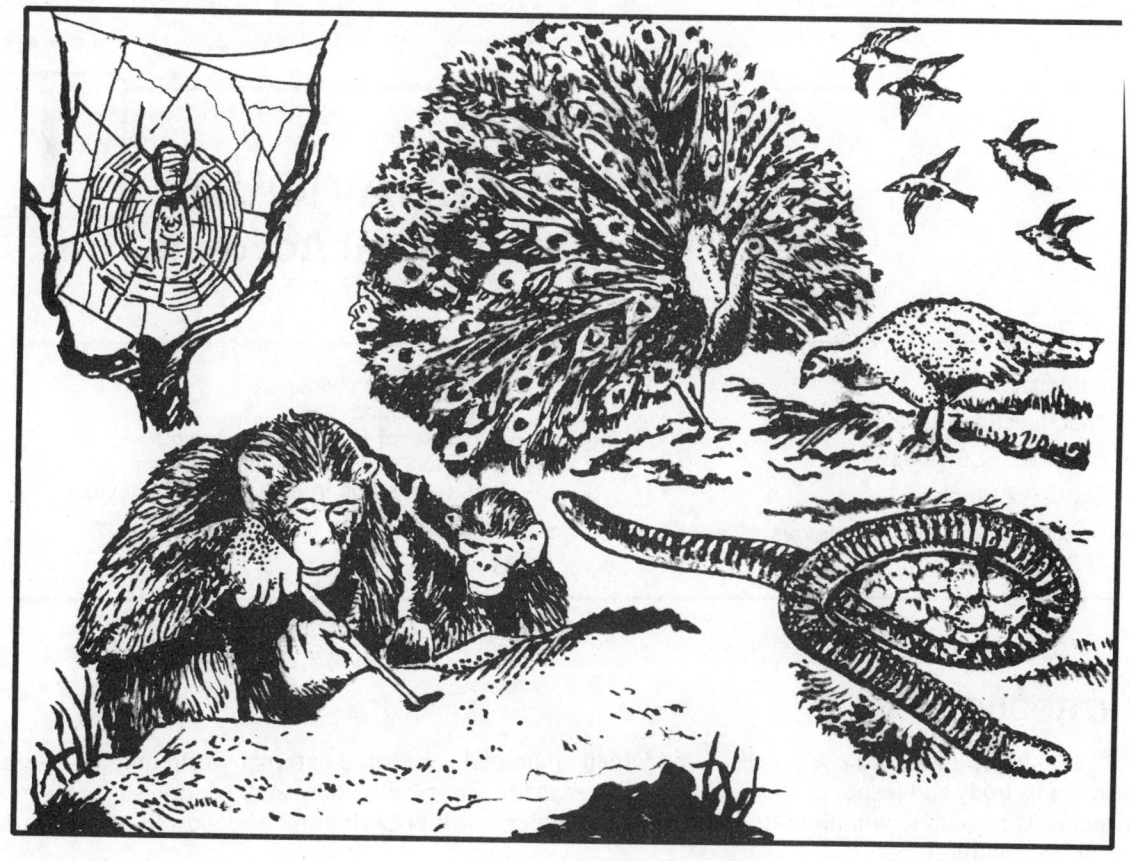

Behaviour and various ways of life of animals have always fascinated man for a myriad reasons, both of practical as well as academic. Modern man has taken keen interest in ethology to gain many useful knowledge. For example, an understanding of the reproductive behaviour of agricultural insect-pests may help control them, while a knowledge of the migrating pattern of an endangered species may enable conservationists to design adequate reserves to save the animal from extinction. But even if there were absolutely no practical benefits to be derived from the ethology, the topic would still be worth learning about for the simple reason that it is fascinating and of academic interest. Animals are capable of extraordinary feats. Dance of peacock, chirping of birds, spectacular ballet of dolphins, different activities of monkey, cat, dog, rat etc. have some meaning in terms of behaviour. Popularity of cartoon show, Mickey and Minnie mouse, Donald duck etc. is the results of human interest in animal behaviour. Now-a-days channels like "Discovery" and "National Geographic" are popular to TV viewers because such channels mostly telecast programmes on animal behaviour. This book describes interesting examples of animal behaviours in more understandable manner.

ANImAL BEHAVIOUR :
A General Account

1

- Introduction
- Importance of Ethology
- Branches of Ethology
- History of Ethology
- Proximate and Ultimate levels of analysis of behaviour

- Evolution of behaviour
  - Origin of behaviour
  - Evolution of Divergent behaviour
  - Evolution of convergent behaviour
  - Important steps in evolution of behaviour
- Some old and new concepts of ethology
- Exercise

INTRODUCTION

Behaviour includes all those processes by which an animal senses the external world and the internal state of its body and responds to stimulations it perceives. Thus behaviour can be defined as the way an organism responds to stimuli in its environment. In other words behaviour may be viewed as a "stimulus response relationship."

The study of animal behaviour is known as *ethology*. The term ethology is made up of two Greek words *ethos* means habit and *logos* means study. Thus ethology is a branch of life science and has made most notable advances during last five decades of twentieth century and first decade of new millennium.

Numerous questions concerning Animal Behaviour arise in the mind of even a layman, such as What is behaviour? What composes behaviour? How many kinds of behaviours are found in animal world? How evolution of behaviour has taken place? Why ants move a single line? Why birds sit on eggs and feed their young-ones? Why peacock dance before a peahen in rainy season? How honeybees communicate to their immates about feeding site? We may get answers to these questions in different chapters of this book.

IMPORTANCE OF ETHOLOGY

Due to various reasons study of animal behaviour has become one of the most important branches of life science.

Animal keepers are supposed to know behaviour of animals for proper care and to get maximum benefit from them. Hale (1969) made an attempt to list characteristics of species that are easily domesticated. Domestication of animals and the industries dependent on them (Dairy, Poultry, Piggery, Horsemanship, Pisciculture, Sericulture, Apiculture, Lacculture etc.) is possible only by knowing behaviour of concerned animals. Insect-pests and rodent damage our crops and stored grain and cause economic felt loss. Biological control of insect-pests and rodent is possible only by knowing their behaviour.

The diagnosis of diseases of humans and pet animals by doctors and veterinarians often involve observation of the patient's behaviour and recognition of abnormalities. In order to assess abnormal behaviour, it is essential for the observer psychiatrist to have precise knowledge of normal behaviour of the animal concerned. Homoeopathic doctors prescribe different medicines to different patients of different temperament even for the same disease.

It is vital in any job to know about the behaviour of colleagues, sub-ordinates and boss. For better family and social life, it is essential to know the behaviour of relatives, friends and neighbours. Human beings are undoubtedly the most critical resource and no matter what the degree of sophistication we arise in our technologies, we still depend on human touches and sentiments. Study of child Psychology is very important for their education and proper growth of personality and maintenance of social cohesiveness.

Ethology answers many intricate questions as, why animals take care for their children? Why sexually aroused males fight with conspecific during breeding season? Why same stimulus given to the same animal at different times does not always evoke the same response? What is the purpose of altruism in animal world? etc.

In some cases behavioural patterns are the only means of discriminating different species of one genus. Different species of crickets living in one habitat are so identical morphologically that they cannot be discriminated by inspection. Different species of male crickets are identified only by recording the different kind of songs produced by them called mating call or mating song (See Chapter 3, Fig. 3.3). Male crickets attract females of its own species over long distances by mating call. A high-pitched sound is produced not by mouth but by rhythmic opening and closing of specialised fore wings that carry friction mechanisms. Each closing stroke of the wings produces a sound pulse, while the opening stroke is silent. The songs differ considerably from one species to another.

BRANCHES OF ETHOLOGY

Ecoethology : Relationship between behaviour of a species and its environment.

Ethogenetics : Genetical basis of behaviour.

Neuroethology : Sensory process and Central Nervous System that initiates and controls a particular behaviour.

Ethoendocrinology : Relations between hormones and behaviour.

Behavioural embryology : Prenatal development of behaviour pattern.

Human ethology : Study of human behaviour.

HISTORY OF ETHOLOGY

Behaviour and various ways of life of animals have always fascinated human beings. Due to continuous efforts of individuals and group of behaviourists a vast wealth of information about animal behaviour is available now-a-days.

Aristotle (340-322 B.C.) was keen observer of animal behaviour. He gave excellent description of animal behaviour in his book *Historia Animalium* meaning by the history of the animals. He collected a great deal of information on pet animals and concluded that animals also possessed INSIGHT and LOVE for families and their masters. The knowledge of animal behaviour was forgotten in next 400 to 1200 years of dark ages.

After a long dark ages, first thought about animal behaviour came into existence by a book *Utopia* written by Thomas More in the year 1518. He mentioned various behavioural patterns of animals in this book.

In 17th century the word ETHOLOGY was used for stage actors. In the year 1859 Geoffroy Saint Hillaire used this term (Ethology) to describe the relationship of animal with environment, family and society. Since the beginning of 20th century the term 'Ethology' is restricted only to the study of behaviour of animals.

The scientific study of animal behaviour has its origin in the work of Gilbert White (1720-1793) and Charles Leroy (1723-1789).

Foundation of Modern ethology was laid down with the evolution theory given by Charles Darwin in the year 1859 through a book *On the Origin of Species by means of Natural Selection*. It is said that this book is only next to the holy *Bible* on its impact on human thinking. Darwin's first book published in the year 1871 on behaviour *The Descent of Man in Relation to Sex* deals with various emotions and imitation in human beings. His second book on animal behaviour *The Expression of the Emotion in Man and the Animals* published in the year 1873 explains the bristling of hair under the influence of terror and uncovering of the teeth under that of furious rage. He also made studies of the body postures of pet animals as a means of communication. His view on instinctive behaviour can be regarded as a direct forerunner of those of the founder of classical ethology. Darwin also tried to explain the role of internal factors, for example, stimulated nervous system in composing animal behaviour.

Darwins friend and disciple Romanes continued Darwin's work on animal behaviour. He published a

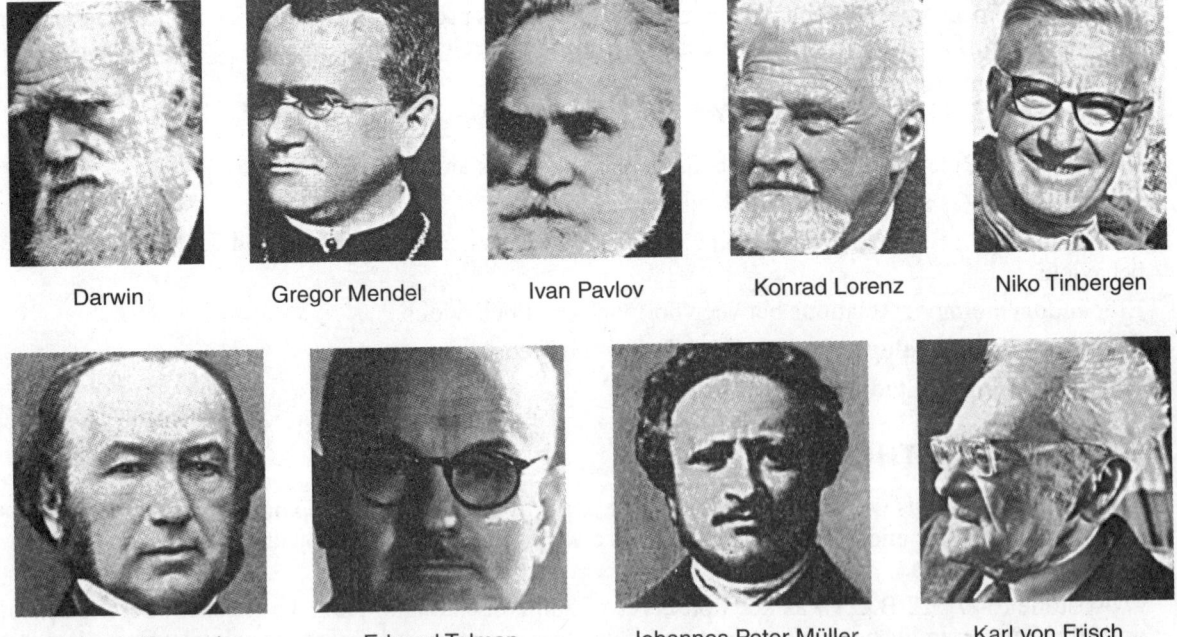

Darwin   Gregor Mendel   Ivan Pavlov   Konrad Lorenz   Niko Tinbergen

Claude Bernard   Edward Tolman   Johannes Peter Müller   Karl von Frisch

Fig. 1.1. The founders of ethology : (i) Charles Darwin, (ii) Gregor Mendel, (iii) Ivan Pavlov, (iv) Konrad Lorenz, (v) Niko Tinbergen, (vi) Claude Bernard, (vii) Edward Tolman, (viii) Johannes Peter Muller, (ix) Karl von Frisch.

comparative analysis of mental function and evolution in his books : *Animal Intelligence* (1882), *Mental Evolution in Animals* (1884) and *Mental Evolution of Man* (1889).

The further basis for the development of ethology was provided by the works of Charles Whitman (1842-1910), Wallace Craig (1876-1954) and Oskar Heinroth (1871-1945).

Three scientists, Karl von Frisch (1886-1983) from Germany, Nikolaus Tinbergen (1907-1988) from Holland and Konrad Lorenz (1903-1989) from Vienna, played a primary role in the development of the modern approach to animal behaviour. These three founders of ethology got the Nobel Prize in the year 1973 in physiology and medicine for their path breaking contributions to behavioural science. The Nobel committee was probably influenced primarily by the proximate component of their research. But an equally important goal of ethology was to understand the adaptive (Ultimate) function of behavioural characteristics in animals. Lorenz emphasized the importance of direct observations under natural conditions. Tinbergen examined the functional significance of behaviour. He published a concise book *The Study of Instinct* suggesting that most of the behaviours of animals are innate and instinctive. Frisch's greatest contribution was his work on honeybee communication (1943) and sensory biology.

Description and contribution of every ethologist is beyond the scope of this book. Details can be found in Warden (1927), Waters (1951), Boring (1957), Jaynes (1969), Klopfer (1974) or other historically oriented works.

PROXIMATE AND ULTIMATE LEVELS OF ANALYSIS OF BEHAVIOUR

Automeris (Sphnix moth) bear large circular patches on their hind wings. The patches look like eyes. The moth keeps its fore wings over hind wings and abdomen so that patches are not visible in normal position. It abruptly open its wing to expose eye like spots which startle the predator, allowing moth to escape.

A snake-mimicking caterpillar resembles the Mexican vine snake. When threatened by predator the caterpillar lowers the anterior part of its body and changes its body shape to create a triangular *snake head complete* with realistic eyes.

This simple act of moth and snake-mimicking caterpillar is a forceful example of behaviour developing in step with the evolution of body marking, allowing the moth and caterpillar to escape.

Many questions about moth wing-flipping and snake-mimicking caterpillar can arise, but all questions can be kept under two categories "how questions", about the proximate causes of the behaviour and "why questions", about its ultimate causes.

How questions may be : What is the causal relationship between the animal's genes and its behaviour? Is the behavioural trait inherited from the parents? How has the development of the moth/caterpillar from a single cell to a multi-million-celled adult affect its behaviour? What stimuli trigger the response and how are those stimuli detected? How are the animal's nervous and muscular systems integrated to enable it to react to predator.

These questions seems to be diverse but they all have one common point within the moth/caterpillar that cause it to pull its fore wings forward in case of moth and lowering the anterior part of body and changing triangular SNAKE HEAD in case of caterpillar, and revealing the eye spots in both cases. The diversity of proximate questions is great enough but we can reduce them into two complementary groups, one dealing with effect of heredity and development of the construction of the mechanism underlying wing-flipping/changing triangular snake head and the other dealing with how the fully developed neural mechanisms actually work to cause with respect to the influence of heredity on development. One question arises that how the special touch receptors brain cells, and muscle controllers used in the wing-flipping reaction arise in an individual. The adult moth began life as a single cell (zygote) that

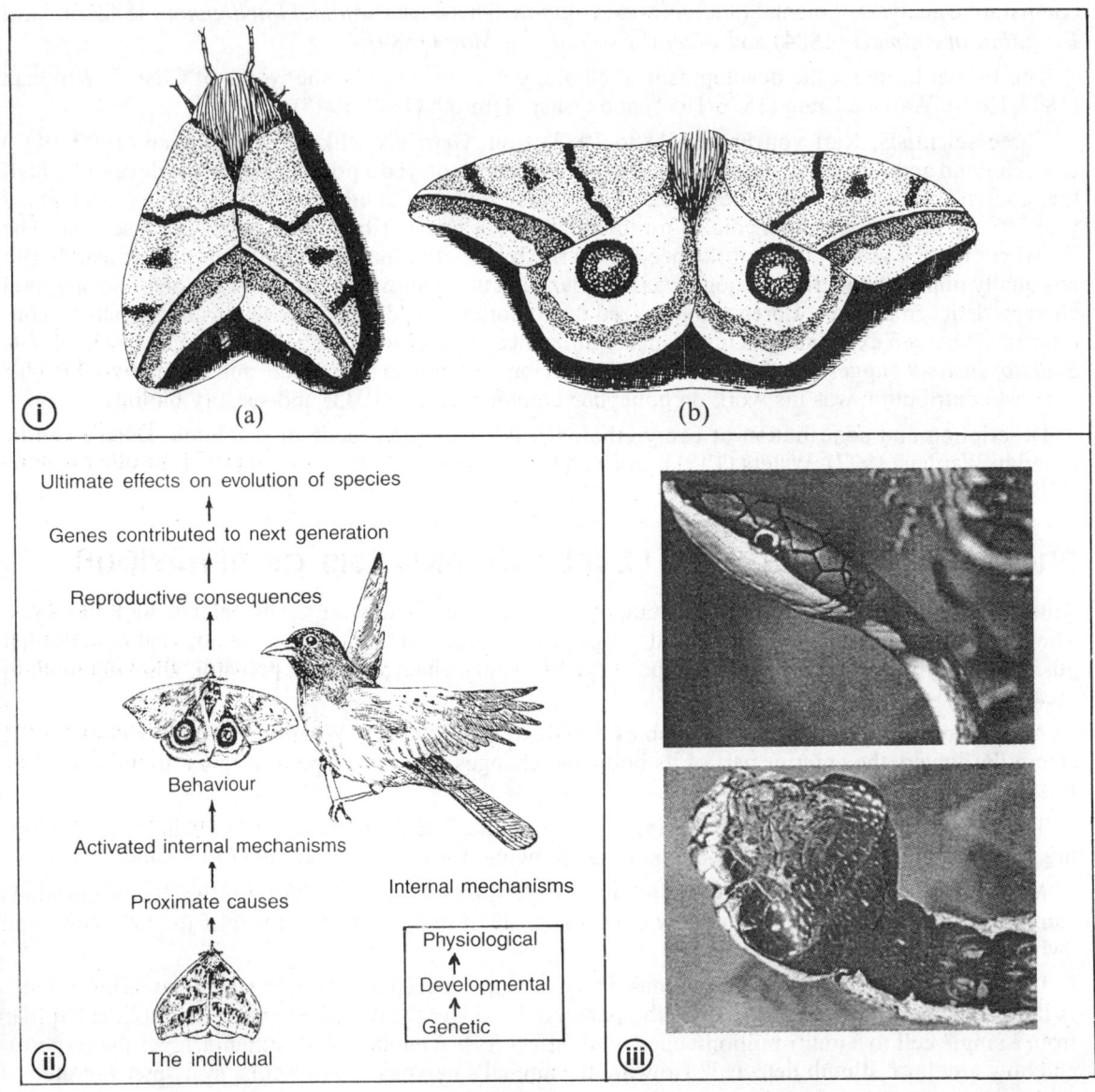

Fig. 1.2. Automeris moth from Costa Rica. (i) (A) Moth is in its resting position with the fore wings held over the hind wings. (B) After being Jabbed in the thorax, the moth pull the fore wings forward to expose the *eyes* (spots) on the hind wings. This is startling behaviour. Sudden appearance of the eye spots scares the predator (small birds) and they do not attack the moth. (ii) Proximate and Ultimate causes of behaviour as illustrated by numerous moths (Sphinx moth-*Automeris*), wing-flipping. At the proximate level numerous mechanisms internal to an individual moth enable it to execute the behaviour. At the ultimate level, the moth's response to potential predators helps in survival and also affects its reproductive success as measured by the number of copies of its genes that are passed on to the next generation. The history of differential reproductive success among individuals determines what genes survive from generation to generation and therefore what genetic information is available to influence the development of moths in the current generation. (iii) A snake - Mimicking caterpillar (above) resembles the Mexican Vine snake (lower) when the caterpillar lowers the anterior part of its body and changes its body shape to create a triangular "snake head" complete with realistic eyes. It is another example of proximate and ultimate causes of behaviour.

contained genetic instructions donated by its mother and father. These genetic instructions affected the development of the moth, channeling the proliferation and specialization of cells along certain path way that produced a nervous system with special features in the adult insect. This is an astonishing complex process, still poorly understood for any organism.

The other part of the proximate questions that how the fully developed neural mechanisms within the adult moth detect certain kinds of stimulation and how messages are then relayed to activate a muscular response is poorly understood. There is great need of neurophysiological foundation of the behaviour of *Automeris* and other organisms under study.

Why questions may be : What is the purpose of the behaviour? How does the behaviour assist the individual in overcoming obstacles to survival and reproduction? How has the behaviour evolved and how has it changed over evolutionary time? What was the original step in the evolutionary process that led to the existence of the current behaviour?

These are all questions about the *ultimate causes* of behaviour. Why does the moth suddenly lift its fore wings or caterpillar shrink or expand its skin to show eye spots when they are threatened. The action become common because it protects the moth and caterpillar from predator, startling and frightening away predatory birds that mistake the eye spots for the eyes of their enemy, predatory owl.

Eye spots showing behaviour of moths and other animals has remained life saving device in the past and the evolutionary process is partly responsible for the behaviour of individual today. The genes that exist in contemporary moths, caterpillars mentioned above are a tiny subset of all the genes that have ever existed. Those that have managed to persist to the present are genes that have in some way contributed to their own survival. If the gene influenced the behaviour of a moth or caterpillar in ways that helped them frighten away predatory birds, that gene would presumably have a better chance of being passed on to descendents of animal concerned. This process could help explain why these animals (moths, caterpillars) have inherited genetic mechanisms that promote the eye spot showing behaviour. The developmental plan, and therefore the behavioural abilities, of each member of the species alive today has been defined by differences in gene survival that occurred during the evolution of the species. Thus studying the current ways of behaviour can give us insight into the ultimate or evolutionary causes of behaviour. Table 1.1 summarizes and Fig. 1.2 (i), (ii) & (iii) illustrates the above discussion about the two fundamental levels of analysis, *proximate* and *ultimate*, in the study of behaviour.

Table 1.1. Levels of analysis in the study of animal behaviour

Proximate causes
1. Genetic - development mechanisms
   Effects of heredity on behaviour
   Genetic - environmental interactions during development that produce
   Sensory - motor mechanisms
   Detection of environmental stimuli : operation of nervous systems
   Adjustment of internal responsiveness : operation of endocrine system
   Carrying out responses : operation of muscular systems

Ultimate causes
1. Historical pathways leading to a behaviour
   Origin of the behaviour and its alteration over time
2. Past effects of natural selection in shaping a current behaviour
   Past and current utility of the behaviour in reproductive terms

EVOLUTION OF BEHAVIOUR

A fundamental ultimate question about behaviour is, what was the sequence of events over evolutionary time that led to the behaviour that we observe today? The phylogeny of behaviour can sometimes be accomplished by finding the appropriate fossils in a lineage leading to a modern species and deducing how the extinct species behaved by analogy with living animals. Alternatively the phylogeny of behaviour can be established via the comparative method. If a clusture of related species exists, one can sometimes trace the pathway leading to the unusual behaviour of one of these species by using a set of logical assumption. One assumption is that if a trait is widespread in a group of related species, the character is likely to have been present in the ancestor of those species. A second assumption is that if a trait is represented in only one or few species, it evolved relatively recently. Studies of fossils and application of the comparative method to modern species support the intuitively reasonable argument that behavioural evolution proceeds gradually, by degrees, with changes building upon and limited by past evolutionary events. The cumulative effect of natural selection can slowly produce great changes in evolutionary lineage.

At *proximate level*, an individual's genetic make up develop behavioural abilities through biochemical action. At the *ultimate level*, we expect alleles with reproduction enhancing information to spread through population. But is there any evidence that evolution of this kind has occurred in nature? Arnold showed how it is possible to integrate proximate and ultimate levels of analysis in context of food preference behaviour between Coastal and Inland Garter snakes (detailed in Chapter 3).

1. Origin of Behaviour

Virus is an interesting transitional group between non-living and living. They do not exhibit any sign of life in independent condition i.e. non-parasitic state. In terms of ethology no behavioural trait is apparent in viruses in non-parasitic state. For the performance of fundamental living activities, viruses need a potential host. The host may be a bacteria, plant cell or animal cell. We are aware that viruses recognize their host-cell with the help of their tail fibers. The response of viruses to their host-cell may be considered as *sensitivity* or *irritability*. After recognizing host-cell, viruses enter into it and start multiplying by utilizing DNA strand of the host-cell. Thus, viruses exhibit two kinds of behaviour. (1) *Sensitivity* and (2) *Multiplication* or *Reproduction*. The first kind of behaviour i.e. sensitivity exhibited by virus may be considered as the origin of behaviour in living being. The second kind of behaviour i.e. reproduction performed by virus may be considered as the appearance of second behaviour in living world.

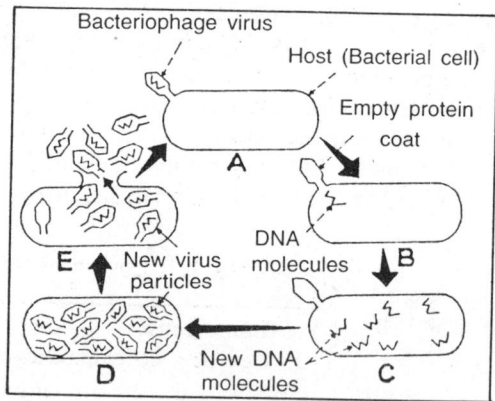

Fig. 1.3. (A-E) Origin of two behaviours in living world : (i) Sensitivity and (ii) Multiplication (reproduction) exhibited by Bacteriophage virus.

Comparative study of behaviour tells that species from different phylogenetic lineages are expected to behave differently because they have different ancestors that endowed them with distinct genetic-developmental characteristics. If, however, two unrelated species have been subjected to similar selection pressures, they should have independently evolved similar behavioural traits through convergent evolution - if the trait truly is an adaptation to that selection pressure.

to the perfect social behaviour. The research of Dilger on the behaviour of love-bird of the genus *Agapornis* provide excellent example of divergence in nest material carrying behaviour. He studied eight of the nine forms that makes up the genus *Agapornis*. All forms displayed stereotyped and easily elicited behavioural patterns in the laboratory. On the basis of behavioural studies, reconstruction of the course of evolution of the forms of this genus can be prepared, right from the more primitive Madagascar, Abyssinal, and red-faced love-birds through peach-faced love birds to form with distinct white rings about their eyes.

The phyletic level is comparison of behaviours of two different groups (genera, families, orders, classes or even phyla) in constructing the broad evolutionary history of behaviour.

Alexander (1964) traced the history of the evolution of mating behaviour of some arthropods and came to the conclusion that it is related to the evolution of spermatophores, adoption of aquatic or terrestrial habitats and more specific environmental conditions within particular groups. Allison and vane Twyver (1970) proposed that sleep behaviour must have evolved independently among birds and mammals. Paradoxical sleep (apparently deep sleep, with actual increased brain activity) in mammals developed after slow wave sleep, a proposed divergence of eutherians from non-eutherians. Heffner et al. (1969) stated that selective pressures responsible for sound waves of low frequencies must have characterized the evolutionary lineage leading to humans. Nottenbohm (1973) is of the opinion that there is a general trend in the evolution of patterns of the ontogeny of bird's song from "*self centered strategies*" to more environmental dependent patterns. The trends toward environmental dependence appears to have evolved independently at least three times.

3. Evolution of Convergent Behaviour

The independent acquisition over time of similar behaviour in two or more unrelated species as a result of natural selection stemming from shared environment

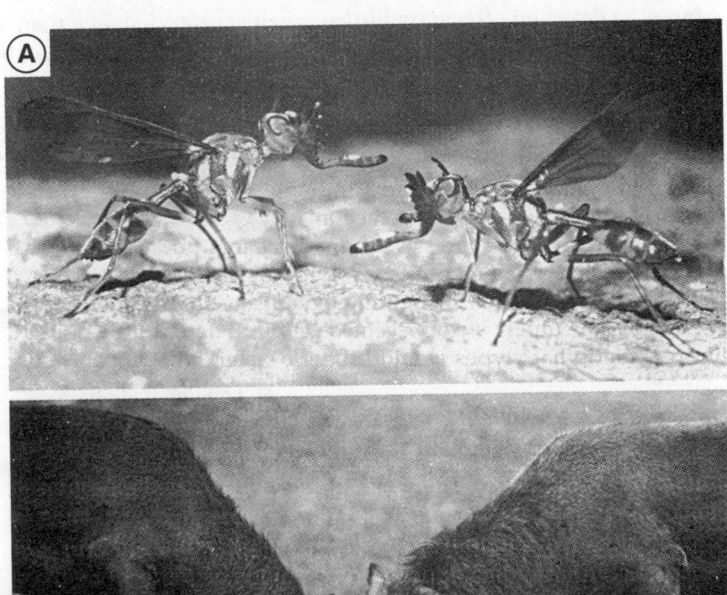

Fig. 1.6. Convergent evolution of territorial behaviour (A). Two male "antlered flies" (note the bizzare projection from their heads) lung at each other. They fight by using their bizzare projections from their head (B). Male red deer have aggressive displays in which opponents lock antlers. The fight help in assessing the rival's strength. These two examples of two very different types of species exhibit convergent behaviour.

pressure is called convergent evolution of behaviour. Divergent evolution of behaviour is the general rule of nature but many cases of convergent evolution of behaviour also occurs in animal world. Different species with same necessities may lead to similarities in not only appearance but also in behaviour.

Threat displays of many unrelated species exhibit convergent behaviour. In the red deer, for example, stags compete to remain with herds of females during the fall of rutting seasons. One male withdraws after fight, judging the strength of rival stag. Two male "*antlered*" flies lung at each other like red deer. Bizzare projection arising from flies head perform the role of horns. Here both red deer and antlered flies are exhibiting similar behaviour in context of threat displays for competing females of their own species though they belong to two quite different species.

Convergent evolution in a communication signal is evident in great tit and other unrelated song-birds when they spot an approaching hawk. If a great tit (small European songbirds) spots a flying haws at some distance it gives the SEET ALARM. This seet alarm call, warn mates and offsprings of possible danger. Seet call is a much softer and much higher-frequency call (in the 7 to 8 kHz range). This signal cannot be detected after travelling a much shorter distance than the mobbing signal (a laud signal in the 4.5 khz range attracting other birds to the site to join in harassing the predators). Thus the probability of informing the hawk is reduced because the hawk cannot hear relatively high-pitched sounds very well, whereas the great tit has high sensitivity to acoustical stimuli in the 7 to 10 kHz range. As a result, a great tit can hear a SEET call given by another tit 40 meters away, whereas a sparrow hawk no more than 10 meters distance will fail to detect the same signal.

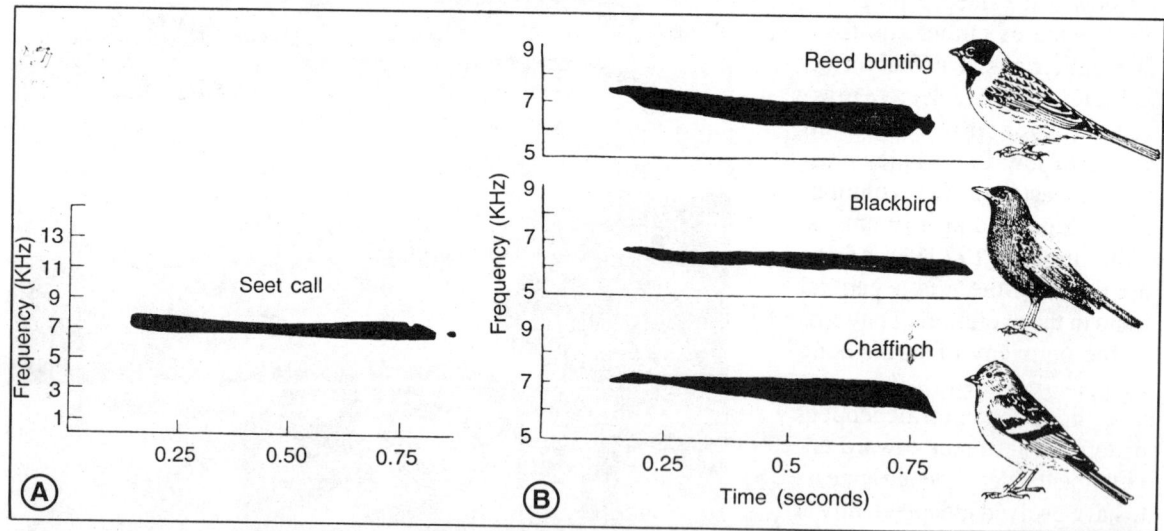

Fig. 1.7. Convergent evolution in a communication signal. (A) A sonogram of the *"seet"* alarm call of great tit. (B) The great tit's high-pitched *"seet"* alarm call is very similar to the calls given by other unrelated song-birds when they spot an approaching hawk.

The remarkable similarity in the "seet" calls of many unrelated European song-birds suggests that selection by bird-eating hawks has favoured the evolution of alarm calls that were hard for hawks to hear. There are many convergent cases of unrelated species whose females live in permanent groups and in which males defend clustered females, thereby exhibiting female defence polygyny. (Detailed in Chapter 6).

4. Steps in Evolution of Behaviour

It is not possible to frame an evolutionary tree of behaviour like organic evolution because recording fossils tell us about physical evolution of animals but unfortunately they do not give us direct knowledge of the course of evolution of behaviour that followed in the past. Yet, studying the current function of behaviour can give us insight to frame actual steps of evolution from primitive to higher form. Thus animal behaviour covers wide range of activities and is applicable from simple irritability to high grade of communication through language, reasoning and cognition. Major modes of adaptive behaviours in phylogeny of organism may be mentioned as follows :

Irritability → Tropism → Nasties → Taxis → Kinesis → Reflexes → Instincts → Motivation → Habituation → Imprinting → Trial-and-error learning → Conditioned learning → Operant learning → Insight → Cognition

During organic evolution, many morphological changes took place in the body of animals and there were both appearance and disappearance of organs. But most probably no behavioural trait disappeared completely during course of evolution of behaviour. We get VESTIGIAL ORGANS due to loss of organs but VESTIGIAL BEHAVIOUR does not exist. Like organic evolution, new behavioural traits did not take place by sudden leaps and bounds but slowly through natural selection. In terms of behaviour, individuals behave suitably to increase their own genetic fitness. It is a measure of the numbers of copies of genes, an animal contributes towards the hereditary composition of the generation. Genetic fitness means individual should behave in such a way as to maximise its reproductive success.

Some stereotyped behaviour within a population can be maintained by nongenetic cultural transmission. Certain aspects of bird song stand within this kind of evolution of behaviour. Among Japanese macaques, patterns of eating candy and wheat, washing sweet potatoes have been propagated by cultural transmission. In human beings cultural transmission embraces customs, beliefs and the acquisition and communication of knowledge. Evolution of behaviour can be far more rapid than by genetic alteration. Such behavioural patterns transmitted across species should not be confused with homologous behaviour.

Though like organic evolution we are not able to make a proper evolutionary tree of behaviour, but we can definitely say that insight, reasoning, cognition and power of speech are top branches of evolutionary tree of behaviour and are present only in highly evolved mammals (in terms of brain) such as primates, elephants and dolphins. Man shows many peculiar behaviours by combining reasoning and learning which are not available in any other group of animals. This suggests that with the evolution of brain many new patterns of behaviour evolved.

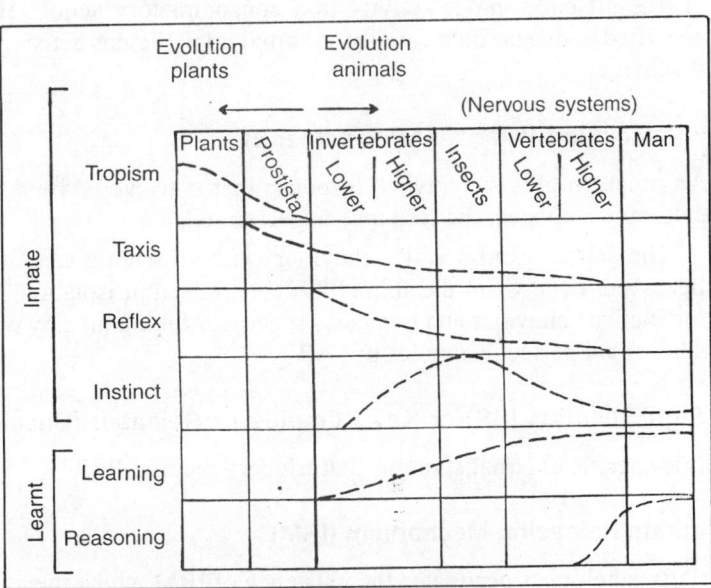

Fig. 1.8. Line figure showing evolution of phylogenetic behaviour.

SOME NEW AND OLD CONCEPTS OF ETHOLOGY

From the work of different ethologists a number of concepts have been formulated to explain the behaviour of animals. Some of them are relevant but many of them have become obsolete. However some important concepts have been dealt in short.

Appetitive and Consummatory Behaviour

On the basis of observation and description of complex behaviour pattern of animals given by different ethologists, Wallace Craig came to the conclusion that each complex behaviour pattern has two parts : *Appetitive* and *Consummatory*. Appetitive part is variable in which animal is excited by external or internal stimulation and orients itself towards the stimulus. Rest part i.e. consummatory part is definite and stereotyped. Morris has considered appetitive part as an accelerator of car, which when pressed, the speed continuously increases, and consummatory part is like bell of *telephone* which remains unaware about the importance of message and always rings in the same manner.

A change in the animal's internal state is sensed by the brain and it leads to buildup a drive to perform the appropriate behaviour. The drive gives rise to appetitive part of behaviour followed by consummatory part. For example, dehydration of the body tissue is sensed by the brain and results in building-up thirst drive, the drive induces the animal to search for water (appetitive behaviour), and when animal finds water, it drinks it (consummatory behaviour) and becomes satiated. Same is the case in context of sexual behaviour or other behaviours. High level of male hormone, present in the body make the male animal sexually aroused and it become satiated after mating.

Konrad Lorenz (1950) outlines the ethological view about appetitive and consummatory components of a complex behaviour pattern in three successive processes : (1) Accumulation of action-specific energy giving rise to appetitive behaviour; (2) Appetitive behaviour struggle to attain the stimulus situation activating the innate releasing mechanisms; and (3) Setting off the releasing mechanism and discharge off endogenous activity in a consummatory action. He postulated that some sort of energy, specified to one definite activity, is sorted up while this activity remains inactive and is consumed in its discharge.

Fixed Action Pattern FAP (Chapter 2)

An innate, highly stereotyped response that is triggered by a well-defined, simple stimulus; once the pattern is activated, the response is performed.

The animal exhibit FAP behaviour, without having seen or learnt from conspecific or perform a behaviour even when the animal has been raised in isolation. In other words, Fixed Action Pattern is instinctive behaviour and is species specific. Making hive by worker honeybees, weaving net by young spiders are perfect examples of FAP.

Sign Stimulus (SS) or Key Stimulus or Releaser (Chapter 2)

It is specific external stimulus that triggers specific FAP.

Innate Releasing Mechanism (IRM)

Early ethologists postulated the existence of IRM which they thought was responsible for the recognition of sign stimuli. The IRM concept is no longer acceptable.

Action Specific Energy (ASE) or Specific Action Potential (SAP)

ASE or SAP Concept was advanced by Lorenz in 1950. He proposed a model known as "*Psycho-hydraulic Model*" or "*Flush toilet model*" to explain the correlation between SS, IRM, ASE (Action Specific Energy) and FAP. This hypothesis of Lorenz could not gain acceptance due to lack of neurological evidences in support of it.

EXERCISE

1. Define animal behaviour and write a short note on ethology.
2. Who coined the term "Ethology" and in what context he used it.
3. Give a brief account of history of ethology with special reference to Darwin, Karl von Frisch, Niko Tinbergen and Lorenz.
4. Throw some light on "levels of analysis of behaviours".
5. Phylogeny of behaviour? Try to trace the "Origin and evolution of behaviour" giving suitable examples.
6. Write short notes on divergent and convergent evolution of behaviour. Mention interesting points in context of Phylogeny of behaviour.
7. Mention important contributions of following ethologists : (i) Lindaur, (ii) Dilger, (iii) Alexander, (iv) Allison and Twyver, (v) Heffner, (vi) Ottebohm, (vii) Charles Darwin, (viii) Konrad Lorenz, (ix) Niko Tinbergen, (x) E.O. Wilson, (xi) King.
8. Describe Darwin's work other than evolutionary theory i.e. in the field of ethology.
9. Write short notes on behaviours of bacteriophage virus (a transitional group between non-living and living), sensitivity and multiplication - which can be regarded as origin of behaviour in living world.
10. Give a brief idea of concepts of ethology.
11. Throw some light on importance of ethology in context of 21st Century.

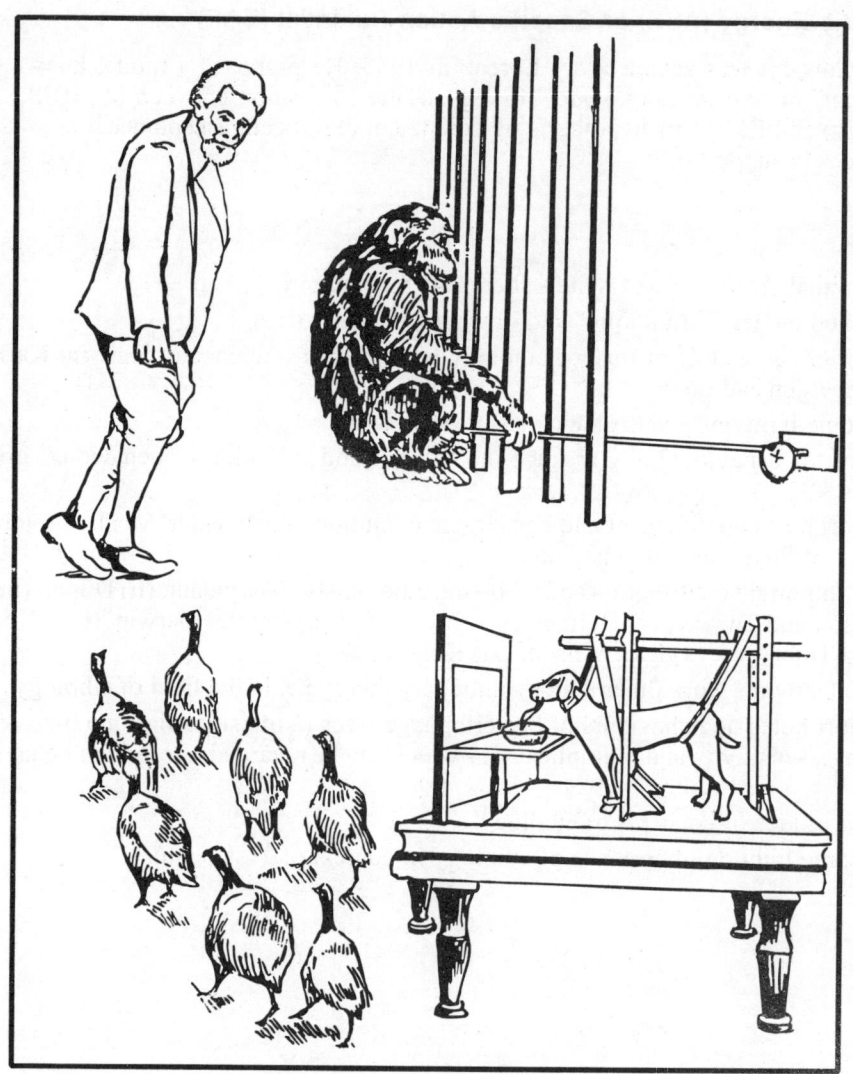

The variety of behaviours in living world is bewildering. However, Animal behaviour may be broadly classified into two types : (1) Innate and (2) Learned. Innate behaviour is claimed to be genetically controlled, whereas learning is believed to be largely dependent on experience. Many behaviours may not fit distinctly under the label of either "Innate" or "learnt" because innate behaviour is often modified by experience, and learning is often constrained in interesting ways. One of the central goals of this chapter is to define Innate and Learned behaviour and to examine the diversity that exists in these two categories.

THE DIVERSITY OF BEHAVIOUR 2

- Introduction
- Classification of behaviour
- Innate behaviour
  - Irritability
  - Tropism
  - Nasties
  - Taxes
  - Kinesis
  - Simple reflex action
  - Instinct and motivation
- Learned behaviour
  - Habituation
  - Imprinting
  - Conditioned reflex
  - Trial-and-error learning
  - Latent learning
  - Insight
  - Reasoning and cognition
- Exercise

INTRODUCTION

The variety of behaviours in living world is bewildering. However, students of animal behaviour have classified all behaviour as either *innate* or *learned*. These two traditional categories are created to acknowledge supposed differences in the proximate mechanisms underlying different kinds of behaviour. Innate is claimed to be genetically controlled, whereas learning is believed to be largely or entirely dependent on experience. Each Innate and Learnt behaviours can be classified into 8 types.

Behaviour

Innate behaviour
1. Irritability
2. Tropism
3. Nasties
4. Taxis
5. Kinesis
6. Simple reflexes
7. Instinct
8. Motivation

Learnt behaviour
1. Habituation
2. Imprinting
3. Conditioned reflex
4. Trial-and-error learning
5. Latent learning
6. Insight learning
7. Reasoning
8. Cognition

INNATE BEHAVIOUR

Innate behaviour is inborn and also called acquired, inherited, inherent, stereotyped. Innate behaviour is independent of the experiences of the individual. It is determined by heredity and is a part of the animal's original genetic makeup. Fries of fish, tadpole of frog, ducklings of duck etc. can swim as soon as they hatch from egg. Young spiders without any previous experience weave a web as fine as constructed by those of older ones. These are a few examples of innate behaviour. Innate behaviour is of eight major types.

1. IRRITABILITY

The ability of an organism to respond to a stimulus is called sensitivity or irritability. Protozoans and Poriferans lack nervous system but protoplasm of these organisms is capable of receiving the stimuli and respond accordingly. By virtue of irritability they maximise their chances of survival. With the help of irritability, Protozoans and Poriferans can distinguish between an edible and non-edible particle, enemies, conspecific etc. Environmental factors such as light, heat, gravity, chemicals, touch etc. function as stimuli to which Protozoans and Poriferans respond in definite manner.

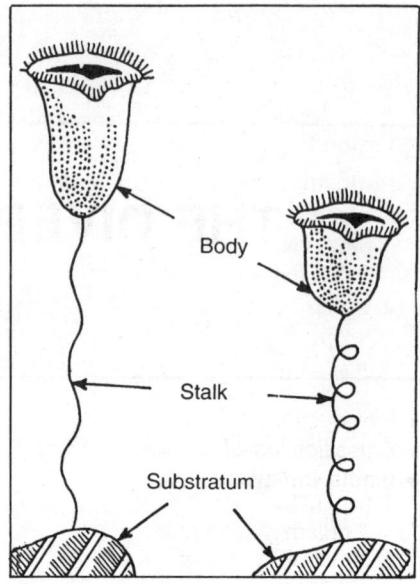

Fig. 2.1. Irritability in vorticella. In normal condition (left), when touched by a microneedle (right).

[Now let us take up two types of innate behaviours or movements found in plants. The reaction of a plant to a stimulus is called response and movements exhibited in response to external stimulus are known as *paratonic* or *induced movements*. Two types of movements : *Tropism* (directed movement) and *Nasties* (undirected movement) are found in plants.]

2. TROPISM

A well directed growth-mediated response of a plant or part, to a stimulus is called tropism. In tropism curvatures are produced due to growth or turgor changes under the effect of stimulus.

Types of tropism

The suffix tropism is used in relation to responses to particular stimuli.

- **Phototropism** : Response of a plant to the stimulus of light.
- **Geotropism** : Response of a plant to the stimulus of gravity.
- **Chemotropism** : Response of a plant to the stimulus of chemical.
- **Thigmotropism** : Response of a plant to the stimulus of touch.
- **Rheotropism** : Response of a plant to the stimulus of water current.
- **Trantnatropism** : Response of a plant to the stimulus of atmospheric pressure

In context of tropism one question is very common to us *why and how does the sunflower always face the sun*? Sunflowers begin the day facing east and then follow the sun. This is because of a phenomenon called ***phototropism***. The response is stimulated by a hormone called AUXIN present in the stem of sunflower plant. Auxins promote lengthwise growth of plants. The AUXIN, beta-indyl acetic acid (IAA), is formed either from the amino acid, tryptophan or from the breakdown of carbohydrates known as glycosides. They promote growth by acting on the chemical bonds of carbohydrates on the cell wall.

In positively phototropic plants when one side of the plant is shaded, greater quantities of auxin are produced on the darker side. This causes that side of the plant to grow fast. In the case of sunflower, the phenomenon is pronounced so as to make the flower turn towards the sun. To show the phenomenon of positively phototropism a simple experiment was performed and represented by Fig. 2.2.

3. NASTIES

A nasty (adj. Nastic) is the movements of a plant organ to a non-directional external stimulus.

Mimosa pudica (touch-me-not) shows paratonic variation type of movements which are brought about in response to external stimulus of touch. If leaflets of *Mimosa* plant are touched, they fold in seconds. If the stimulus is strong, successive pairs of leaflets fold up and the stimulus eventually passes through the whole leaf, resulting in the petiole drooping. If the stem is stimulated the stimulus will pass in the reverse direction. Fig. 2.3 shows

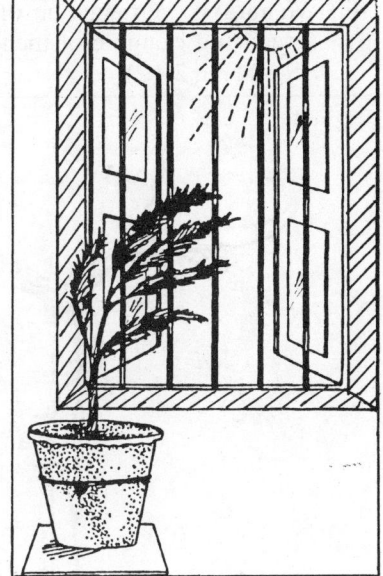

Fig. 2.2. Phototropism. A green plant on a window still in a room grow towards sun light coming through the window.

the two sites at which pulvini are found. The stimulus is transmitted by a hormone, moving through the xylem, electrical changes are associated with its passage, though there is no nervous system. *The sleep movements* i.e. the opening and closing of flowers (*nictinasty*) of certain flowers and leaves, whereby they open and close in response to stimuli, are nastic.

4. TAXES

Orientation of the organism in a straight axis with respect to the source of stimulation is called taxis. Taxis movements may be towards or away from the stimulus. Like tropism, taxis is also named after the stimulus. Following types of taxes are recognised.

  (i) **Klinotaxis :** Movement of an animal in response to a stimulus where the animal compares the intensity of the stimulus to lateral side of its body. Klinotaxis response was observed when *light* was thrown on blow-fly larva (Maggote) from different angles (Fig.2.4A).

 (ii) **Telotaxis :** When there are two sources of stimulation, the animal moves towards one and never in a median direction showing that the influence of one stimulus is ignored. Fraenkel and Gunn (1940) demonstrated telotaxis in hermit crab. It follows any one track (not median) when two light sources L_1 and L_2 were projected on it (Fig.2.4B).

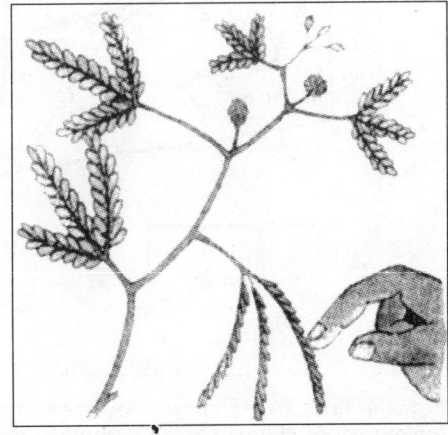

Fig. 2.3. Nasty. Twig of a plant of the genus *Mimosa pudica* in normal condition (left) and in response to a slight touch (right).

(iii) **Menotaxis :** Orientation of animals taking place at an angle to the direction of stimulus. An interesting example of menotaxis is the light compass response shown by homing ants (Brun, 1914) (Fig.2.4C).

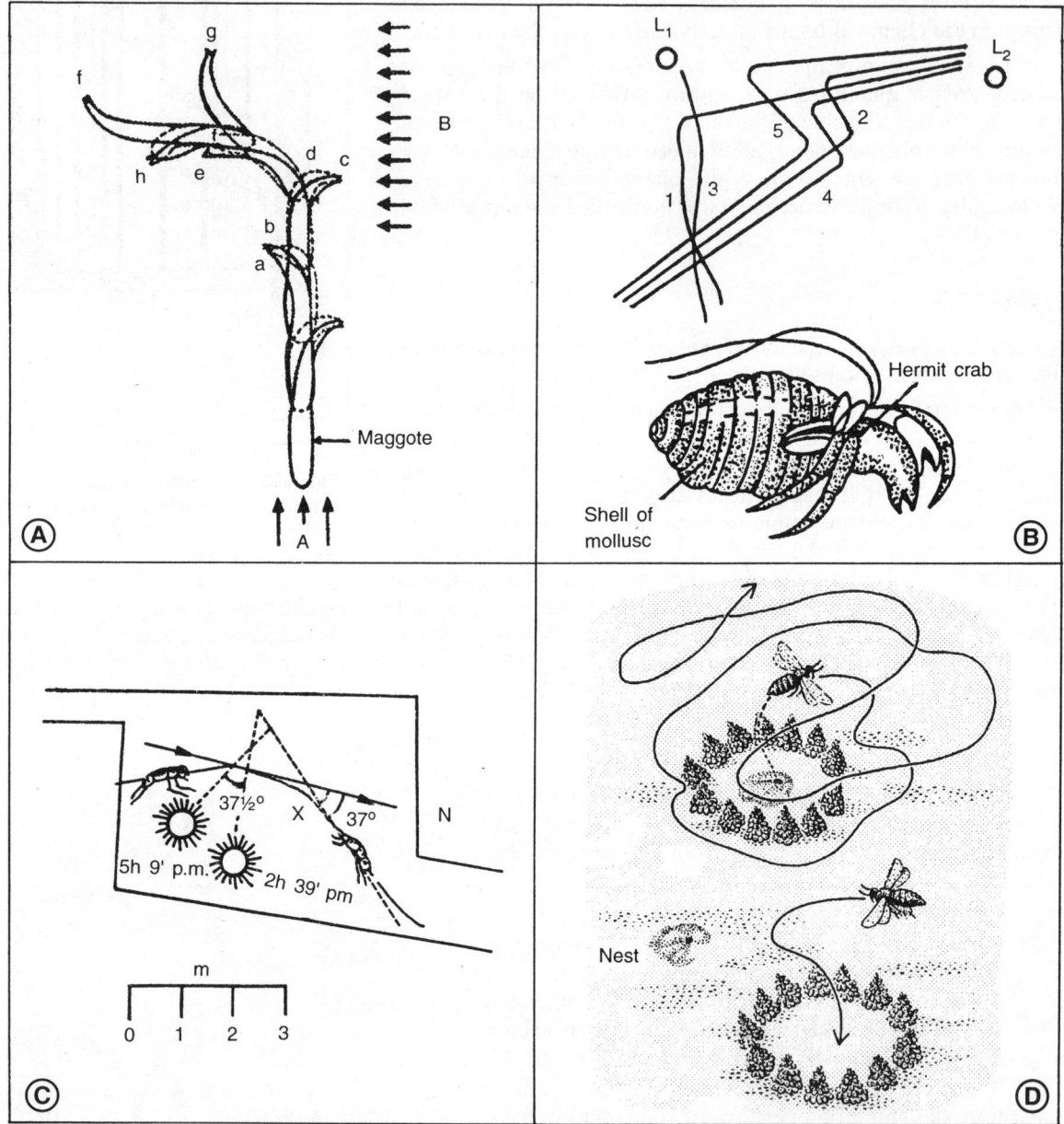

Fig. 2.4. Taxis. (A) Klinotaxic movement shown by Maggote : When light is thrown from two angles. (B) Telotaxic movement of Hermit Crab : When two sources of light L₁ and L₂ was thrown on it. (C) Menotaxis or light compass : An ant (*Lasius niger*) returning to its nest N, with the sun shining from the right at an angle of 90° to the animal's path. At the place X the ant was imprisoned for 2½ hours. When released it deviated from its former path by an angle which was the same as that through which the sun had travelled during this period, so that the sun's rays again made an angle of 90° which is the animal's path. (D) Mnemotaxis : (A) Digger wasp or Hunter wasp (*Philanthus triangulum*) remembers and uses land marks while homing.

(iv) **Mnemotaxis :** It depends on complex stimulus situation and memory of the animal. The hunting digger wasp (*Philanthus triangulum*) uses a number of landmarks simultaneously while returning to its nest. Removal of any of the landmark disturbs the hunting digger wasp to find the path of the nest. (Fig.2.4D).

(v) **Tropotaxis :** A complex case of taxis in which orienting locomotory movement of whole body is influenced by both external stimulation and internal state of organ of the animal.

One set of control fishes A, B and C and another set of ear removed fishes A^1, B^1 and C^1 were taken and kept in different aquarium. When light was thrown from above to both sets of fishes (normal A and ear removed A^1), no change in position in any set of fishes take place. When light was thrown from one side to control fish B and ear removed B^1 fish, both sets of fishes orient on some angle to the source of light. When light was projected from lower side to normal fish C and ear removed fish C^1 different results were obtained. There was no change in the position of normal set of fishes C but ear removed fishes C^1 lose their equilibrium and overturn. Here locomotory movement of whole body of fish is influenced by both external stimulation i.e. *light* and internal state of organ i.e. *ear*. (Fig.2.4E).

Types of taxes

- Klinotaxis :
- Telotaxis :
- Menotaxis : ⎫ Described above.
- Mnemotaxis : ⎬
- Tropotaxis : ⎭
- Phototaxis : Locomotory movement caused by light.
- Thermotaxis : Response to temperature.
- Chemotaxis : Response to chemical stimuli.
- Geotaxis : Response to gravity.
- Rheotaxis : Response to water current.
- Thigmotaxis : Response to touch.
- Galvanotaxis : Response to electric current

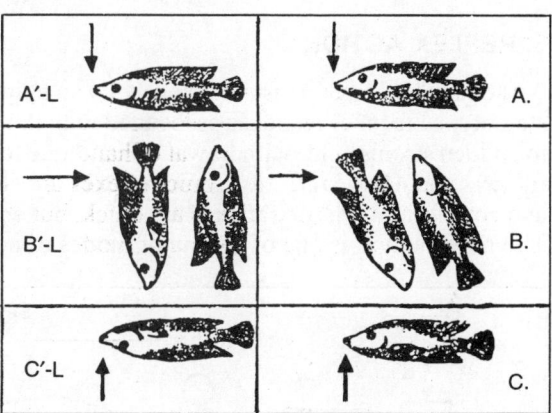

Fig. 2.4(E). Tropotaxis shown by fishes. It is a complex case of taxis in which orientation of animal depends on both stimulus and an internal organ. Two sets of fishes (CONTROL and EAR REMOVED) were used.

5. KINESES

It is a non-directional orientation movement in which velocity of movement or turning depends on the intensity of a particular stimulus. Movement of tentacles of *Hydra* in search of food is random and slow but if water flea (food) comes near the *Hydra*, the rate of movement of tentacles increases. This is the example of kinesis. Two following types of kineses have been recognised.

(i) **Orthokinesis :** The non-directional movement of the animal is straight and velocity of its movement is proportional to the strength of the stimulus. Culture of *Paramecia*, taken on a glass slide, move away (in any direction) from a drop of acid. The rate of movement away from acid depends on the concentration of acid. Low concentration of acid induce *Paramecia* to move away slowly but high concentration of acid exert fast orientation. Ammocoet larva exhibit the phenomenon of orthokinesis in intense light.

(ii) **Klinokinesis :** Velocity of turning of animal in response to a stimulus is proportional to the strength of stimulus. Planaria (flatworm) changes its direction of movement according to the intensity of light thrown on it. In dim light it turns occasionally but in bright high light, the rate of turning of the worm increases accordingly.

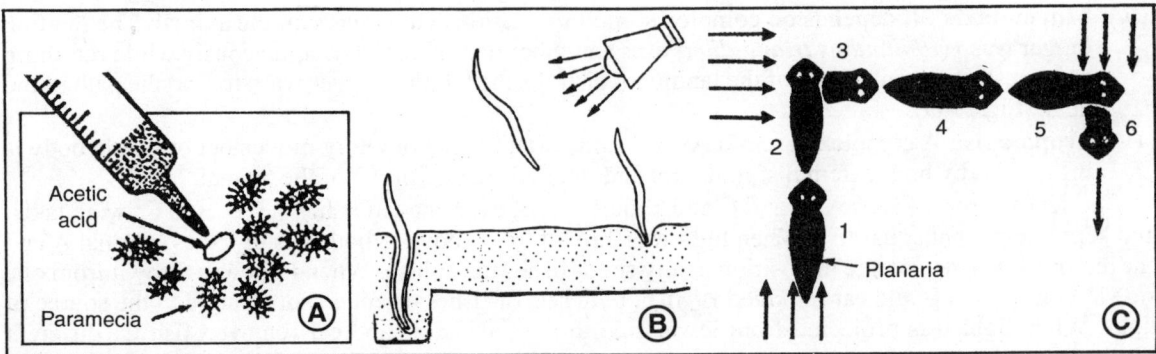

Fig. 2.5. Kinesis. (A&B) Orthokinesis : Paramecia and Ammocoete larva show orthokinesis according to intensity stimus (acid and light respectively). (ii) Klinokinesis shown by planaria : Planaria takes sharp turn in bright light.

6. REFLEX ACTION

An action that is made instantaneously by an animal in response to a stimulus is called reflex action. It is stereotyped form of response associated with the nervous system. Flexion response, blinking of eye due to sudden strong light, withdrawal of hand due to needle pinch etc. are examples of reflex namely *tonic reflexes* and *phasic reflexes*. Tonic reflexes are slow, long lasting adjustments like muscle tone, posture and equilibrium. Phasic reflexes are quick, but short lived adjustments as found in the flexure response. The reflex action is one of the major modes of adaptation in animals.

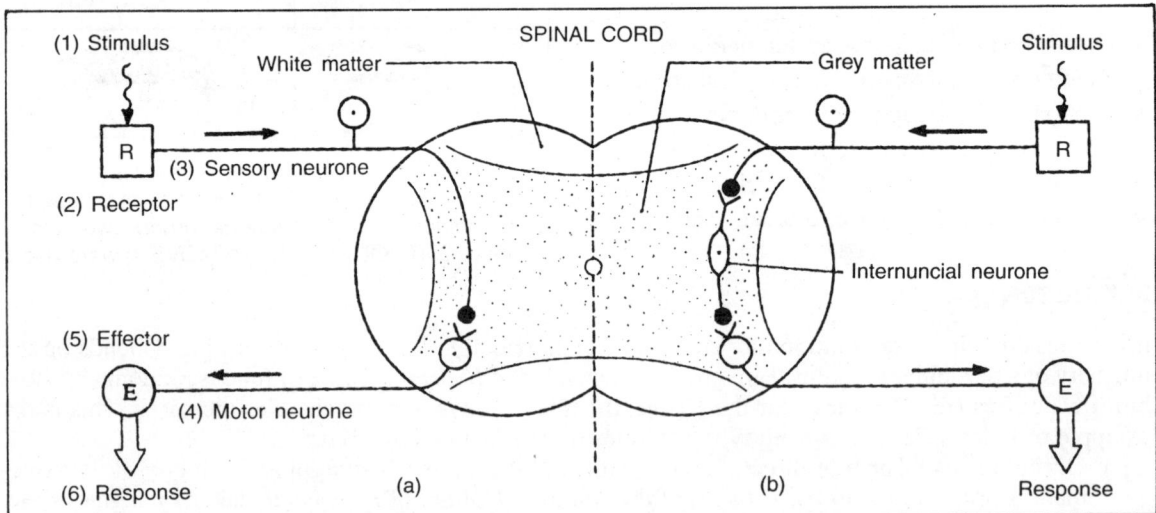

Fig. 2.6. A reflex arc involving the spinal cord in reflex action.

The neurones forming the pathway taken by the nerve impulses in reflex action make a reflex arc. *Afferent sensory neurones* (*a*, towards) carrying impulses from a receptor and an *efferent neurone* (*e*, away from) or motor neurone carrying impulses from away nervous tissue to an effector make a reflex arc. Reflexes are important for survival of the individual and it is not species specific. It is found in nervous system bearing animals.

7. INSTINCT

A genetically inherited character that impel animals to behave a certain fixed ways (i.e. a Fixed Action Pattern : FAP) is called instinct. Each instinct is initiated by a particular stimulus called *sign stimulus* or *releaser*. Instinct is inborn, complex and species specific behaviour patterns. Instinct forms a kind of *species memory* passed on from each generation to its offsprings. Social behaviour, parental care, migration, etc. found in different species of animals are instinctive behaviour.

Instinct is the most controversial term in ethology and is frequently understood as an innate behaviour mechanism expressed in ordered movement sequences. The notion of FAP was formulated by Konrad Lorenz. A FAP is a specific and stereotyped sequence of activities that is triggered by a specific stimulus called a sign stimulus or releaser. A classic example of FAP is provided by the study of egg-rolling behaviour of the greylag goose (*Anser anser*). The greylag goose builds shallow nest in the ground and it uses a stereotype set of behaviour in bringing back the egg that roll out of the nest. The sight of an egg outside the nest acts as a sign or key stimulus and that elicits egg-rolling behaviour.

Occasionally responses (FAP_S) occur in the absence of the appropriate stimulus called Vacuum behaviours. Insectivorous birds deprived of flying insects, for example, may fly out and go through all the motions of catching, killing and eating an imaginary insect.

Many behaviours do not fit neatly under the label of rigid *instincts* because instincts are often modified by experience. Thorpe observed that chaffinches reared in isolation or made deaf by destroying internal ear in young, sing only rudimentary song. Chaffinches reared by their parents, listening to the songs of parents and conspecific, develop up to mark song. The differences of *rudimentary song* and *up to mark song* is not detectable to the human ear, but sound spectogram clearly distinguishes rudimentary and up to mark song.

External factors that signals to trigger instinctive acts are called *Sign stimuli* (Russel, 1943). Definite sign stimulus or releaser works and initiates like a right key. In three-spined stickleback fish, one stimulus, *red belly* of male, is specific stimulus, responsible for releasing territorial defence and other reproductive activities. Tinbergen (1952) used some models to study the specificity of sign stimulus releaser in a three-spined stickleback fish (Fig. 2.7. iii). One fish was real but lacked a red belly, other models were odd-shaped. Only one odd-shaped model was with red spot. Model with a red spot underside acted as sign-stimuli for releasing attack behaviour, required for territorial defence. Here remarkable thing is that the real fish was not attacked by a male three-spined stickleback fish but a model was attacked bearing red spot on belly. Here red spot on belly is "sign stimulus" or releaser.

A herring gull's chick pecks at a red spot present on its parent's bill and that acts as sign stimulus which induced the parent to regurgitate food called crop milk. Chicks of song bird respond to the jerk on their nest for begging food. When the parents arrive on the nest, a jerk is created, which acts a sign stimuli for begging behaviour of chicks.

8. MOTIVATION

It is a common observation that the same stimulus given to the same animal at different times does not always evoke the same response. Presenting food to a starving dog will produce an immediate response from that shown by a dog that has been fed. Female of many species of mammals (with few exceptions) and birds are receptive to mating attempts by males only at certain times of the year. These times coincide with the breeding period. When a male European robin (*Turdus migratorius*) was presented with stuffed robin with red feathers in mid-winter, no response was observed. But if stuffed robin with red feathers was presented in the spring, the male robin exhibited threat displays.

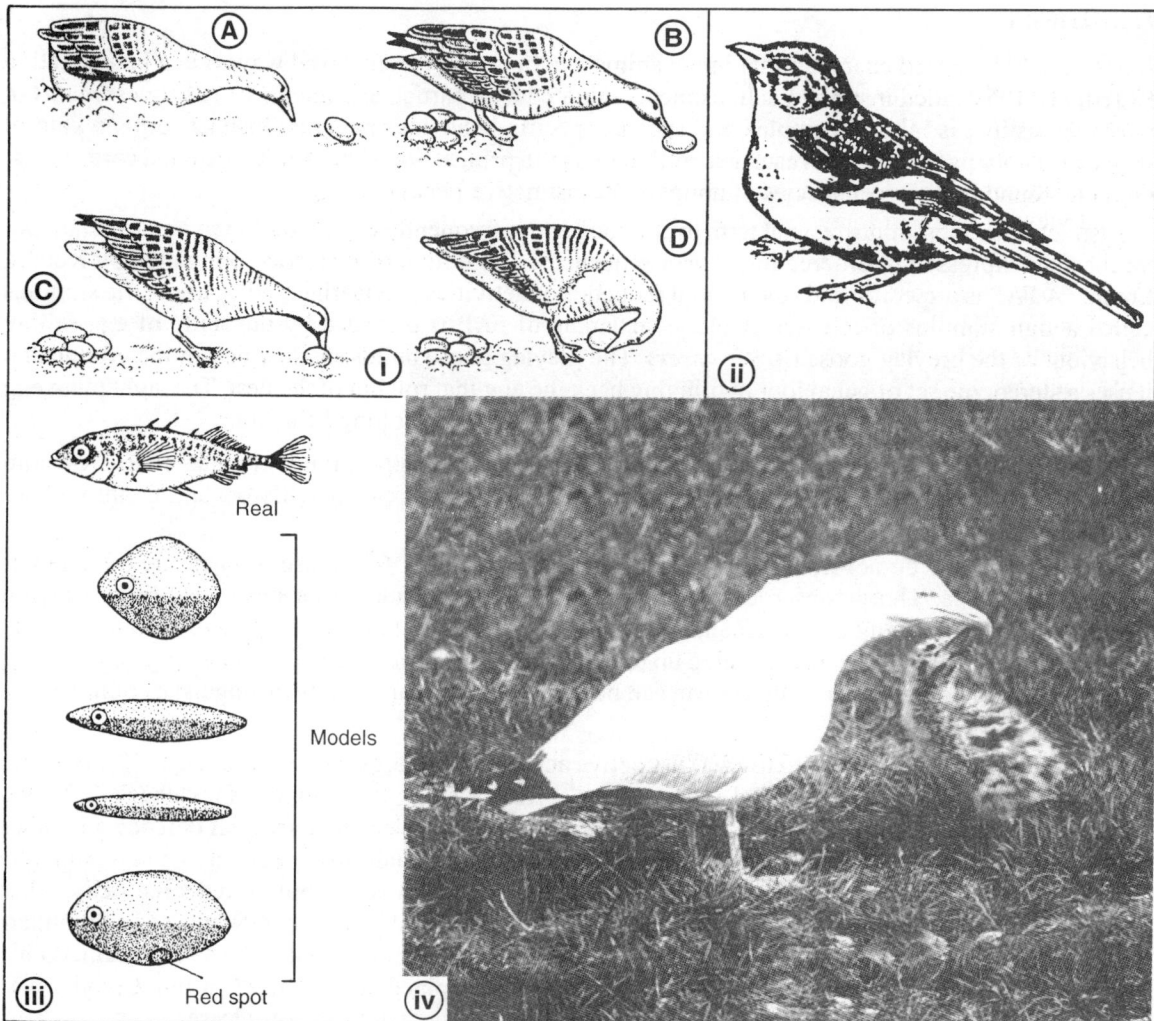

Fig. 2.7. (i) Instinctive behaviour. Grey-lag goose exhibiting instinct by egg-rolling behaviour. (A) It looks at the egg which has rolled out. (B) Rises and tries to drag it with the beak. (C) Places the underside of its beak on the top of the egg. (D) Bends the neck and swings it laterally in a rhythmic movement to pull the egg back to the nest. (ii) Instinct modified by experience: In chaffinches (a singer bird) sings simpler song when reared in isolation. But young chaffinches reared by their parents and living with conspecific, sing complex song. (iii) Releaser for instinctive act in fish: A male three-spined stickleback fish and four models of fish different in shape and size. One odd shaped model bear red spot on belly. The real three-spined stickleback male fish attacked odd shaped model bearing a red spot on belly. (iv) Releaser for instinctive act in bird : Herring gull's chick pecking at red spot present on parent's bill. After pecking parent regurgitate food for chick.

Female rats exhibit differences in general activity levels at different phases of the oestrous cycle. In human beings, special motivational states are often associated with strong subjective feelings or emotions. Something inside the animal must be there for response to the given stimulus. This internal state of the animal is called motivation. An ethologist define motivation as "the cause for a spontaneous change in the behaviour of animal which occur independently outside any stimulus", or a change in the threshold or responsiveness of an animal to a stimulus and which is not due to fatigue or learning.

A specific motivation is often called a *Drive*. The term drive was introduced by Robert Woodworth (1918) as an alternative to William Mc Dougall's (1908) concept of instinct. Woodworth distinguished between the energizing (drive) and the *directing* aspect of motivation. Primary drives resulted from tissue needs, and other (secondary) drives were learnt habits. Konrad Lorenz (1950) outlines the etho-logical view in terms of three successive processes :

1. Accumulation of action-specific energy giving rise to appetitive behaviour.
2. Appetitive behaviour striving for and attaining the stimulus situation activating the innate releas-ing mechanism.
3. Setting off of the releasing mechanism and discharge of endogenous activity in a consumatory actions.

Lorenz assumed that "some sort of energy, specific to one definite activity, is stored up while this activity remains quiescent, and is consumed in its discharge." The view of hunger and thirst as homeo-static drives implies that feeding and drinking are initiated as a result of monitored changes in the animal's physiological state. Food deprived dog (hungry dog) is an example given above, might be described as having a high feeding drive. Osker Heinroth (1950) called the drive as *mood*. Mechanism of motivation can be mentioned as follows :

High motivational level → Appetitive behaviour → Search for goal → Orientation toward goal → Achieving the goal by the consummatory behaviour of FAP → Fall of motivational level to a minimum level → Quiescent period showing refractory behaviour → Motivational level starts rising after a lapse of time and again the same steps are followed.

There are basically four motivational systems - *feeding, reproducing, fighting* and *fleeing* or escap-ing. Each motivational system is made up of many subunits. These subunits usually remain interrelated with each other. For example, reproduction motivational system consists of sexual behaviour, nest building behaviour and parental care subunits.

There is biological significance of drive. This directs the animals to search goal and after achieving the goal animal is satiated. This forces animal to perform some task which is essential for survival and continuation of the race.

LEARNT BEHAVIOUR

Learning is a process through which life experiences leave their mark in the form of memory on the individual. Eight major types of learnt behaviour are recognised.

1. HABITUATION

A gradual decrease in behavioural responsiveness which occurs when a stimulus is repeated frequently with neither reward nor punishment is called habituation. This involves learning to ignore insignificant stimuli. Habituation is important in development of behaviour in young animals in helping to understand neutral stimuli such as movements of things due to wind or gravity.

The escape response of young birds to a cloud-shadow passing over head diminishes progressively. Scarecrows erected to deter birds in crop fields are effective for short time. Birds soon become habitu-ated to this harmless scarecrow. There are several examples of habituation in our day to day life. People living near railway track sleep without any disturbance but a new comer cannot sleep due to noise.

2. IMPRINTING

Imprinting is a kind of learned behaviour. It is the imposition of a stable behaviour pattern in a young animal by exposure to particular stimuli during a critical period (early receptive period) in the animal's development. Stimuli may be a person, an odour, an event or something else. The early sensitive period for imprinting varies species to species and it may vary few hours to few days to months and even years. It is a common observation that the younger we adopt and rear a litter of mammals or birds the easier is to tame them. Circus animals are trained right from the young age. Young animal associate themselves with their master during brief sensitive period of imprinting. In other words imprinting is a kind of learning that reveals "Preprogrammed" nature of learned behaviour.

Osker Heinroth (1871-1945), a German zoologist, is given the credit for being the first to use the term *Imprinting*. Konrad Larenz (1937) was first to study imprinting objectively and systematically. He showed that baby ducks and goslings, which normally follow their mother away from the nest shortly after hatching, could be induced to follow a substitute. Lorenz reared the birds himself and newly hatched ducklings followed him. The baby bird formed an immediate attachment to Lorenz and followed him everywhere for days, thereafter instead of following an adult female of their own species or another human being. They had evidently learned to recognise him as an individual, just as they would normally learn to identify their mother. Presumably a baby duck can do these things because its nervous system is *primed*

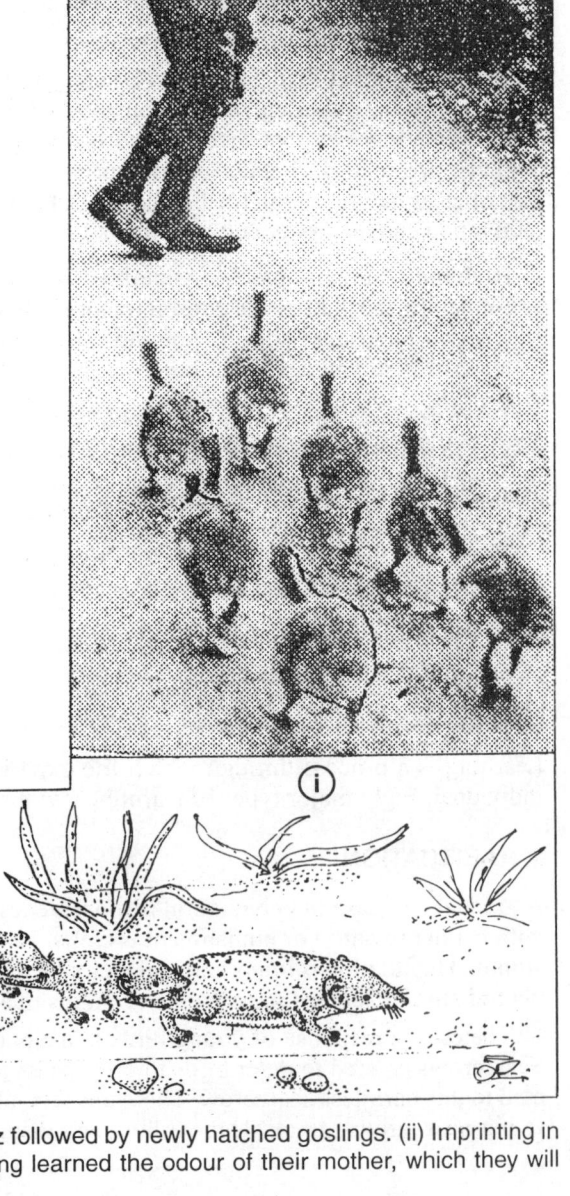

Fig. 2.8. Imprinting. (i) Imprinting in duck. Konrad Lorenz followed by newly hatched goslings. (ii) Imprinting in shrews. Young shrews form a *caravan* early in life, having learned the odour of their mother, which they will follow.

to be altered in a narrowly defined way during the first few hours after hatching. Imprinting-like behaviour are known to occur in many other precocial birds.

Maximum work on imprinting is carried out in ground-nesting birds but it also has been observed in other vertebrates ranging from moles to hoofed mammal. Young shrews can be stimulated by their mother (when she desires to lead her brood from one place to another) to hold onto the fur of another shrew (either the mother or a sibling). The mother then sets off with a conga line of babies trailing behind her.

Experiments have shown that between 5 and 14 days after birth, the baby shrews become imprinted on the odour of the individual that is nursing them. Their caretaker is their mother. If 5 or 6 day-old shrews are given to a substitute mother of another species, they will become imprinted upon her, and when returned to their real mother at 15 days of age will not follow her on any siblings that had left with her. They will follow a cloth impregnated with the odour of the replaced mother, a response that demonstrates that they became imprinted for the odour of the replaced mother that nursed them when they were younger.

3. CONDITIONED REFLEX

It is a form of reflex action where the response is modified by past experiences. These reflexes are co-ordinated by the brain. Our understanding about the mechanism of conditioned reflex, derived from the work of I.P. Pavlov on dog.

Pavlov placed a hungry dog on a strand, restrained by a harness and presented food in powder form at regular intervals. When he signalled the delivery of food by proceeding it with an external stimulus, like the sound of the bell, the reflex of the dog towards the stimulus gradually changed.

The dog began responding to the bell alone licking its lips and salivating. It appeared that the dog had learnt to associate the bell with the food. He referred to the bell as the *conditioned stimulus* (CS), the food as the *unconditioned stimulus* (UCS), salivation in response to presentation of food as *unconditional response* (UCR), salivation in response to the bell as *conditioned response* (CR).

In the case of conditioned reflex, the type of response is modified by past experience and reflexes are co-ordinated by the brain. In this context an interesting example can be mentioned which happens in our day to day life. If an empty tin is picked up and found to be extremely hot, burning the fingers, it will be dropped immediately (simple reflex action) whereas a boiling hot cooked casserole in an expensive dish, equally hot and painful, will probably be put down, quickly but gently (conditioned reflex). The reason for the difference in degree of response reveals the involvement of conditioning and memory followed by a conscious decision by the brain.

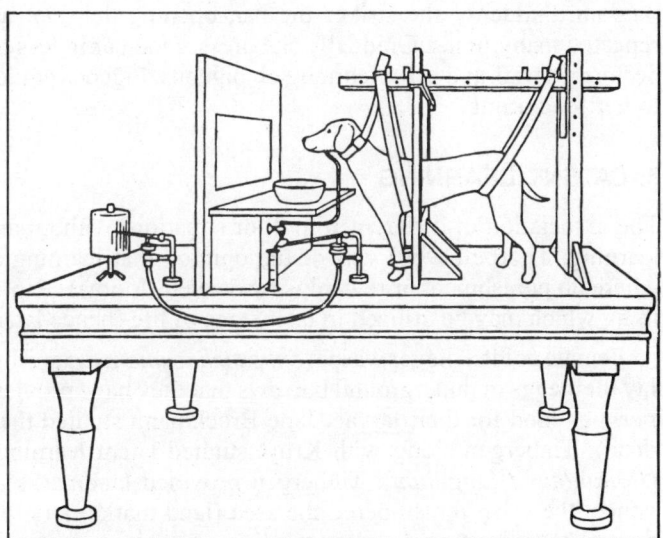

Fig. 2.9. Reflex action : Pavlov's arrangement for the study of conditioned reflex action (salivary conditioning) on dog.

4. TRIAL-AND-ERROR LEARNING

It is a common observation that animals learn things in day to day happenings of life by trial-and-error method. By trial-and-error an animal tries each alternative and learns gradually to solve the problem through successes and failures.

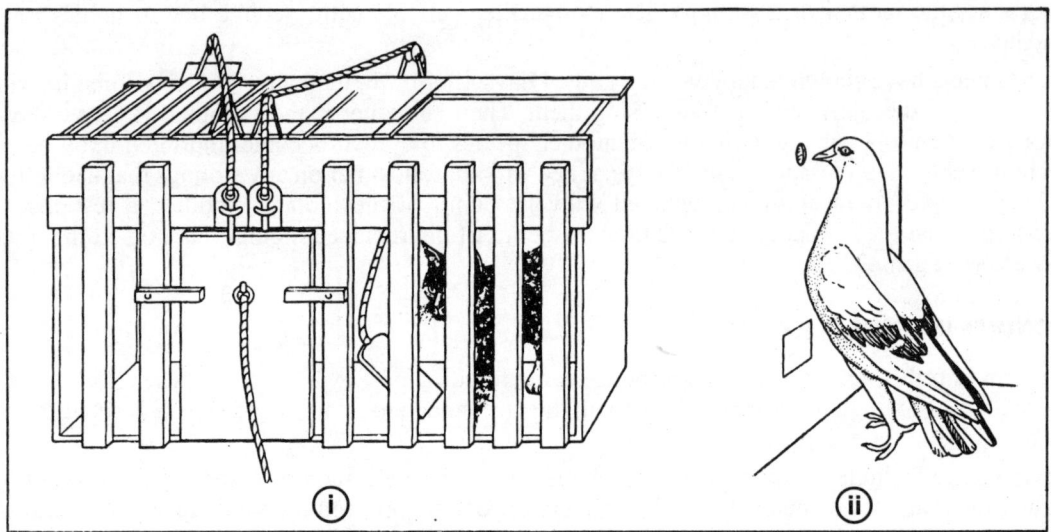

Fig. 2.10. (i) Trial-and-error learning by a cat : The cat gradually learns to press the bar and open the box to get fish. (ii) Trial-and-error learning by a pigeon : Pigeon learnt to press lever to open box and to get foodgrains.

Thorndike (1910) devised a box for investigating trial-and-error learning in cat. A bar in the box opens the door when pressed. A fish placed in the box. Cat tries to get the fish placed in the box, at random. Suddenly she strikes the bar, opening the door and getting the fish. Same experiment was repeated many times. Gradually she presses the bar in less time interval and finally in no time. Skinner performed trial-and-error learning on pigeons. Pigeons could learn to press lever to open the door of box to get foodgrains.

5. LATENT LEARNING

The association of different stimuli or situations without any immediate patent reward is called latent learning. Thorpe (1960) was of the opinion that learning also takes place even in those happenings where no punishment or reward is associated. Animals explore new experience and always learn something which may be utilized in later stage of life (hence latent).

Female golden digger wasps (*Sphex ichneumoneus*) and other species of wasp (*Philanthus triangulum*) lay their eggs in underground burrows that they have provisioned with katydids (*long-horned grasshoppers*) as food for their larvae. Jane Brockmann studied the female golden digger wasp's behaviour in detail. Tinbergen along with Kruyt studied latent learning in predatory digger wasp or hunter wasp (*Philanthus triangulum*). Tinbergen provided landmarks around the wasp's nest holes. Upon emergence, the wasp remembered the area (land marks) and then flew off. If Tinbergen removed or rearranged some land marks, the returning wasps become disoriented to varying degrees. Numerous other studies support the conclusion that the entire configuration of land marks is used by the returning wasp as a guide to the location of its burrow (Fig. 2.4D).

Tolman studied the phenomenon of latent learning in rat. He took a maze having many blind paths and a single open path leading to the goal. A rat's home cage was placed in such a fashion that rat could wander into the maze aimlessly. Rat moves through different paths without any patent reward. Does he learn anything about the maze as he explores? Tolman is of the opinion that learning has taken place. This learning is latent and may be utilized at the time of need. This can be confirmed by giving a food reward at the end of the maze. Two rats were placed before the maze. One previous rat, having experience of blind paths of maze and a new rat. The previous one, the experienced rat, reaches to food in much shorter time than the second newly introduced rat. It indicates that previous *latent* learning of first rat was utilized in the hour of need.

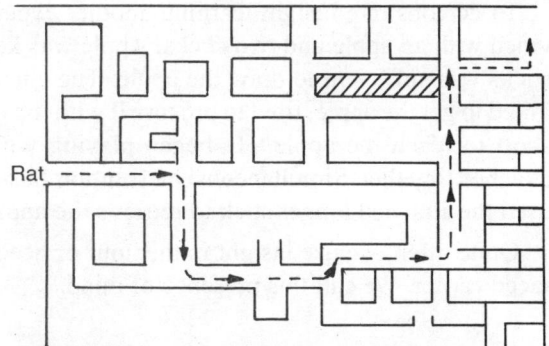

Fig. 2.11. Latent learning : Latent learning by a rat in maze.

Metzgar (1967) has shown how latent learning process might work in nature for the deer-mouse (*Peromyscus leucopus*). One group of mice was given exposure to and experience in an enclosed very big hall containing natural things like plants, twigs, logs etc. A second group was kept in laboratory cages without any experience of natural things. Now mice from each group were placed in the enclosed room with an owl which is a predator to deer-mouse. Metzgar found that only two of twenty deer-mouse with prior experience in the hall were caught by the owl, while eleven of twenty mice with no prior experience in the habitat were captured. Latent learning apparently provided the experienced deer-mouse (residents) to avoid predator the owl.

6. INSIGHT

Ability to respond correctly to a situation that is experienced for the first time in life, and that is different from any experience encountered previously is considered as insight.

Kohler's work on chimpanzees demonstrate *insight*. When a chimpanzee named "X" was presented with a few wooden boxes kept on ground and a few bananas too high from the reach of the chimpanzee, it tried to get banana by jumping. But he failed and sat quietly. After sometime something flashed in his mind and suddenly he stacked up the wooden boxes and climbed up to get bananas. This response appeared after a period of apparent thought and is called insight (Fig. 2.12).

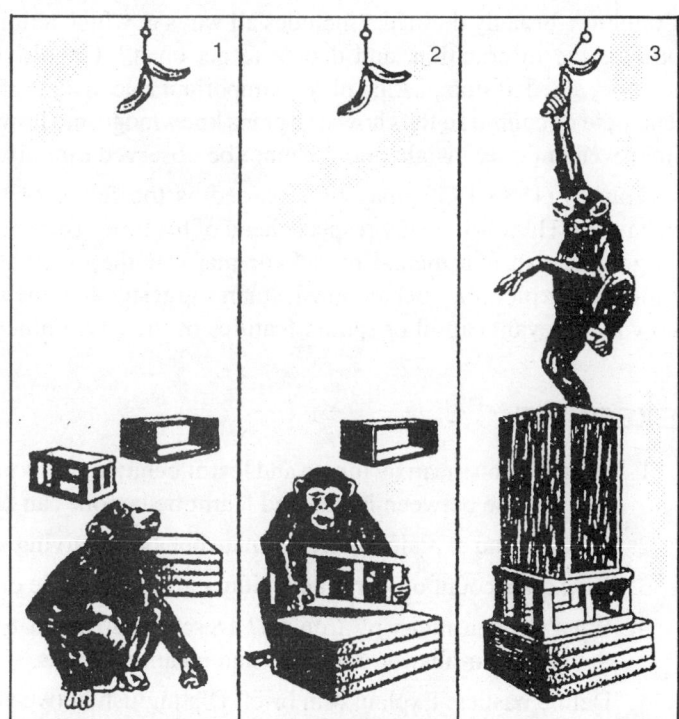

Fig. 2.12. Insight in Chimpanzee. Kohler's experiment on a Chimpanzee. Chimpanzee applied the faculty of insight to get banana which was beyond his reach.

To demonstrate insight learning another experiment on a hungry ape was performed. He was provided with an apple and two sticks. Apple was kept out of the reach of the chimpanzee. Length of two sticks was sufficient to draw the apple. The chimpanzee first tried to get the apple by hand. When he failed to get the apple, tried to procure it with the help of one stick, again he failed because one stick was short to reach the apple. He began playing with both sticks. Suddenly, by chance, both sticks got attached together. Simultaneously a solution flashed in the mind of chimpanzee to obtain the apple. He used the attached longer stick to retrieve the apple.

Quite often, we use insight in the hour of need to solve some intricate problems which we have not faced earlier. We call this presence of mind.

7. REASONING

Reasoning is very evolved form of behaviour perhaps found only in Apes, Dolphins, Killer whale and Human beings. The reasoning is the mental process of drawing inferences from the two on more than two statements or happenings. Reasoning may be defined as "the ability to combine spontaneously two or more separate experiences to form a new experience which is effective for obtaining a desired goal". Reasoning is the mental process of solving problems, when we are in dilemma. Much is yet to learn about neural mechanism of reasoning.

8. COGNITION

Cognition, broadly defined, "includes all ways in which animals take in information through the senses, process the information, and decide to act on it". Cognitive processes such as perception, learning, memory and decision making play an important role in mate choice, foraging and many other behaviours. The field of cognition tells how one gains knowledge and how one uses that knowledge. Cognitions is an improvement over insight and it cannot be observed directly.

Tolman (1886-1959) may be regarded as the father of the modern cognitive approach to animal behaviour. He was in many respect ahead of his time. Tolman also pioneered the idea of cognitive maps. Cognitive map is a mental model (or map) of the external environment which may be constructed following exploratory behaviour. Tolman suggested that the animal acquires a cognitive map indicating how the relevant causal or spatial features of the environment relate to each other.

EXERCISE

1. What do you mean by innate and learnt behaviour? Explain your answer with suitable examples. A distinct line between innate and learnt behaviour can be drawn or not. If not explain it in brief.
2. Mention and explain different innate behaviour giving suitable example and diagrams?
3. Give an account of learnt behaviours giving suitable examples and diagrams.
4. What do you mean by tropism? Describe different types of tropism giving suitable examples. Support your answer with neat and clean diagrams.
5. Define nastics. Explain it in brief. Distinguish between Nastics and Tropism.
6. Taxes? Classify taxes giving suitable examples and diagrams.

7. Kineses? Describe different types of kinesis. Explain your answer with suitable examples and diagrams.
8. Reflex action? Describe Pavlov's experiment on dog demonstrating conditioned reflex.
9. Instinct? Mention some interesting cases of instinct. "Explain how most of the instinctive behaviour is initiated by a right key (sign stimulus or releaser).
10. Motivation? Explain motivation with suitable examples.
11. Habituation? Describe habituation with suitable examples.
12. Imprinting? Explain Lorenz's experiment demonstrating imprinting in ducklings.
13. Describe imprinting in shrew and other mammals.
14. Trial-and-error learning? Describe contribution of Kohler in this field.
15. Define latent learning. Describe Tolman's experiment on rats demonstrating latent learning.
16. Define insight. Explain it by giving suitable examples.
17. Write short notes on memory, habituation, impriting, cognition and conditioned reflex.
18. Define cognition and explain Tolman's contribution in this field.
19. Differentiate between (i) Tropism and Taxis, (ii) Taxis and Kinesis, (iii) Irritability and Reflexes, (iv) Reflex action and Instinct, (v) Insight and Trial-and-error learning, (vi) Insight and Cognition, (vii) Simple reflex and Conditioned reflex, (viii) Habituation and Accommodation, (ix) Klinotaxes and Telotaxes, (x) Menotaxes and Mnemotaxes, (xi) Orthokineses and Klinokinesis.

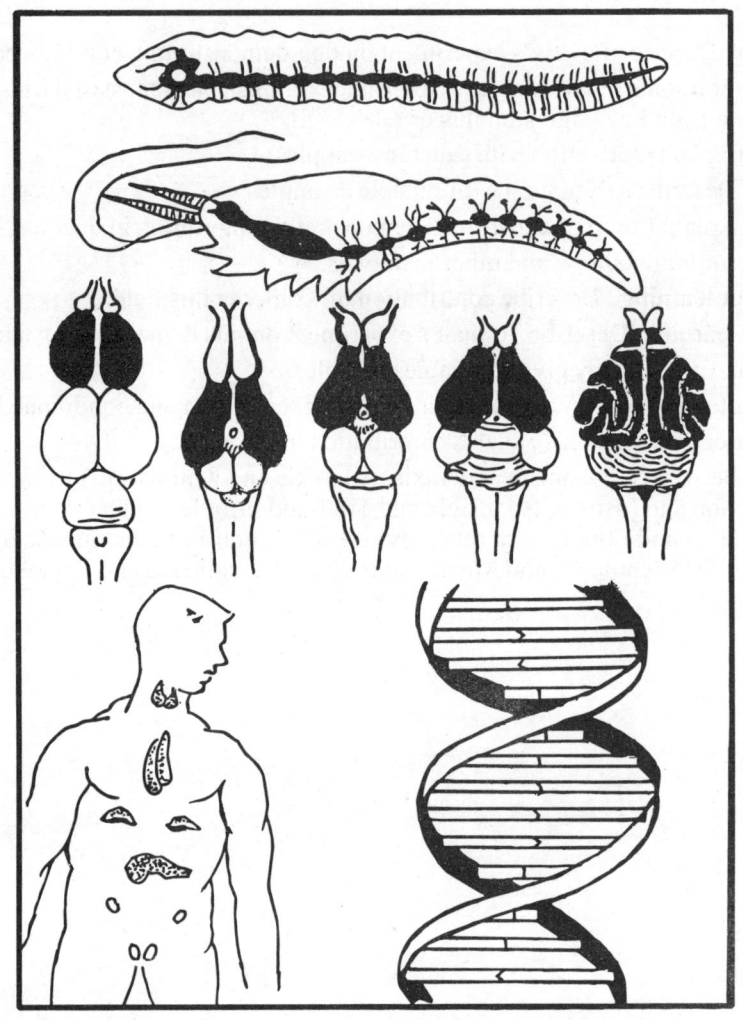

Behaviourists often face a very pertinent question "what composes behaviour"? The question seems to be very simple but the answer is not so simple and straight because development of an organism's behaviour depends on the interaction between internal "biotic factors" and environmental "abiotic factors." Since the influence of heredity and environment are integrated during the development of behaviour, and therefore one cannot draw a sharp line to separate behaviour into genetically controlled versus environmentally determined categories. One of the central goals of this chapter is to deal with major internal factors (genetic material, nervous system, endocrine system, pheromones etc.) composing behaviour.

FACTORS COMPOSING BEHAVIOUR:
Ethogenetics, Neurothology, Ethoendocrinology & Pheromones

ETHOGENETICS

• Introduction • Gene action and egg laying behaviour of *Aplysia* • Genetic differences responsible for behavioural differences - Prey catching behaviour of funnel web spider - Nest cleaning behaviour of honeybees - Geotaxic behaviour of *Drosophila* - Mating call of male crickets - Nest material carrying behaviour in love - birds - Crowing postures in fowl - Migratory and non-migratory behaviour of blackcap warbler - Genetic basis for food preference difference between coastal and inland garter snakes • Behavioural differences caused by a single gene difference - The fruitfly (*Drosophila*) - Alcoholism in mice due to single gene action • Genes and Human Behaviour - Behaviour of identical twins - Autosomal and sex-linked diseases - Schizophrenia, maniac-depression and alcoholism in humans - The gene for pleasure • Exercise

INTRODUCTION

Learning how an individual's genes influence its behaviour is an exciting and challenging part of the study of the *Proximate cause* of animal behaviour. All behaviour patterns require genetic information for their development. But how do genes affect behaviour? This is a question of great interest to behaviour geneticists, who have tried to explore the link between genetic information and the development of the Proximate mechanisms that underlie animal behaviour. Hamer and Copeland mentioned that "genes are not switches that say 'happy' or 'shy' or 'sad' rather genes are simply chemicals that direct the combination of chemicals." What genes do is to order up the production of proteins in organs including the brain, which might seek to stimulate the personality.

Behaviour development involves an interaction between an individual's Genotype and the Environment in which it exist to produce that individual's phenotype (Fig. 3.1).

GENE ACTION AND EGG LAYING BEHAVIOUR OF APLYSIA

How genes of *Aplysia* (a shell-less marine snail) influence its egg laying behaviour is interesting to note.

Aplysia lays over a million eggs. All eggs remain connected in a long strip. The snail picks up the end of strip in its mouth and performs a series of head-waving motions. By doing this snail frees the strip of eggs from its own reproductive duct. *Aplysia* secrete mucous from mouth which wraps over eggs to make a ball of eggs. Finally, the snail presses the egg mass onto a substratum, where the eggs adhere until hatching. The entire series of egg-processing actions is tightly stereotyped pattern of behaviour. Scheller and Axel (1981) found the behaviour sequence to be the result of gene action at a number of levels. The cells that give rise to Aplysia's entire nervous system are descendents of a few cells in the embryo's body wall. Early in the development of *Aplysia* a subset

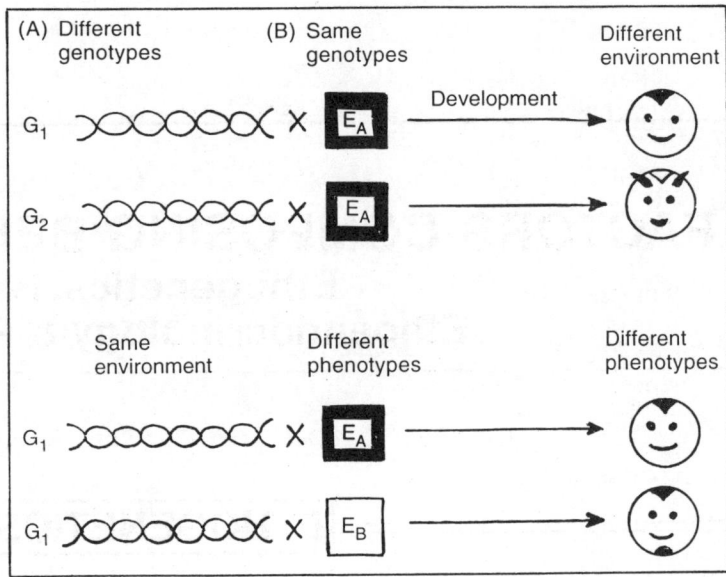

Fig. 3.1. What causes individuals to differ in behaviour? The development of an organism's behaviour depends on the interaction between genetic information and environmentally supplied materials. Differences between individuals in either (A) their genes or (B) their environments can lead to the development of different phenotypes and behaviour.

of these pre-nerve cells produces a specific protein called ELH (egg-laying hormone). All these pre-nerve cells are daughters of a single cell in the very early embryo that has the ability to use the appropriate gene to make ELH. All other cells in the embryo possess this gene but are non-functional. The ELH producing cells divide further and migrate to their final locations in the developing organism, where they differentiate into adult nerve cells. In the adult snail, therefore, certain nerve cells have inherited the ability to produce ELH while others have not.

By the time of maturation of the snail, all these systems are in place. At a specific movement another hormone is released that causes the ELH-producing cells to go into full production. ELH then acts as a neurotransmitter and neighbouring nerves are stimulated. ELH also acts as a hormone, circulating in the blood and causing specific muscle fibres to contract, a response that results in the co-ordinated behaviour pattern observed as egg extraction and deposition. In this sequence; embryogenesis, genes, neurotransmitters, nerves and muscles—all play important role acting in co-ordination to generate a behaviour pattern critical to the reproduction of the snail.

The above example suggests that in *Aplysia* the action of the gene is of direct importance in guiding the production of a stereotyped behaviour pattern.

GENETIC DIFFERENCES RESPONSIBLE FOR BEHAVIOURAL DIFFERENCES

Genetic differences are responsible for behavioural differences among individuals.

PREY CATCHING BEHAVIOUR OF FUNNEL WEB SPIDER

Two different populations of funnel web spider of the same species exhibit different behaviour in context of prey catching. Funnel Web Spider found in a relatively lush streamside habitat in Arizona are *slow to respond to prey* that land on their webs, whereas individuals of the same species that happen to live in the dry desert grassland of New Mexico, *catch their prey very fast*. One can assume that different response behaviour in catching prey between two groups of spiders might be due to environmental differences. To test this possibility Hedrick and Reichert brought few spiders from both areas into the lab and reared a new generation to maturity under identical condition. The offsprings of the streamside parents still were slow to respond to prey and offsprings of grassland parents were very fast in prey catching even

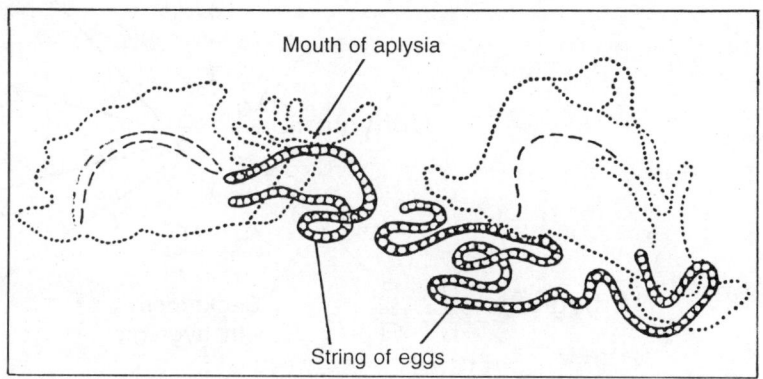

Fig. 3.2. Influence of gene on egg laying behaviour of *Aplysia*. The string of egg cases is expelled from the reproductive duct in the side of the body. The animal grasps the egg string in its mouth (left) and fixes it to the substrate (right).

though they had received just as much food as the laboratory descendants of streamside spiders. These results support the view that genetic differences are responsible for the different speeds of attack exhibited by individuals from the two areas and not the environmental differences.

NEST CLEANING BEHAVIOUR OF HONEYBEE

The best known and most convincing example of simple Mendelian transmission of single-gene behaviour pattern involves honeybee's nest cleaning behaviour.

Rothenbuhler (1964) carried out genetic analysis of the nest cleaning behaviour of three strains of the European honeybee *Apis mellifera*. The larvae of honeybee are some times killed by a bacterial disease called American foulbrood. This bacteria (*Bacillus larvae*) affects the larvae and kills the pupae. To maintain a hygienic environment within the hive, one strain of the worker bees-genotype uurr-normally open the comb cells that contain diseased larvae/dead pupae and remove them. Second strain of honeybees with genetic make up - UURR- are unhygienic i.e. they neither uncap the comb cells nor remove dead pupae. When unhygienic strain (UURR) of honeybee was crossed with hygienic strain (uurr), first generation (F_1) was unhygienic (UuRr). This indicate that unhygienic is dominant. When hybrid (UuRr) was crossed with hygienic bee (uurr) i.e. back cross was done, second generation (F_2) gave four types

Table 3.1 Result of a cross between hygienic (uurr) and unhygienic (UURR) strains of honeybee

UU	=	Do not uncap the comb chamber.
RR	=	Do not remove the diseased larvae.
uu	=	Uncap the comb chamber.
rr	=	remove the diseased larvae or dead pupae.

Rothenbuhler's analysis of hygienic behaviour in honeybees. U and u indicate the dominant and recessive genes for uncapping behaviour respectively and R and r indicate the dominant and recessive genes for removing dead pupae respectively.

of individuals (UuRr; Uurr; uuRr and uurr). Out of 23 progeny; 9 uncapped the comb chambers (containing infected larvae) but did not remove diseased larvae, 6 did not uncap the comb chamber but remove the infected larvae if the cap of the chamber were uncapped by any person, and 8 would neither uncap comb chamber nor would remove infected larvae.

Result of above cross indicate that different genes control the uncapping of the comb chamber and removal of diseased larvae or dead pupae. Results can be explained on the basic of two pairs of alleles, of which the unhygienic alleles U and R are dominant. Thus, worker bees with UU or Uu will not uncap the comb chamber (containing diseased larvae) and those with RR or Rr will not remove diseased or dead larvae or pupae.

No physical or physiological differences have been discovered among totally hygienic, partially hygienic or totally unhygienic worker bees. This suggests that the alleles U and u act as a switches that release the uncapping behaviour, provided there is a certain threshold of stimulation.

GEOTAXIC BEHAVIOUR OF DROSOPHILA

Hirsch and Kimling selected three population of *Drosophila melanogaster* for the study of geotaxic behaviour and its link with the genetic make up of the individual. Out of three population, one was *positive geotaxic*, second was *negative geotaxic* and third was an unselected *control population*.

These were crossed with a special stock that carried various chromosomal inversions and marker genes. The marker genes were used to identify the three large chromosomes. They were dominant genes controlling phenotypic features by which their presence in the genotype is made visible. By means of a special mating design, females were produced that were either homozygous or heterozygous for the chromosomes to be investigated.

The three chromosomes were identified by marker genes : chromosome X by bar eyes (B), chromosome II by curly wings (CY), and chromosome III by stubble bristles (sb). Tester females carrying these markers were mated with males from one of the stocks to be investigated. Of the progeny, only those carrying all three marker genes were used in the subsequent part of the experiment. These were back crossed with the original male population, producing eight possible genotypes. From the eight classes of genotype, the individual effects of the chromosomes and their interactions can be studied. Hirsch and Kimling (1962) found that, in an unselected population, chromosomes X and II contributed to *positive geotaxis* and chromosome III contributed to *negative geotaxis*. In a strain selected for *negative geotaxis*, the negative contribution of chromosome III was increased, while the positive effects of chromosomes X and II were reduced. When the effects on the three chromosomes were taken together, the magnitude of the effect was greater for *negative geotaxis*. This is not surprising because the total response to selection is greater for *negative geotaxis*.

These results suggest that *geotaxic behaviour* in *D. melanogaster* is controlled by a number of genes, which are distributed over all three of the major chromosomes (X, II and III).

MATING CALL OF MALE CRICKETS

You must have heard the sound produced by crickets. This sound may be annoying and meaningless for us but in fact male cricket attracts female of its own species over long distances by a calling song. The difference in songs of different species are not distinguishable by human ear but by oscillogram. **Leroy** (1964) obtained hybrids between two species of the Australian field crickets, *Teleogryllus commodus* and *Teleogryllus oceanicus*. David Bentley and Ronald Hoy (1972) recorded the songs of parents and hybrids in oscillogram and observed that the song of F$_1$ hybrids are distinctly different from either parental song. In particular, the intrachirp and intratrill intervals of the hybrids are intermediate between those of the parents.

NEST MATERIAL CARRYING BEHAVIOUR IN LOVE-BIRDS

Love-birds are members of the parrot family (Psittacidae) which breed easily in captivity. Within the genus *Agapornis* many species are present. Peach-faced love-birds *Agapornis roseicollis* species is one of the most beautiful of the love-birds. In the wild, it breeds in the nests of weaver birds. In captivity, this spe-

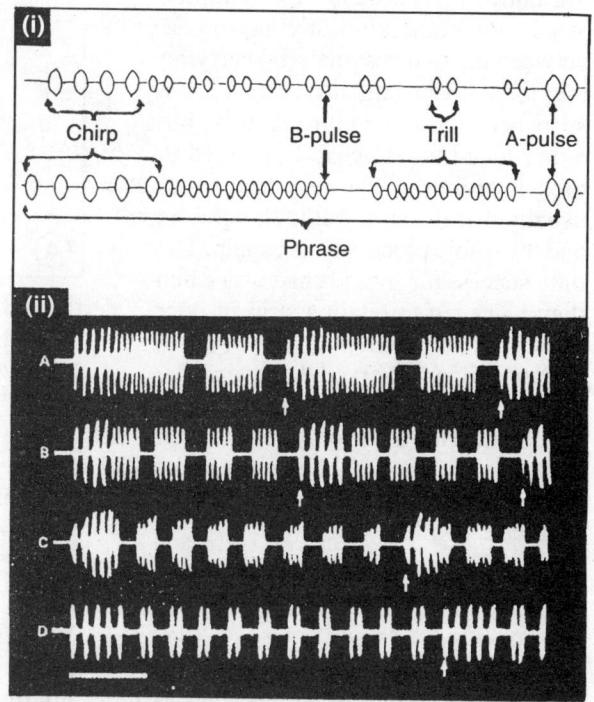

Fig. 3.3. (i) Phrases structure of the calling song of the cricket *Teleograllus*. (ii) Mating Call of Male Cricket : Oscillogram of calling songs of *T. oceanicus* (A) and *T. commodus* (D); and their hybrids *T. oceanicus* (female) × *T. commodus* (male) (B) and *T. commodus* (female) × *T. oceanicus* (male) (C). (Arrows mark the beginning of phrases).

cies can breed in wooden nesting boxes. The hen peels the bark from plant twigs and uses it to construct her own nest inside the box.

A very interesting case of influence of genetic make up on nest material carrying behaviour of lovebirds have been studied by Dilger. Within the genus *Agapornis* two types of nest-material carrying behaviour are represented. All species tear strips of material from plants to build nest. One species

Agapornis roseicollis tuck the strips into their rump feathers and fly back to the nest carrying several pieces. Other species *A. fisherei* carry the strips singly in their beak.

Dilger (1962) crossed these two species *A. roseicollis* and *A. fisherei* (which differed in nest carrying behaviour) and watched the nest-building behaviour of the hybrids. For some time hybrids were incapable of building a nest at all because they attempted to perform some kind of compromise between the two nest material carrying methods. They might start to tuck a strip between the rump feathers, but either failed to let go of it or failed to tuck it properly. The end result was usually that the strip fell to the ground and the whole process began again. The only success the hybrids had was when they managed to retain a strip in their beak after the attempted tucking procedure. Dilger observed that even after months of practice, hybrids managed successful carrying in only 41% of their trials. Two years later they were successful in nearly all trials, but before carrying a strip in their beak they still made the turning movement of head which is the preliminary to tucking it to their rump feathers.

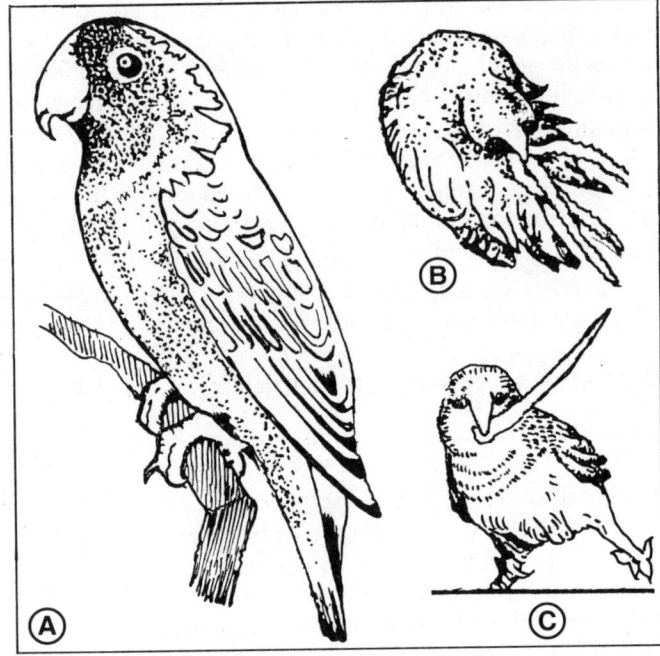

Fig. 3.4. (i) Love-bird : (A) *Agapornis roseicollis*. Transportation of Nest material in two species of genus *Agapornis*: (B) *A. roseicollis* carry nest material into their rump feathers (C) *A. fisherei* carry stripes singly in their bill.

CROWING POSTURES IN FOWL

The Roosters of two different species crow in different postures. Ring necked pheasant crows by stretching its neck and pointing its head upward. Domestic rooster crows stretching its neck but looking down. A hybird of both species assumes intermediate position while crowing.

MIGRATORY AND NON-MIGRATORY BEHAVIOUR OF BLACKCAP WARBLERS

The migratory behaviour of members of different blackcap warbler populations varies from region to region. Blackcaps that breed in Germany migrate great distances twice a year moving between Europe and Africa via Spain in the spring and fall. But there are non-migratory blackcaps as well. Non-migratory blackcaps live in Cape Verde, an archipelago off the west coast of Africa, where they stay throughout the year. Berthold crossed Female German migratory blackcap warbler with male Cape Verdean non- migratory blackcap warbler and vice versa in laboratory aviaries and got *"hybrid"* offsprings. He measured migratory behaviour in the parent birds and the hybrids. He did so by placing the blackcaps in special cages with electronically activated perches that record whenever a bird lands upon them. During the migratory period, caged German migratory blackcaps jumped back and forth between perches every night for many weeks, averaging about 370 hours of migratory restlessness. Contrary to this, during the same period, caged Cape Verdean non-migratory Blackcaps slept quietly throughout the night without exhibiting any restlessness. As expected hybrid blackcap offsprings showed a much reduced migratory tendency compared with their German parent but much more migratory activity than their Cape Verdean parent. They averaged about 250 hours of night - time hopping. This result supports the hypothesis that the hereditary genotype of a blackcap influences its tendency to migrate.

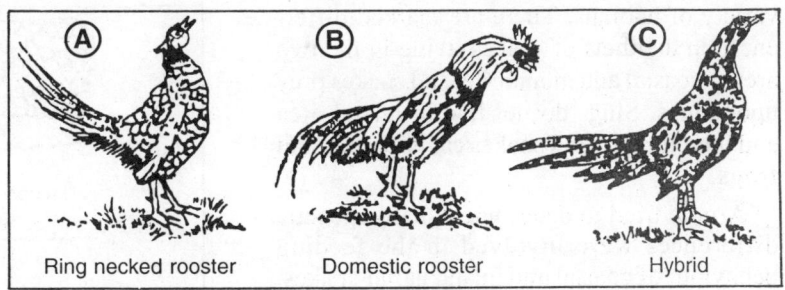

Fig. 3.5. (A & B) Different postures exhibited by two different species of Roosters while crowing. (C) A hybrid of two species assume intermediate position while crowing.

Halbig extended the Berthold's experiment and added one more dimension by examining whether hereditary differences also cause birds from two different migratory populations to follow different flight paths while migrating. German blackcaps fly in *southwesterly direction to Spain* and then on to Africa. But Austrian blackcaps follow a totally different migratory route that takes them *southeast across Turkey to Lebanon* and *Israel* before turning south to Ethiopia and Kenya (Fig. 3.6). Migrating route choices of hybrid offspring (German and Austrian blackcaps) was found to be intermediate with those of their German and Austrian parents.

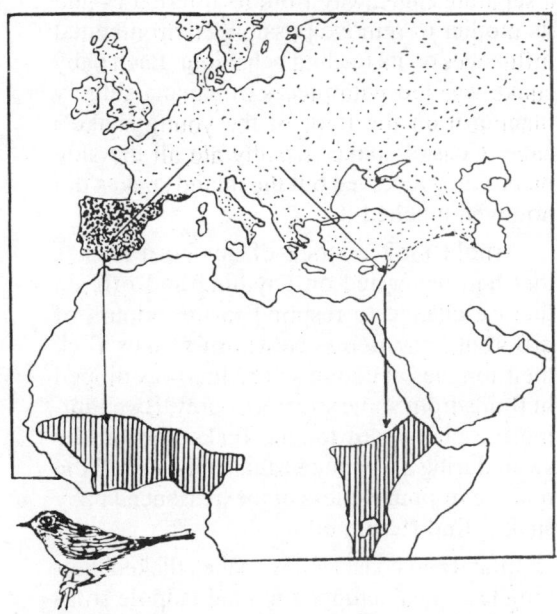

Fig. 3.6. Different Migratory Paths of German and Austrian Blackcap Warblers : Hybrid of German and Austrian blackcap Warbler follow an intermediate route.

GENETIC BASIS FOR FOOD PREFERENCE DIFFERENCE BETWEEN COASTAL AND INLAND GARTER SNAKES

Of all the creatures known to mankind, the snake may be regarded as occupying a position which is held in the utmost respect. The respect probably arose from fear. But Arnold's respect for snakes is not due to fear but for studying genetic basis of snake behaviour.

For most snakes, the sense of smell is the most important. They depend mostly on the tongue to pick up scent particles from the air and ground and transfer them to the Jacobson's organ present in the roof of the mouth that analyzes odours carried to it by the tongue [Fig. 3.7 (A)]. This is the reason why snakes are seen flicking out their tongue all the time. Thus, they are able to track their food, locate suitable mates, and seem to smell and also avoid predators, such as mongoose and man.

Arnold worked with a garter snake, *Thamnophis elegans*, that is found in North America in a wide variety of habitats. There are marked differences in the diets of snakes living in the two areas - coastal and inland. Coastal snakes prey upon slugs. Slugs do not live in inland area and therefore, inland snakes eat upon fish and frogs.

Arnold tried to determine whether genetic differences were involved in the feeding behaviour of coastal and inland garter snakes. He took pregnant female snakes from the two populations in the laboratory, and kept them under identical condition. When the females gave birth to babies, each baby was placed in a separate cage away from its littermates and its mother to remove possible environmental influences on its feeding behaviour. Each baby snake was fed with pieces of banana slug by placing it on the floor of the young snake's cage. Coastal snakes usually ate all the slug pieces they received but the inland snakes did not even touched it.

Arnold took a stock of newborn snakes that had never fed on anything and offered them a chance to respond to the odours of different prey items. Newborn snakes flick their tongues at cotton swabs that was dipped in fluids from some species of prey. By counting the number of tongue flicks that hit the swab during a 1 minute trial, he measured the relative responsiveness of inexperienced baby snakes to different odours.

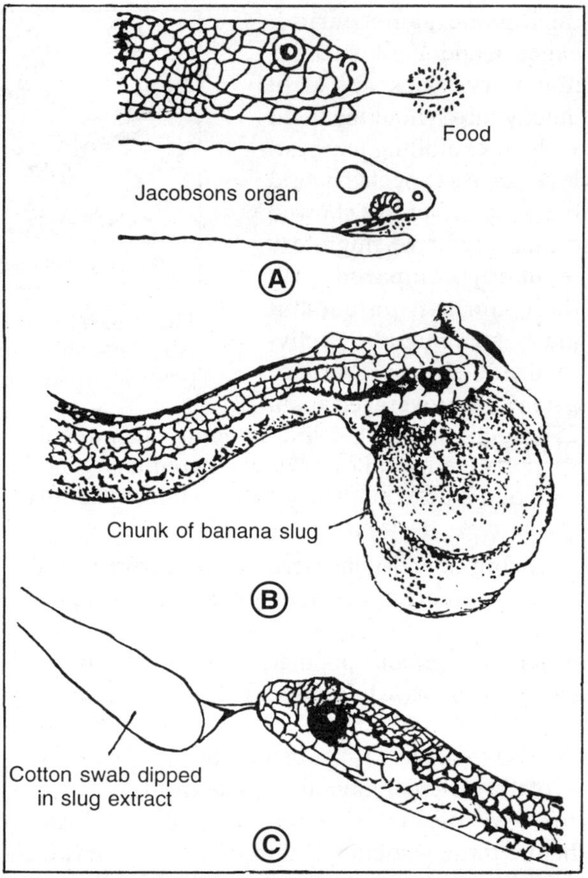

Inland and coastal baby snakes flicked their tongue to swabs dipped in toad tadpole solution (toad tadpole is a prey of both groups) but behaved very differently towards swabs

Fig. 3.7. Genetic Basis for food preference in snakes : (A) Jacobson's organ present in the roof of mouth of snake. (B) Coastal Garter Snake : Consuming a chunk of banana slug, a favoured food of these snakes. (C) A tongue flicking baby garter snake : Senses odour from a cotton swab that has been dipped in slug extract.

dipped with slug scent. Inland snakes ignored the slug odour, whereas coastal snakes responded to it. All the baby snakes experienced the same environment but showed differences in their willingness to eat slugs had to have been caused by genetic differences among them.

Arnold not only identified genetic basis for differences in food preference between coastal and inland garter snakes but also tried to analyze evolutionary basis for these differences. He assumed that among the original colonizers of the coastal habitat were a very few individuals that carried the then rare allel (s) for slug acceptance. These slug eater were able to take advantage of an abundant food resources in their new habitat. If, as a result, their reproductive success was little higher than that of their slug - rejecting fellows, the coastal population could have attained its present state of divergence from the inland population in less than 10 millennium.

It is clear that slug - accepting alleles enjoyed an advantage and spread rapidly in coastal populations. But why they have been nearly eliminated from inland populations? Arnold found that slug - eating snakes also consume aquatic leeches. These leeches are absent in coastal area but are abundant in inland lakes. He assumed that slug eater snakes die because leeches damage the alimentary canal of snakes. Therefore, snakes with leech - eating alleles reproduce less in inland area, eliminating from this population the alleles that also lead to the development of the ability to detect and attack slugs.

Thus, the geographic differences in the feeding behaviour of the snakes can be explained in terms of their proximate genetic basis (different alleles predominate in the two population). Their proximate physiological basis (the Jacobson's organ that detect certain molecules associated with both slug and leeches are more prevalent in coastal populations), and their ultimate ecological and evolutionary basis (inland snakes must contend with potentially dangerous leeches whereas coastal snakes are exposed only to edible slug). Arnold's finding of snake behaviour genetics provides a model of how to integrate proximate and ultimate levels of analysis in behavioural sciences.

BEHAVIOURAL DIFFERENCES CAUSED BY A SINGLE GENE DIFFERENCE

Hybridization studies like those done with funnel web spider, honeybee (*Apis mellifera*), crickets, some species of birds etc. have proved that behavioural differences between individuals living in different populations are caused by genetic differences between them. But what about behavioural variation within a single population due to single gene difference?

THE FRUITFLY (*DROSOPHILA*)

Ethogeneticists have used *Drosophila* for the study of genetic differences and behavioural difference within a single population.

Bastock (1956) studied the influence of single gene upon behaviour of fruitfly, *Drosophila melanogaster.* She crossed a sex-linked recessive yellow mutant with wild stock for several generations and observed that males with the yellow mutation were less successful in mating with wild females. The yellow mutated males had an altered courtship behaviour that failed to attract females reducing their mating success.

Some larvae of *Drosophila melanogaster* called *rovers* are highly active while feeding on yeast cells. Others called *sitters* are not active while feeding. Marie *et al.* crossed adults of these two strains and obtained first generation. Individuals of first generation were *rovers during the larval phase*. When these larvae matured, they were inbred, producing F_2 generation with a ratio of rovers to sitters of 3 : 1. The results suggest that rovers carry one or two copies of the dominant form of a gene affecting larval foraging behaviour, whereas sitters have two copies of the recessive form of this gene. This is a case in which the difference between the two behavioural types stems from a difference in the information contained in a single gene, located on the IInd chromosome.

Some mutant alleles have been named to reflect their behavioural consequences, among them *bang-sensitive* (a sudden jolt causes the mutant fly to become paralyzed), *stuck* (males with the mutant gene fail to dismount after the normal 20 minutes of copulation), *Coitus-interruptus* (males with this allele disengage after just 10, not 20 minutes of copulating).

Wild fruit flies bearing period gene (per^+) exhibit circadian rhythm characteristic of wild-type flies. Other mutant alleles affect the circadian rhythm of fruit flies. Flies with the allele per^0 are arrhythmic. Flies with the per^s allele have a cycle of 19 hours, while flies with per^L exhibit a cycle of 29 hours.

Molecular geneticists have shown that each of the mutant alleles differs from the wild type period gene (per^+) by just one pair of nucleotides in a chain of DNA composed of more than 3500 such pairs. For the per^0 allele of the gene, the single alteration in the DNA molecule results in the production of a

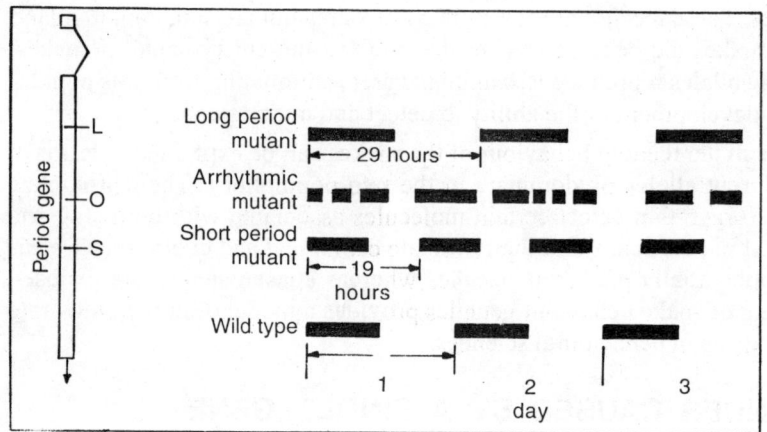

Fig. 3.8. Single Gene Effects in Fruit flies : Many alleles of the period gene of *Drosophila*. On the left is shown the strand of DNA that constitutes the period gene. Each mutant allele has a characteristic effect on the activity pattern of fruit flies, shown on the right (dark bars represent time when the flies are active). The normal pattern of wild - type flies appears at the bottom of the diagram.

protein chain that contains about 400 amino acids, instead of the 1200 appearing in the wild-type protein. This mutation causes the cellular activities to stop "*reading*" the gene's information prematurely.

The information hidden in the per^S and per^L alleles is used by the cells of *Drosophila* to make a protein chain with the full 1200 amino acids. However, the mutant chains differ from the wild - type protein by a single amino acid. Even this small mutation causes behavioural differences in the circadian rhythmic pattern of the *Drosophila*.

per^+ form of the gene is responsible for the development of normal circadian rhythm and per^0 form is responsible for the arrhythmic cycle. Gene engineers were able to insert per^+ allele in arrhythmic individuals that had per^0 allele. As a result of this gene engineering, arrhythmic flies restored the normal circadian rhythm i.e. 24 hours cycle.

ALCOHOLISM IN MICE DUE TO SINGLE GENE ACTION

Behavioural geneticists of USA have found a gene said to be responsible for the alcoholism in mice. They demonstrated in knock out mice that the loss of the individual gene is enough to turn healthy

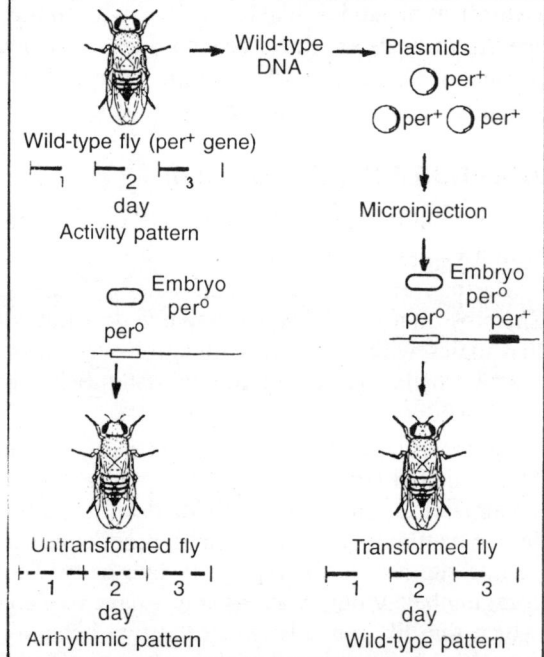

Fig. 3.9. Genetic Engineering : Wild type DNA from *Drosophila* can be taken up into a tiny virus like entity called PLASMID, some of which will then carry the per^+ allele. The plasmids can then be collected and microinjected into the embryos of fruit flies with the per^0 allele. These individuals would have developed into arrhythmic adults, but by receiving the wild - type (per^+) allele via the plasmids they become genetically transformed; transformed flies regain the circadian rhythm characteristic of wild-type flies.

rodents into heavy drinkers. The gene is said to affect the neurotransmitter serotonin, a protein that sits on the surface of neurons and controls serotonin release. Humans having low levels of serotonin are generally alcoholic and prone to violent behaviour.

GENES AND HUMAN BEHAVIOUR

Molecular Biologist, Dean Hamer tried to explain how genes govern our individuality. He studied specific strips of DNA that appear to influence our behaviour, from mood (drive) to sexual behaviour. In 1986, Hamer seconded on Israeli Group's finding that linked a gene on chromosome 11 to personality trait. Some year later this team pinpointed another gene on chromosome 17 that appears to play a role in controlling anxiety.

Unlike the genes that are responsible for different traits, Hamer opines that biology of personality is much more complicated than anticipated. According to him the genes appear subtly bias the psyche so that different individuals react to similar experiences in surprisingly different ways. Identifying the genes that influence personality is a daunting task. Most of these vary from individual to individual by way of only one base out of four - Adenine, Thymine, Guanine and Cytosine. It is precisely these minute differences that ethogeneticists are trying to identity.

BEHAVIOUR OF IDENTICAL TWINS

Hamer's conclusion about the role of genes in composing behaviour of human beings were based solely on the studies of twins. Studies of human twins have confirmed that certain behavioural differences among people are indeed caused by genetic differences. Dizygotic twins are different in genetic make up because they have developed from two different fertilized eggs. But monozygotic twins are identical in their genetic make up because they have developed from the very same fertilized egg which divides and give rise to two genetically identical embryos.

A comprehensive study of identical twins reared apart demonstrates that genetic differences are responsible for a significant part of the differences among humans in personality, temperament, and social behaviour. For example, when identical twins filled out elaborate questionnaires designed to provide quantitative measures of personality traits (e.g., degree of co-operativeness, sociability, and so on), the scores of monozygotic twins brought up apart were nearly as similar as those of monozygotic twins who were reared together.

Ethogeneticists of last few decades of twentieth century and first decade of 21st century have studied that chromosomal abnormalities in human beings cause behavioural disorders such as low intelligence, sterility, schizophrenia, maniac- depression, alcoholism etc.

Change in the genes that lead to genetic diseases and mentally defective individuals are : Gene incompatibility, Gene alteration, over or under doze of genes and chromosomal aberration.

AUTOSOMAL AND SEX-LINKED DISEASES

Autosomal recessive disease occurs in sibling brothers and sisters because it is related with the autosomes so both males and females are equally affected. Many diseases such as Cat cry Syndrome, Down Syndrome (Mongolism or Mongolian idiot), Edward's Syndrome and Patau Syndrome are due to autosomal chromosome alteration. Some Syndrome such as Klinefelter's Syndrome, Turner's Syndrome and Criminal Syndrome are evident due to chromosomal aberration in sex-chromosome.

SCHIZOPHRENIA, MANIAC-DEPRESSION AND ALCOHOLISM IN HUMANS

We often find schizophrenic people in our society. It is a mental illness in which a person is unable to link her or his thoughts and feelings to real life. He suffers from delusions and withdraws increasingly from social relationship into a life of the imagination. Persons suffering with schizophrenia have an excess of dopamine, a *Neurotransmitter* that relays messages in certain parts of the brain. One study found that some schizophrenic people have unusually low levels of an enzyme that breaks down dopamine molecules. The shortage of the enzyme should result in a buildup of dopamine molecules, which could them disrupt normal signal processing in the brain, resulting in the behavioural symptoms of schizophrenia. Various drugs used to control schizophrenic symptoms bind with receptor molecules on nerve cells that normally bind with dopamine. By blocking these receptors, antipsychotic drugs apparently prevent dopamine from reaching the receptors, which behave abnormally when subjected to excessive amounts of this neurotransmitter. Like schizophrenia another common mental disorder is maniac-depression. Alcoholism is also supposed to be the genetically determined behaviour.

The children of a schizophrenic, maniac-depressive, or alcoholic parent have half that parent's genotype and are at much greater risk of developing the condition than are children of parents who do not have these diseases.

An alternative to the hereditary explanation for these conditions is that living with a person suffering from schizophrenia or maniac-depressive or alcoholism creates an environment that induces the trait in others. Once again, ethogeneticists can test and reject this possibility by examining the life histories of children reared in foster homes away from their genetic parents. Adopted children with a schizophrenic/ alcoholic genetic parent show a four or five times greater incidence of the illness than adopted individuals whose parents were not schizophrenic.

Whether schizophrenia is a single disease or a group of diseases is a subject of debate. It is clear that schizophrenia is inherited, but how it is not clear. A possible cause of the disease is the presence of single dominant mutant allele. A possible biochemical basis for this disease has been indicated by the finding that the blood platelets of schizophrenic have a *lower monoamine oxidase activity* than normal people.

Maniac-depression is a common mental disorder. This appears to be caused by a dominant gene on the human X chromosome. This mutant allele exhibits incomplete action. A drug *lithium salt* can cure or control this genetic disorder.

Ethogeneticists of 21st millennium disagree to the statement that schizophrenia, manic - depression and alcoholism are purely hereditary diseases. These are neither "Genetically determined" nor "Environmentally determined". Although a child of a schizophrenic or maniac depressive or alcoholic parent may have inherited certain key alleles from the affected parent, he or she may not be affected because development of the condition depends on the environment as well as heredity. Most carriers are behaviourally normal; but they have great chance of developing the disease, because of greater susceptibility to environmental factors that triggers the syndrome.

THE GENE FOR PLEASURE

According to a team from the university of Texas, "*a pleasure gene*" encoding the receptors on brain cells for the neurotransmitter dopamine, is crucial to the nicotine - ingesting habit, as well as other deleterious substance abuse, including that involving alcohol, cocaine, opiates etc. According to the study, a person's sensorial experience depends on the form of the particular gene that he or she inherits.

Dopamine is an important chemical messenger between brain cells for life - serving functions. However, when a person ingests pleasure - inducers, such as nicotine or alcohol, additional dopamine is released, enhancing the feeling of well - being.

A gene encoding these protein molecules has two components - *A* and *B*, always occurring in pairs and persons with A_1 or B_1 have fewer dopamine receptors. Studies tells that about 10% of the entire population inherits a gene pairing that includes either A_1 or B_1, raising a challenge to psychiatrists as well as ethologists. Are all these individuals so genetically affected that they have a problem quitting smoking? Can it help them to learn early on their inheritance? Is some sort of genetic therapy conceivable? These questions need further research for answer.

NEUROETHOLOGY

• Introduction • Different kinds of nervous system in animal world • Moths evading bats • Human Brain and Behaviour - Planum temporale - Basal ganglia - Pons and medulla oblongata • Psychiatric disorders of humans and nervous system • Homosexuality in human males • Size of selected brain cells and territorial behaviour of cichlid fish • Stimulus filtering and behaviour • Sound perception in bats • Central pattern generators.

INTRODUCTION

The simplest form of reactive behaviour is the reflex. Initially it was considered that many behavioural patterns are brought about by long and complex chain of reflexes. Erich von Holst (1932) and Lorenz (1935) independently stated that behaviour is not just a reaction to external stimuli but is also based on internal physiological conditions and spontaneous reactions controlled by nervous, hormonal and muscular systems. On the basis of this finding innate and acquired behavioural patterns could be separated. Apparently behaviour is a result of *co-ordinated muscle activity* and it is very well known to us that muscles do not contract unless stimulated by nerves. Behaviour may be viewed as the "symphony of muscle contraction, guided by messages from the central nervous and hormonal systems". Animal senses its external world through sense organs, which in turn send nerve impulses to brain, where it is interpreted and message is sent to respective muscles to act accordingly. Sense organs form an integral part of animal's behaviour, because these organs receive external stimuli from environment and keep adjusting to changes accordingly. The brain plays the most important role in inducing a behaviour. Thus behaviour and physiology are inseparable, interdependent and interacting with each other.

In the light of above discussion Animal behaviour may be defined as *"Behaviour is the product of an integrated series of changes in cell chemistry, initiated by receptor cells and carried on by sensory interneurons and motor cells and muscles"*. Here, one thing is remarkable that nervous system not only respond to stimuli but also possesses a remarkable ability to preserve the effect of previous stimuli for a shorter or longer period.

Neuroethologists aim at giving an explanation of the behaviour in term of the functioning of the nerve cells. It is true that ultimately one can be able to explain behaviour in terms of the functioning of the basic unit of the nervous system, the nerve cells (neurones). But neuroethologists should not forget that study of any behaviour, in terms of the action of the individual nerve cell would be equivalent for trying to read a page of a book with a high - powered microscope. Therefore, while studying behaviour of a species we should take into account the entire nervous system of the concerned species.

DIFFERENT KINDS OF NERVOUS SYSTEM IN ANIMAL WORLD

Let us have some basic knowledge of nervous system of animals which will enable us to understand the intricate relationship of nervous system and different behaviour of animal world.

There are two types of nervous system in animals, *Protosome* and *Deuterosome*. *Protosome* type of nervous system is found in Non-chordates. This is represented by paired ventral solid nerve cord having swellings (ganglia) at certain intervals. Big ganglions in anterior region is called brain. *Deuterosome* type of nervous system is found in Vertebrates. This type of nervous system have a dorsal, hollow tubular spinal cord. The anterior swollen end of spinal cord is differentiated into large convoluted brain. The brain is composed entirely of groups of cell bodies, nerve tracts and blood vessels. The nerve fibre tracts form the *white matter* of the brain. Bundles of neurones called nuclei or centres composed of group of cell bodies and synapses collectively form the *grey matter* of the brain.

Reflex action is the basic form of response to stimulation and all animals bearing nervous system show this response. Ethologists have found conditioned reflex action right from coelenterates to mammals. Lower animals with protosome type of nervous system (coelenterates to annelids) exhibit only primitive behaviours like taxis and kinesis. Higher animals with protosome type of nervous system (arthropods to hemichordates) exhibit some classical behaviours. Let us study one of the classical behaviours in which moths evade bats and save themselves from this predator.

MOTHS EVADING BATS

Let us study the causal relationship between nerve cells and behaviour with respect to how certain nocturnal moths avoid their predator, insectivorous bats. This case tells that, how activity in a particular nerve influences an animal's behaviour.

Bats hunt moths in its tail membrane and fly off with its catch. Some flying moths turn abruptly even before a bat come rushing into view. Moths drive out of the grasp of an approaching bat. They have the ability to detect a bat at a distance and can make themselves difficult to capture.

How do they do this? One possibility is that moths hear the vocalizations that bats produce as they dash through the ear of moth. Some moths can detect the pulses of ultrasound (some frequencies higher than 20 kHz, which we cannot hear) produced by their nocturnal predators. This detection mechanism consists of a pair of ears, one on each side of the thorax of moth (Fig. 3.10).

A moth ear has an outer tympanic membrane. This membrane remains attached to two nerve cells, the A_1 and A_2 fibers, that act as sensory receptors. When pressure waves strike the moth, they may cause the tympanum to vibrate. These vibrations reaches the receptor cells and induce them to respond.

A neurone, responds to stimulation with a change in the permeability of its cell membrane to sodium ions. In the moth ear, positively charged sodium ions enter the receptor cells at a point near the tympanum, altering the electrical charge differential or membrane potential of the receptor cell membrane. This change affects the permeability of neighboring portion of the membrane, so that sodium ions enter at those sites and repeat the effect, causing changes in membrane potential to sweep around the cell body (Fig. 3.11). Depending upon the intensity of the activating stimulus, the change in membrane potential may be great enough to induce a brief, stereotyped, all-or-nothing reverse in the electrical charge cross the nerve membrane. These changes, called *action potentials*, are the means by which neural messages are transmitted. An action potential travels the length of the neurone to the synapse with the next neurone in the network.

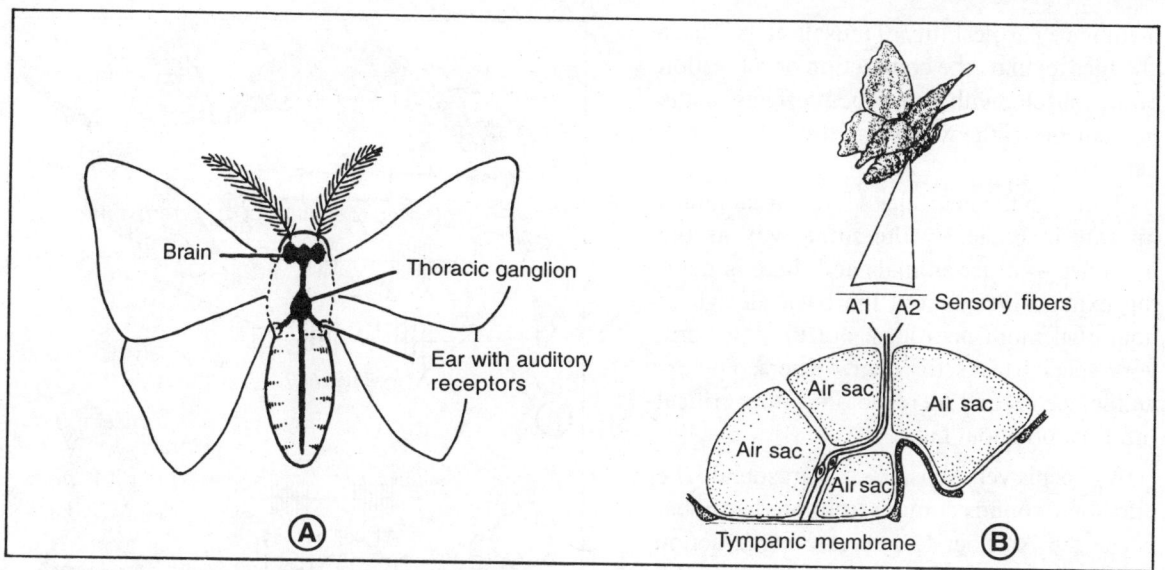

Fig. 3.10. Nocturnal Moth Ears : (A) The location of the ear. (B) The ear's design, which features two sensory fibers (A_1 , A_2) connected to a tympanic membrane

Neurones communicate with one another in a number of ways. A common method is for the arrival of an action potential at a synapse to cause the release of a neurotransmitter chemical by one cell that diffuses across the gap separating it from the neighboring cells. These neurotransmitter substances may affect the membrane permeability of the postsynaptic cells in ways that increase or decrease the probability that they will produce their own action potentials.

The neurones that relay receptor information to the brain are called *sensory inter-neurones*. These messages can change the activity of other cells in the central nervous system, which in the nocturnal moth consists of aggregates of neurones in the thoracic ganglia and other ganglia in the head. These cells not only receive information but also analyze sensory inputs and make decisions about which reactions to order.

Certain patterns of activity in the thoracic ganglia affect *motor interneurones*, whose action potentials in turn reach nerve cells that are connected with the wing muscles of the moth. When a motor neurone fires, the *neurotransmitter* it releases at the synapse with a muscle fiber induces changes in the

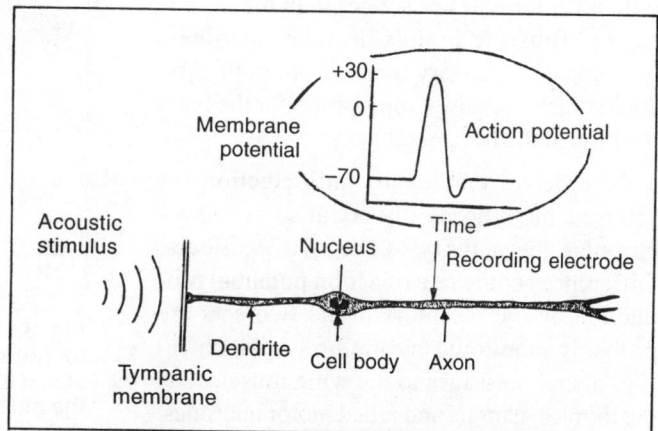

Fig. 3.11. Structure of a nerve cell : The electrical activity of this acoustical receptor depends first on the effect of acoustical stimuli on the dendrite. Changes in the electrical charge differential of the dendrite's membrane can trigger an action potential that begins near the cell body and travels along the axon of the receptor toward the next cell in the network.

membrane permeability of muscle cells. These changes regulate the contraction or relaxation of the muscle, with consequent effects on the movements of the wings and thus, the moth's behaviour.

Although the neurones of nocturnal moths operate in basically the same way as the neurones of other animals and there is nothing extraordinary about the basic design of nocturnal moth neurones, but they perform very special tasks for their owners. For example, the A_1 and A_2 receptors gather critical information about bats.

A_1 fiber is very sensitive to ultrasound. The ultrasonic sounds coming from predatory bat cause the A_1 fiber to generate some action potentials when the predator bat is 25 meter away, long before the bat can detect the moth. In addition, the moth's ears gather information that could be used to locate the bat in space (Fig. 3.12). For example, if a hunting bat is on the right, the A_1 receptor in the right ear will be stimulated sooner than the A_1 receptor in the left ear, which is shielded from the sound by the moth's body. As a result, the right receptor will fire sooner than the left receptor. Thus the brain's decoder neurones, by comparing sensory inputs from both ears, could order responses appropriate for the bat's position in the horizontal plane.

In order to employ its antidetection response a moth need only orient so as to synchronize the activity of the two A_1 fibers. Differences in the rate of action potential production by the receptors in the two ears are probably monitored by the brain, which relays neural messages to the wing muscles via the thoracic ganglia and allied motor neurones. The resulting changes in muscular action steer the moth away from the side of its body with the ear that is more strongly stimulated. As the moth turns, it will reach a point where

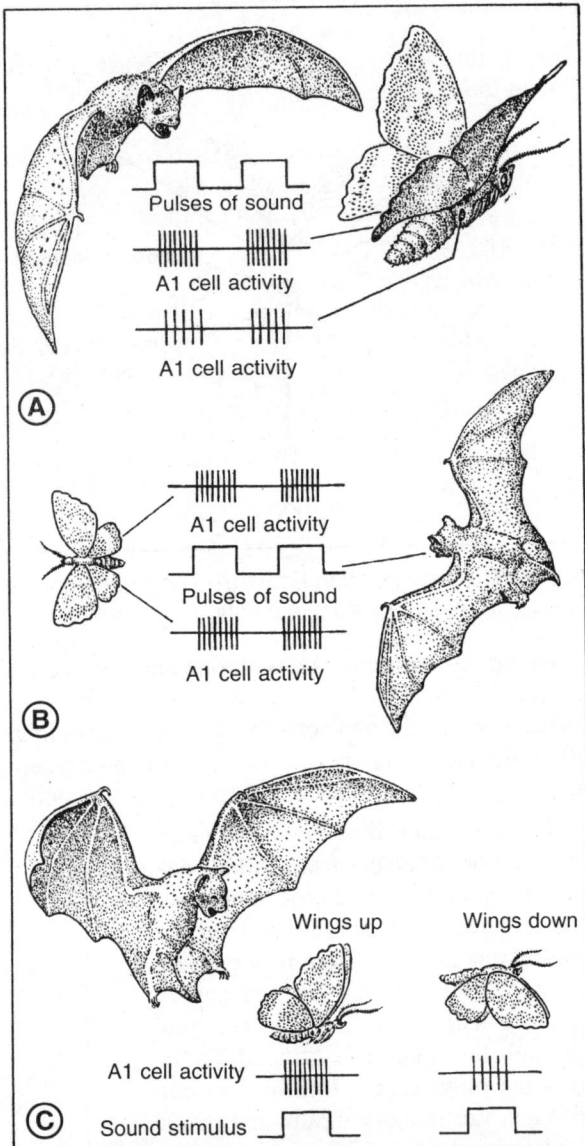

Fig. 3.12. How moths locate bats in space : (A) A bat is to one side of the moth; the A_1 receptor on the side closer to the predator fires sooner and more often than the shielded A_1 receptor in the other ear. (B) A bat is directly behind the moth; both A_1 fibers fire at the same rate and time. (C) A bat is above the moth; activity in the A_1 receptors fluctuates in synchrony with the wingbeats of the moth.

both A_1 cells are equally active. At this time moth will be facing away from the bat and flying away from predator bat.

HUMAN BRAIN AND BEHAVIOUR

Brain is the controlling center of almost all behaviours. The brain of vertebrates has evolved as adaptation to the ecological niche just as having other organs. Animals that have specialized sensory systems and forms of behaviour, must have correspondingly specialized brain mechanisms. The adult vertebrate brain has five regions, and they assume a particular significance within each class, associated with the mode of life and level of structural and functional complexity attained by the group.

Human brain is most advanced in function and has tremendous ability to learn and remember things. Human brain is capable of remembering more than 50 thousand characters but elephant has sharpest memory in animal world. Let us have some current knowledge of activities of important parts of human brain.

1. FORE-BRAIN (Prosencephalon)

It is anteriormost part of brain and concerned with advanced behaviours like *reasoning, planning, emotion* etc. It consists of three major parts.

 (i) **Olfactory lobe :** It is simple in humans but well developed in fishes. Olfactory lobe of scoliodon is well developed and have great power of smell and hence they are commonly called dogfish.

 (ii) **Cerebrum :** It is the most important part of brain from function point of view. *Thought* and *feeling* originates from cerebrum. Received information is analyzed and accommodated here. Outer layer of cerebrum is densely packed with nerve cells, forming a region of *grey matter* called the cerebral cortex.

Cerebrum is composed of two cerebral hemispheres, left and right cerebral hemispheres. These two parts remain linked together by nerve fibre tracts called the *corpus callosum*. There are four different regions of cerebral hemisphere and each part controls different behavioural activities:

 (a) **Frontal lobe :** Frontal lobe is supposed to be the centre of *intelligence* because all intelligent animals such as dolphin, chimpanzee, gorilla, bonobo, elephants, including man bear large frontal lobe. Its basic function is concerned with *memory, emotion, wish, judgement, intelligence* and *personality*.

Pre-motor area of frontal lobe controls movement of muscles of learnt skills, such as playing with musical instruments, dancing, driving a car or scooter, flying an aeroplane. Just opposite to it, primary motor cortex controls muscles of general movements. Another part *prefrontal cortex* is responsible for *reasoning, planning, emotion* and *personality* of the individuals. One part of motor cortex is concerned with *memory* and *speech*. The part concerned with speech is called Broca's area which remains present in left frontal lobe. Some part of grey matter of frontal lobe remain suspended. Perhaps this part is the site of *foresight*.

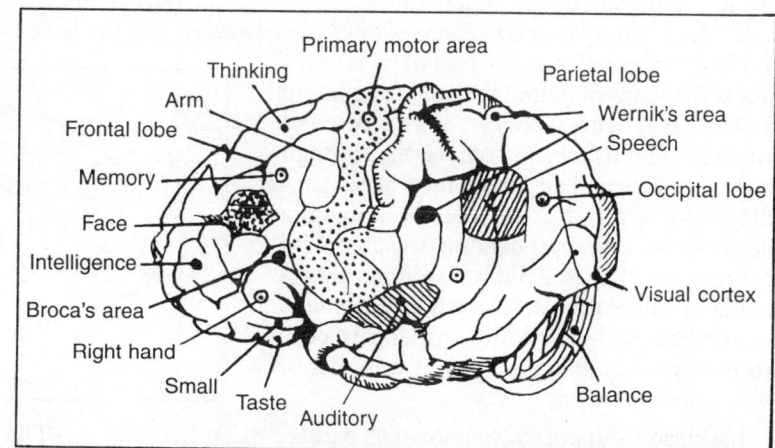

Fig. 3.13. Different areas in Human brain and their different functions.

(b) **Parietal lobe :** It is centre of numerous general sensory functions. For example, feeling of heat, cold, pain, pressure and position of the body. Since this lobe co-ordinates every kind of sensation of body, therefore, this lobe is called *somesthetic area.*

(c) **Occipital lobe :** This is posterior part of cerebrum and is related with *vision.* Sensation received from eye reaches to this part of the brain and perception of the object - shape, size, colour, ugly or beautiful etc. is analysed here.

(d) **Temporal lobe :** This part is concerned with *hearing, olfaction* and *gustation.* Karl Wernic discovered the area of speech and language in the temporal lobe and hence this centre is called *Wernic area.* Wernic area is like a dictionary where learnt words are preserved and are used on the basis of memory in an hour of need. Damage or error in language center (Broca and Wernic area) cause error in language. For example, *Aphasia* – unable to speak; *agraphia* – unable to write; *word deafness* – unable to understand spoken words; *word blindness* – unable to read and understand written text.

Our brain's visual mechanisms may also be specialized to assist us in the recognition of human faces. There is still controversy about whether the temporal lobe of humans contains a face detecting "centre". To detect whether such a mechanism might be present in other animals, David Perrett and Edmund Rolls conducted experiments with a primate, rhesus monkey. They used microelectrodes to record the activity of single neurone in the region of the monkey's temporal lobe that corresponds to the area implicated in face recognition in humans. They discovered that cells in question have something to do with the perception of faces, a task highly pertinent to the lives of these social primates. 21st century ethologists are sure that primates, dolphins and elephants recognize every member of their society individually.

Planum Temporale

Chimpanzees have a structure in their brain that is similar to a so called language centre in human brains.

In most people, the structure, a slender 2.5 cm. long piece of tissue called the Planum Temporale, is larger in the left side of the temporal lobe than the right side. This area is involved in the processing and comprehension of speech sounds and sign language. Until now, no other animal was shown to have the same asymmetry in this brain region, located at the side of the head and connected to the ears.

Basal Ganglia

Inside each cerebral hemisphere there are aggregation of special nerve fibres (nuclei) that is collectively called *basal ganglia* or *basal nuclei* or *cerebral nuclei.* It is made up of head and tail of caudate nucleus and lentiform nucleus. One part of basal ganglia is made up of neural part of amygdaloid nucleus. It remains connected with cerebral cortex, thalamus and hypothalamus through numerous fibres. The function of basal ganglia are varied. Damage to one basal ganglia produces the tremor of hands associated with Parkinson's disease. Sub-conscious movements of skeletal muscles such as automatic movements of limbs while walking is controlled by basal ganglia. Loss of this part of brain cause paralysis.

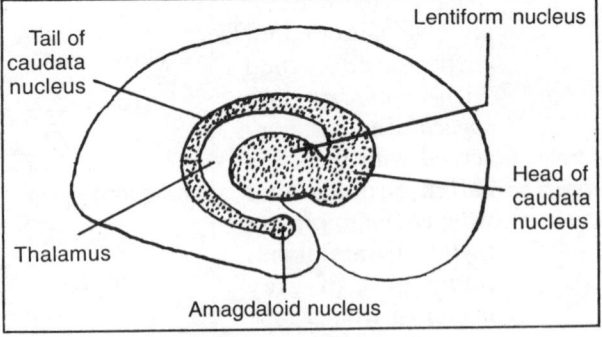

Fig. 3.14. Basal ganglia.

Parkinson's disease also known as paralysis agitants is a progressive neurological disorder that weaken motor skills of sufferers and can ultimately be fatal. It occurs due to destruction of *Substantia nigra* leading to less amount of dopamine secretion. Patients of Parkinson's disease develop muscle rigidity, involuntary tremor and inability to initiate movement called akinesia. Nerve cells of the basal ganglia fire too rapidly resulting in muscle tremors. This continuous firing is caused due to insufficiency of an inhibitory neurotransmitter called dopamine. The treatment, which is meant to replace the chemical dopamin in the brain, was found to have improved the symptoms of Parkinson's by 40 per cent. The worst part of Parkinson's disease is that there is no permanent cure. Now biotechnology shows a ray of hope to patients suffering from this disease. Synder et al. are trying to find a way of stimulating growth of brain cells using gene therapy. They hope to make the brain capable of replacing its dead cells with new ones. US researchers have introduced cells from pig embryos into the brain of patients suffering from Parkinson's disease, with positive result.

Alzheimer's disease is the premature ageing of brain. Recent memory goes first followed by stored memory. This disease occurs due to deficiency in secretion of *acetylcholine, somatostation* and substance from nucleus basalis of brain. Now scientists have shown that adults grow new brain cells even in their 60s and 70s. The new finding is reported in the November (1997) issue of the journal Nature Medicine by Fred Gage of the Salk institute for Biological studies in La jo. The finding raises a hope for treating brain diseases or damage by getting the brain to fix its broken circuitry. The new neurones that form circuits, were found in just small part of the brain, the *hippocampus*, a deep-brain structure that is important for memory and learning. The big question is whether scientists can find ways to make new brain cells appear in the right places to overcome damage from brain injuries and such diseases as Parkinson's and Alzheimer's.

(iii) **Diencephalon :** It is the posterior region of the forebrain. Its dorsal and lateral regions form the *thalamus* and the ventral region form the *hypothalamus*. The *pineal body* arise in dorsal region and *Pituitary* in ventral region.

    (a) *Thalamus :* The majority of sensory neurones carrying impulses to the cortex terminate in the thalamus. Here the origin and nature of the impulses are 'analyzed' and relayed to the appropriate sensory areas of the cortex by neurones originating in the thalamus. It therefore, act as a *processing, integrating* and *relay centre* for all sensory information. It shows similarities to a switchboard in a telephone exchange. Lateral geniculate nucleus is related with vision, ventroposterior nucleus with gustation and general sensation. Rest center is related with somatic motor system such as ventro-lateral nucleus is related with *involuntary motor activities* and ventro-anterior nucleus is concerned with arousal. Thalamus is not only centre of sensation of pain, heat, touch, pressure but it also analyses degree of these sensations. Lateral part of the thalamus is also concerned with *emotions* and *memory*.

    (b) *Hypothalamus :* This is the main co-ordinating and control centre for the autonomic nervous system. Specific regions of the hypothalamus contain specific centres for the initiation of feeding, drinking and sleeping, aggression and sex.

2. MID-BRAIN (Mesencephalon)

It consists of *optic lobes* and *crura cerebri*. All nerve fibre tracts pass through this region which is part of the brain stem. The superior part of *corpora quadrigemina* receive sensory neurones from the eye and muscles of the head and control *visual reflexes*. They control the movement of the head and eyes to fix and focus on an object. The interior part of corpora quadrigemina receive sensory neurones from the ears and muscles of the head and control *auditory reflexes* such as the movement of the head to locate and detect the source and direction of the sound. The floor of mesencephalon bear many nuclei. These nuclei control specific sub-conscious stereotyped muscular movements such as bending forwards and backwards and rotation of the head and trunk. Stimulation of these nuclei, the red nucleus, causes the head and upper trunk to extend backward.

3. HIND-BRAIN (Rhombencephalon)

It consists of *cerebellum* and *medulla oblongata*. The dorsal region of hind brain forms the *cerebellum* and ventral region forms the *pons*. Functionally, the *cerebellum* is concerned with co-ordination of the *actions of muscles* or *motor activities*.

Cerebellum has grey matter on its outer side which contains flask-shaped *Purkyne cells* bearing many dendrites. These cells receive impulses concerning muscular movement from a number of different sources, including sensory receptors in the balance organs (the vestibular apparatus of the ear concerned with balance), proprioreceptors in joints, tendons and muscles and motor centres of the cortex. The cerebellum is thought to integrate obtained information and produce co-ordinated muscular activity in all the muscles involved in a given movement including the reflex control of body posture. The cerebellum is vital to control rapid muscular activities such as swimming, typing and even talking. All the activities of the cerebellum are involuntary but may involve learning in their early stages. During early training periods the cortex directs the control of cerebellum when utmost concentration is required, such as when learning to walk, swimming or riding a bicycle. Once the learning is acquired, reflex control by the cerebellum takes place long life.

Pons and medulla oblongata

Pons contains several 'nuclei' relaying impulses to the cerebellum. Medulla contains important reflex centres for the regulation of autonomic activities such as heart beat rate, blood pressure, ventilation rate, swallowing, salivation, sneezing, vomiting, coughing etc.

PSYCHIATRIC DISORDERS OF HUMANS AND NERVOUS SYSTEM

Psychiatric disorders such as anxiety and depression are believed to be due to unbalanced chemical transmission at synapses. Drugs are used in the alleviation of psychiatric disorders. Many tranquillizers and sedatives, such as the *tricyclic* and *depressant imipramine* and *reserpine* and *monomine oxidase* inhibitors, exert their effects by interacting with transmitter substances or their receptor sites. For example, monomine oxidase inhibitors prevent the activity of an enzyme involved in the breakdown of adrenaline and noradrenaline and, presumably, are effective in treating depression by prolonging the effects of these transmitter substances. Hallucinogenic drugs, such as *lysergic acid diethylamine* (LSD) and *mescaline*, produce their effects by either mimicking the actions of naturally occurring brain transmitter substances or having antagonistic effect on other transmitter substances.

Research into the activity of the pain-suppressing opiate drug, *heroin* and *morphine* in the mammalian brain have revealed the presence of naturally occurring (endogenous) substances having similar effects. These substances which react with the opiate receptors are collectively called endorphins. They reduce pain, influence emotion and are involved with certain types of mental illness. This research has opened up new ideas on brain functioning and offers a biochemical basis for the control of pain and healing by diverse activities as hypnosis, acupressure, acupuncture and faith - healing.

HOMOSEXUALITY IN HUMAN MALES

There is a special neuronal basis for homosexuality in human males. Some human males show little or no sexual interest in females but instead have a preference for their fellow males. Neuroethologist Simon Le Vay discovered that the brains of homosexual men possess distinctive structural and functional attributes different from those of heterosexual men. Le Vay could exhibit the differences in the size of certain nuclei (aggregates of nerve cells) in the anterior hypothalami of homosexual and heterosexual males. It is known that anterior hypothalamus plays a key role in regulating sexual activity in humans and other vertebrates. There is large differences between human males and females in the size of certain nuclei in the anterior

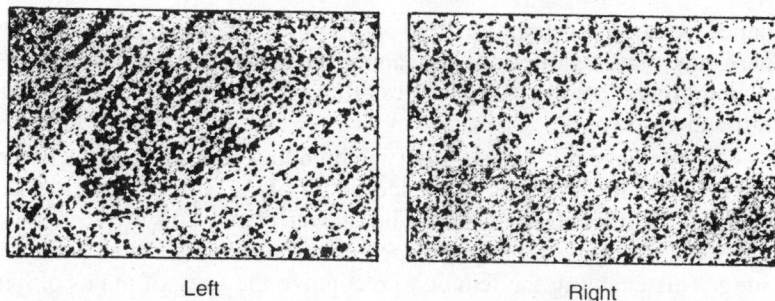

Left   Right

Fig. 3.15. The INAH-3 Regions in Human Brain : On the left, a section through the INAH-3 from the brain of a heterosexual male showing bigger, dense oval collection of cells. In the corresponding area from the brain of a homosexual male, shown on the right the oval structure is absent and INAH-3 was much smaller.

hypothalamus, indicating that these cells act on an important mechanism underlying sexual behaviour.

Le Vay acquired the brains of a number of homosexual men who had died of AIDS. Microscopic examination of anterior hypothalami of these men and measurement of the size of nuclei revealed the fact that a nucleus called INAH-3 was much smaller in the homosexual men (Fig. 3.15). This study provides support for the hypothesis that specific clusters of cells in the human brain have great effect on the sexual behaviour of adults. Still ethologists have to ascertain whether social interactions among homosexual humans cause change in specific neurones within the hypothalamus, or a given set of cells in the INAH-3 cause homosexuality.

SIZE OF SELECTED BRAIN CELLS AND TERRITORIAL BEHAVIOUR OF CICHLID FISH

The behavioural interactions have an effect on the size of selected brain cells has been demonstrated in studies of a cichlid fish. When a male of this species succeeds in acquiring a territory by aggressively dominating other males, specific cells in the preoptic area of his brain become enlarged. If the male lose his territorial status, these particular neurones of preoptic area become smaller.

STIMULUS FILTERING AND BEHAVIOUR

In natural environments, animals face a great variety of stimuli. Most of the informations are meaningless for the animals from survival and reproduction point of view. Therefore, animal nervous systems respond selectively, extracting relevant stimuli and ignoring most of the useless other stimuli. This process is called stimulus filtering.

The nocturnal moth's auditory system provides an example of the operation and utility of stimulus filtering. The moth's ear does not relay information about low-frequency sounds audible to us. Even when the receptors respond to ultrasound, they do not produce different patterns of signals in relation to sounds of different frequency.

The moth's ear is associated to the detection of cues associated with its nocturnal predators. But its auditory capacity is limited, sensitive to pulsed ultrasonic sound but incapable of reacting to most other sound. Its behavioural repertoire of responses is simple and adaptive. It turns away from low intensity ultrasound and dives, flips, or spirals erratically when it hears high-intensity ultrasound.

Vertebrate neural systems generally are composed of numerous neurones than those of insects, but even so, they have their specializations too. Human ear is incapable of hearing ultrasonic sounds and hence we do not respond to ultrasonic sounds like moth or cricket. Our visual and auditory system also performs stimulus filtering. We cannot see things through ultraviolet rays but honeybees are capable of seeing things through it. Colourless flowers seen by us may be colourful for honeybees as they see it through Uv rays.

Consider an adult female canary in breeding condition as she listens to a host of sounds, among them the songs of her own and other species of birds. Sexually excited females react to canary song with a copulation-solicitation display. They never respond to the songs of males of other species. This suggests that they possess a special perceptual mechanism that is activated in a distinctive way by canary song. This enabling the female to recognize the song of males of her own species only.

Eliot Brenowitz discovered that a neural mechanism plays a role in the perception of song by female canaries. Females do not sing but possess in reduced size the same brain regions that make up the song system in males. The caudal nucleus of the ventral hyperstriatum (HVc) is a song system structure responsible for song production by male canaries, but it also contains cells that fire when a male hears a recording of his own song. Brenowitz made a small lesions in the brains of some females in the HVc area. After the recovery, the females could still hear sounds, but they had lost the ability to distinguish canary song from other species' song, as demonstrated by their readiness to give copulation - solicitation displays to both canary and sparrow song. This tells that a particular part of the female's brain causes the bird to identify and respond appropriately to canary song. This suggests that a special point of brain has stimulus filtering mechanism in female canary.

SOUND PERCEPTION IN BATS

Bat's brain is filled with special feature-detection units. Echo detector neurones have been found in the Mexican free-tailed bat. Echo detector cells respond more intensely to the second of two separate pulses of sound, one following the other in close succession, just as an echo would follow the vocalization pulse.

Echo detector nerve cells are also found in the brains of mustache bats as well. Some neurones called "tracking neurones" remain active only if there is a continuing decrease in the interval between the bat's emitted orientation sound and the echo. Continuing activity in these neurones would inform the bat that it was getting closer and closer to an echo-reflecting source. The bat catches the thing if it is edible or returns back at once. Other cells in the mustache bat's brain are

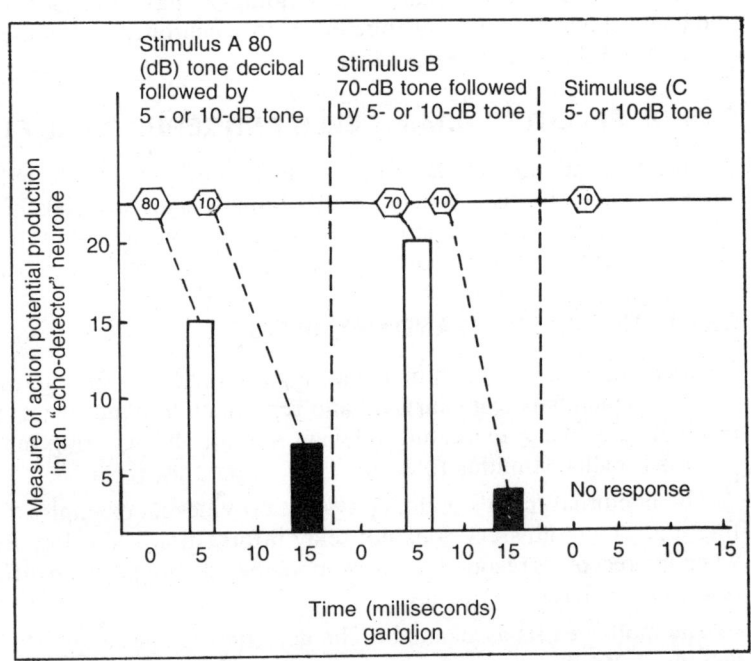

Fig. 3.16. Echo Detector Cells in a Mexican free-tailed bat respond differently to three kinds of stimuli. The cells do not respond to isolated low intensity sounds (stimulus C), but will produce neural impulses when these same tones are preceded by a loud burst of noise (stimuli A and B).

"range tuned". These neurones respond most actively to one constant interval between a vocalization and an echo. For example, one of these cells would fire at its highest rate only when the delay between orientation pulse and returning echo was 3-millisecond; another might be tuned to a 6-millisecond delay; a third might fire most rapidly when the interval was 9-millisecond. These nerve cells are arranged in linear sequence, running from short-delay to long-delay neurones, in the bat's cerebral cortex. In effect sensory inputs are received by neurones on the surface of the central cortex in a manner that corresponds to their location relative to the animal, creating a brain map that decode spacial information contained in the sensory messages. The brain maps of mustache bats help them identify the distance to a flying insect (target range) and the speed with which the prey is moving (target velocity), vital information for catching the prey.

CENTRAL PATTERN GENERATORS

In context of Neuroethology we find a term *Central Pattern Generator* - a functional clusture of cells contained within the central nervous system that can generate the pattern of signals needed to produce particular response. Such system do not require sensory feedback in order to produce their self - generated sequence of signals. For example, if one takes the brain stem and spinal cord from a lamprey (Jawless primitive fish), the living tissue can still play out the rhythmic pattern of signals that would cause swimming motions in an intact lamprey. This experiment exhibit that within the brain stem or spinal cord, a *Central Pattern Generator* exists that controls the swimming behaviour in this species. *Central Pattern Generators* that regulate locomotion are widely distributed through out the animal kingdom and have been especially well studied in certain invertebrates – Grasshopper (*Locusta migratoria*), Tritonia sea slugs, leech etc.

ETHOENDOCRINOLOGY

● Introduction ● Invertebrate endocrine system and behaviour ● Vertebrate endocrine system and behaviour ● Fish - Fanning behaviour of stickleback fish ● Reptiles ● Birds ● Mammals ● Hormones and other factors eliciting specific behaviour in Vertebrates ● Hormone, environment and sexual behaviour ● Hormone, season and migration ● Mechanical stimulation, hormone secretion and milking of cattles ● Gene, environment and hormone in composing aggressive behaviour in mice ● Experience, hormones and behaviour.

INTRODUCTION

Patterns of behaviour controlled by secretion of endocrine glands (hormones) is studied under the title ethoendocrinology or behavioural endocrinology. Sometimes the neurone cells play a dual role of conduction and secretion of neurohormonal substance. These hormones are called *neurohumors*. All nerve cells release a chemical substance, a neurotransmitter (epinephrine) at their terminal synapse but neurosecretory cells are nerve cells that have developed the secretory capacity to a high level.

The direct action of hormones upon the brain is the most important mode of influence upon behaviour. It was first demonstrated by Harris et al. (1948) by implanting minute quantity of oestrogen into certain regions of the brain of female cats. This could induce sexual behaviour in cats even though it was non breeding season and the level of oestrogen in the blood was well below the level normally required for sexual behaviour. When on heat female cats show a very characteristic posture called *lordosis*. The rump is elevated, the tail deflected to one side and the hinder part making treading movements (Fig. 6.34). A female cat will assume this posture as soon as a male cat approaches, and will submit for mounting. An unreceptive female (anoestrus) will lash out viciously if a male gets too close for copulation. A needle tip, coated with oestrogen is placed in certain parts of the hypothalamus or required dozes of oestrogen is injected to a castrated (ovary removed) female cat, she will show strong oestrus behaviour. Same experiment with other vertebrates gives the same result and confirmed the general conclusion that oestrus behaviour is possible by the introduction of oestrogen in castrated females of vertebrate series.

Sexually matured male rat mount on the receptive female rat in a matter of seconds, but a castrated male rat takes much longer time to initiate mounting. Testes secrete male hormone (androgens) which help in initiating sexual behaviour and in absence of testis, male hormone becomes absent, that do not initiate mounting behaviour. Synthetic androgen injection to castrated rat can also develop mounting tendencies to normal level.

INVERTEBRATE ENDOCRINE SYSTEM AND BEHAVIOUR

Lower invertebrates lack organized type of endocrine system and therefore, the role of hormones on behaviour have been studied in higher invertebrates especially in insects.

Two important endocrine glands *Corpora Cardiaca* and *Corpora Allata* are found in grasshoppers and cockroaches. Paired corpora cardiaca lie just behind the brain and paired corpora allata are located alongside the oesophagus. Neurosecretory cells of protocerebrum of brain secrete *prothoracicotrophic* hormone that control these two endocrine glands. Different morphological and regulatory functions such as metamorphosis, moulting, finding hiding place, cocoon formation, feeding activities etc. are coordinated and regulated by hormones produced by above mentioned two glands i.e. corpora cardiaca and corpora allata.

Adult male desert locusts *(Schistocera gregaria)* fail to exhibit sexual behaviour after the corpora allata have been removed. When corpora allata are transplanted into corpora allata

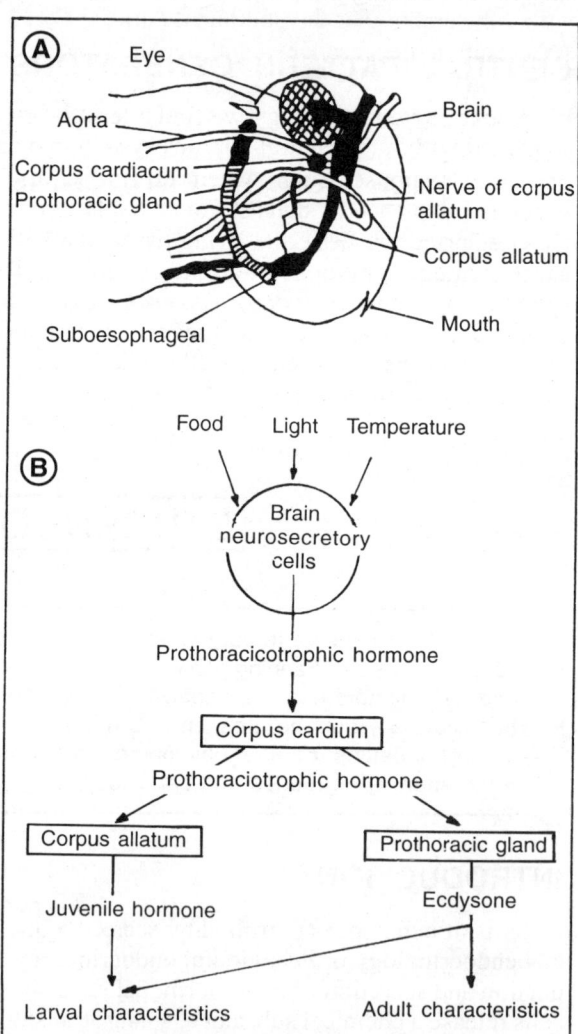

Fig. 3.17. (A) Endocrine system of grasshopper: Neuro-secretory cells and glands of the head region in grasshopper. (B) The hormonal control of ecdysis and moulting in insects.

removed males, sexual behaviour is regained. Some species of locusts are *solitary* while others are *gregarious*. This difference has a hormonal basis. Solitary hoppers have larger prothoracic glands than gregarious species. If prothoracic glands from solitary adults are transplanted into gregarious adults, the gregarious locust become solitary. Reverse is the case when prothoracic glands from gregarious adults are transplanted into solitary locusts then gregarious locusts become solitary i.e. sustained flight activity is diminished.

Role of hormones in invertebrates other than insects have revealed common pattern. Ethoendocrinologists have demonstrated in crustacean and mollusk, the presence of neurosecretory cells whose secretions affect sexual differentiation and reproductive behaviour. Parasitic barnacle, *Sacculina* parasitizes the crab under the abdomen. Parasite *Sacculina* destroys the androgenic gland of the male crab. As a result, in the absence of androgenic gland sex reversal in host crab takes place and ultimately in sex behaviour.

VERTEBRATE ENDOCRINE SYSTEM AND BEHAVIOUR

With some minor variations, all groups of Vertebrate series have similar hormones. However, the same hormone may have quite different functions in animals of different vertebrate classes. For example, the hormone that causes the mammary gland of mammals to secrete milk, causes hens to incubate their eggs. The widespread occurrence of hormonal control of reproduction, particularly in Vertebrates, has led most ethoendocrinologists to accept the view that hormones are the ultimate arbiters of sexual behaviour as they communicate between the animal's various internal organs of reproduction. Key hormones provide the casual basis for reproduction leading to an associated reproductive pattern in which sexual activity associate with increase in a particular hormone or hormones. Influence of hormone on sex-reversal is also found in humans [Fig. 3.18].

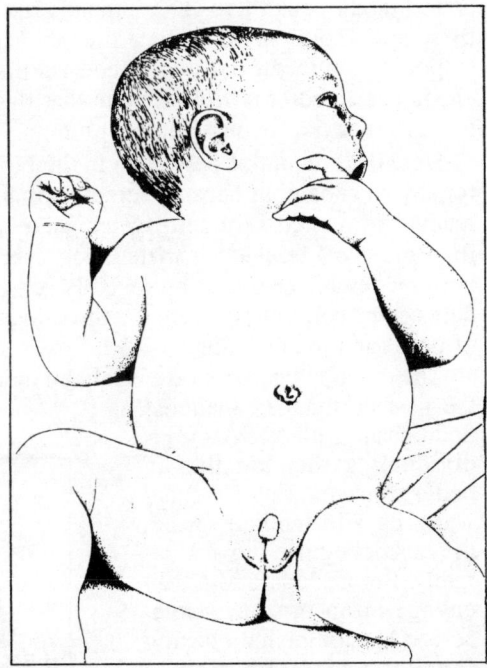

Fig. 3.18. The appearance of a male genital organ (penis) like structure in a newborn baby whose mother had been treated with androgens during pregnancy. The baby is, in fact, a genetic female.

FISH

Like any other vertebrate groups fishes also exhibit different kinds of behaviour composed by different hormones. Ethoendocrinologists have observed many interesting cases of behaviour in fishes, influenced by hormones.

Fanning behaviour of stickleback fish

Male stickleback fishes (*Gasterosteus oceallatus*) perform fanning behaviour as a part of parental care to aerate its eggs. During fanning the male positions himself in front of the nest entrance and hangs there, beating forward vigorously with his pectoral fins, and backwards with his tail. The fish stays still and a current of water is propelled through the nest and over the eggs. This keep eggs well oxygenated (Fig. 3.19). Blum and Fiedler (1969) injected the pituitary hormone '*prolactin*' in an isolated male of a species of fish *Cranilabus oceallatus* and found that this fish fan in a place which is devoid of all the normal stimuli for fanning i.e. nest site, eggs etc. The time they spend in fanning is dependent on the dose of prolactin.

Migration in fishes

Thyroid is implicated in the onset of migration of migratory fishes. Migration of three-spined sticklebacks (*Gasterosteus oceallatus*), from the sea to the river occurs normally even in castrated animals. This migratory behaviour can be elicited, out of season, by T_4 injection.

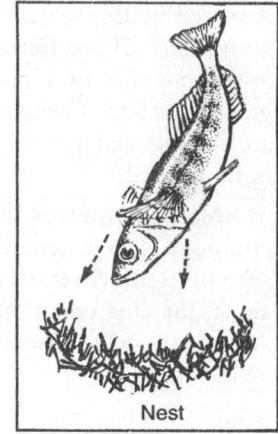

Fig. 3.19. Influence of Hormone in initiating fanning behaviour : Male three-spined stickleback initiate fanning behaviour in non-breeding season and in absence of nest when injected with prolactin hormone.

REPTILES

Let us consider the cyclical regulation of sexual receptivity in the female green anole, a small lizard found in the Southeastern United States. Adult female have a 10 to 14 day cycle of changing receptivity that is linked to the amount of oestrogen released by her ovaries. Oestrogen travels via the bloodstream to the head of the lizard, affecting various endocrine and neural target cells there. The female's brain eventually becomes primed by specific hormone to activate precopulatory neck-arching behaviour in response to a territorial male's courtship signals. Should such a female encounter an adult territorial male that flags her with his extended dewlap as he bobs his head up and down, she is likely to copulate with him.

Here the amount of oestrogen in the bloodstream is a key proximate factor that lowers the threshold for sexual behaviour because removal of an adult female's oestrogen - producing ovaries abolish sexual receptivity. Injection of oestrogen in an ovary removed, nonreceptive female restore her sexual receptivity. But once a female has mated, her receptivity drops precipitously. Within 5 to 7 minutes after copulation, a female ceases to be sexually receptive and will ignore, run from, or even attack any male that dares court her. She will remain unwilling to mate for 10 to 14 days, untill she has regained high levels of oestrogen in her blood.

The red-sided garter snake is inhabitant of South Canada. As a cold blooded reptile it spends much of the year dormant in sheltered underground place. Many individuals gather together in better overwintering sites. On warm days in the late spring, the snakes begin to move separately. Before separation, they engage in an orgy of sexual activity, with males chasing females and attempting to copulate with her. Although males compete for females but they do not fight with one another for the privilege of mat-

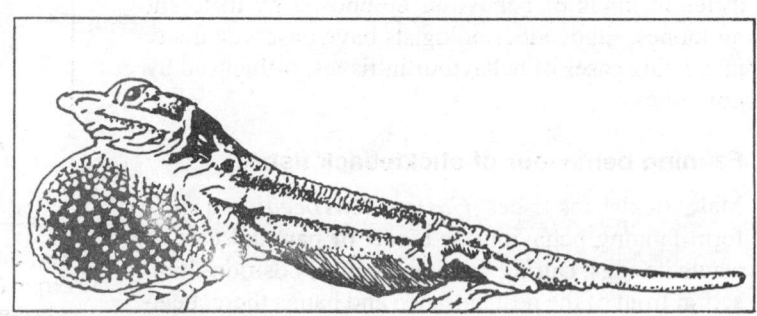

Fig. 3.20. Dewlap Display of male Jamaican anole.

ing. Examination of the sex hormone concentration in their blood reveals that there is no testosterone or equivalent substance in these nonaggressive snakes. Yet they successfully mate. Removal of the pineal gland of male snakes prior to hibernation almost always fail to court the following spring. It does not mean that testosterone has no role to play in the sexual cycle of the snake. High levels of testosterone are present in males in the fall and contribute to the production of sperm. Although temperature increase may be the acti-vational cue for sexual activity, testosterone may play an organizational role in the development of the underlying mechanisms of reproductive behaviour in the red-sided garter snake, as it does in so many other vertebrates. Castrated adult males are unable to produce testosterone but they comfortably show courtship behaviour after a period of hibernation. These findings weaken support for the position that sexual behaviour is mediated by activational hormones in every species. Instead, there are many different mechanisms involved in regulating sexual activity, just as there are numerous external factors known to affect the behavioural priorities of different species.

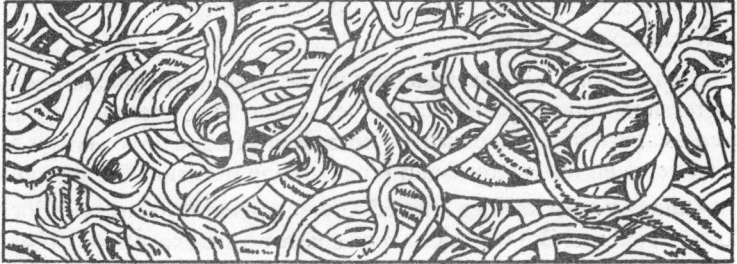

Fig. 3.21. Male red-sided garter snakes in spring mating aggregation. The snakes copulate eagerly and enthusiastically despite having almost no circulating testosterone in blood-stream.

BIRDS

Hormone directed gonadal development and mutual behavioural communication changes can be observed by taking a pair of birds of same species but of opposite sex. In breeding season, most species of birds observe reproductive behaviour stepwise. First of all males perform courtship behaviour, then male or female or both perform nesting behaviour, followed by mating, and then the female lays eggs and eggs are incubated by one or both sex. Hutchinson and Komisaruk used ring doves as an experimental animal and revealed

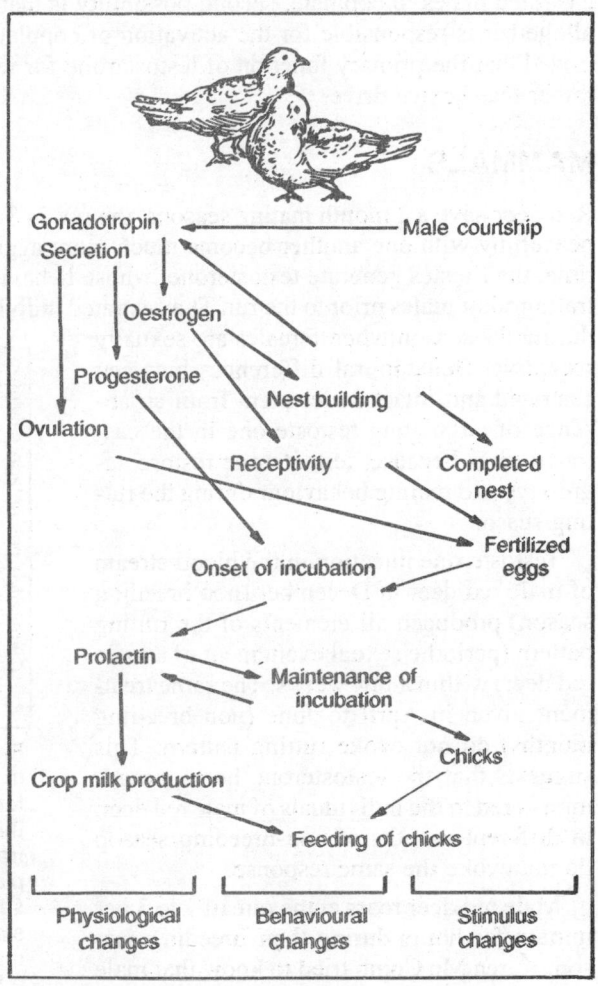

Fig. 3.22. Reproductive Behaviour of Ring Dove in context of hormonal interaction.

that there are regions in the brain of dove which are sensitive to different hormones responsible for different sexual activities.

The introduction of testosterone in the anterior hypothalamus causes castrated male dove to exhibit aggression, courtship and mating behaviour. Progesterone introduced in the same point of brain suppresses aggressive and courtship behaviour of male dove. This is also a direct demonstration of antagonism between testosterone and progesterone in context of reproductive behaviour.

Although most species studied to date appear to possess endocrine hormone associated with reproductive patterns. But white-crowned sparrows are exceptional. Usually the male sexual behaviour should not occur in individuals that have been castrated because removal of the testes eliminates a major source of testosterone production. But even without testes (without testosterone in blood stream), a male white - crowned sparrow will mount on female that finish copulation, provided that he has been exposed to long photoperiod. In this case there are two possibilities : firstly some other organ besides the testes produces testosterone in white-crowned sparrows, providing a hormonal explanation for the ability of castrated males to copulate, second possibility is that in white-crowned sparrows some other hormone altogether is responsible for the activation of copulation. John Wingfield and Michael Moore hypothesized that the primary function of testosterone for white-crowned males is to enhance aggressiveness rather than sexual drive.

MAMMALS

Red deer have a 2 month mating seasons, the rut, in September and October. Stags that have been living peacefully with one another become much more aggressive and sexually active during the rut. At this time, their testes generate testosterone, whose behavioural importance has been demonstrated by castrating adult males prior to the rut. The castrated individuals show little aggression and do not try to mate during the season when females are sexually receptive. Behavioural differences between castrated and intact males stem from an absence of circulating testosterone in the castrated stags because, testosterone restore aggressive and mating behaviour during the rutting season.

Testosterone injection in the blood stream of male red deer in December (non breeding season) produced all elements of the rutting pattern (periodic sexual excitement of a male red deer) within a few weeks. The same treatment given in April to June (non breeding months) do not evoke rutting pattern. This suggests that the testosterone hormone administered to the individuals of male red deer, in different months of non-breeding season do not evoke the same response.

Male red deer roars at the rate of 1 to 3 per minute for hours during their breeding season. Karen Mc Comb tried to know that male roars influence the timing of female sexual receptivity or not. To test the hypothesis that

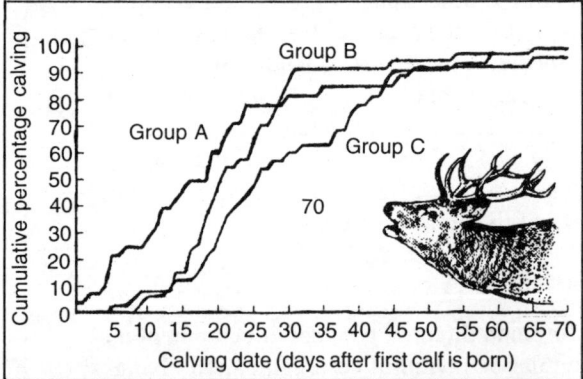

Fig. 3.23. Roaring by stags affects the onset of oestrus in female red deer. The cumulative percentage of female deer giving birth on each date is shown for three groups : females in group A were held in isolation from males and heard no tapes of roaring prior to being placed with a fertile stag; group B females were exposed to tapes of roaring before gaining access to a fertile stag; group C females were held with a vasecto-mized male (which roared regularly) before being placed with a fertile red deer. Females exposed to roaring, even if only on tape, generally calved sooner than females that lacked this stimulation.

they do, she performed some experiments with red deer. She divided a herd of females into three groups: *one group* was kept with a vasectomized male that roared and moved among the females but could not inseminate them; *second group* was held away from all males but was treated to long playing tapes of male roars; and the *third group* was kept in isolation from both males and their calls. Subsequently all females were given access to a number of non-vasectomized males, which impregnated them as soon as they were receptive. The date on which a female gave birth indicates when she came into oestrus. Females that had the company of a sterile but otherwise unaffected male, and also females that listened to tapes of male roars, gave birth sooner on average than females held in complete isolation from males and their roars.

Testosterone also increases the persistence of mammals. This has been extensively studied in young mammals (cat, dog, lion) in a variety of tasks, such as searching, discrimination, and open field tasks. Such effects may be related to various effects of androgens on cognitive performance in human beings. Role of perinatal hormonal conditions in the development of behaviour in rhesus monkeys has been conducted and one of the interesting finding, is the effect of early hormonal make up on active play behaviour. Normal males display much more active play than females. Pseudohermaphrodite females are those who were exposed to androgens prenatally, showed levels of play that were intermediate between those of the normal females and males. Sportsman and athletes use steroids to enhance their ability in sports and other activities.

A female hormone oestrogen has ability to counter dementia i.e. the loss of memory associated with old age. Age related memory loss, clinically known as Alzheimer's disease can be minimised by the administration of oestrogen even in males. A neuroendocrinologist, Victoria Luine and Bruce Mc Ewen were studying how hormones control reproductive behaviour. They observed an increase in the levels of the enzyme *choline acetyltransferase* in certain neurones of the basal forebrain on administering oestrogen to female rats. Choline acetyl transferase is the enzyme, responsible for synthesis of a chemical, that helps to communicate messages between nerve junctions.

Luine discovered a massive loss of acetylcholine - releasing hormone in the basal forebrains of patients with Alzhemer's disease. She correlated this knowledge to her previous observation and speculated that oestrogen might prove to be an useful drug against the disease. Rockfeller's group discovered unique mechanism explaining how oestrogen may assist in the better functioning of neurones, involved in learning and memory. They found that oestrogen actually helps to build and maintain synapses, the junctions through which one neurone communicates to another.

Rockfeller's team found that removal of ovaries from adult female rats caused a loss of spines from certain hippocampal cells. Dominique Toran-Allerand (1970) had demonstrated that oestrogen stimulates the growth of axons and dendrites.

Researchers have also found that oestrogen can directly protect brain cells against damage by toxins. This protective role was first observed by James Simplins when he found that the rate of death of cancerous brain cells was much lower in cell cultures when oestrogen was present. Recent studies show that oestrogen acts as an antioxidant, scavenging destructive free radicals.

HORMONES AND OTHER FACTORS ELICITATING SPECIFIC BEHAVIOUR IN VERTEBRATES

In fact any behaviour exhibited by an individual is the outcome of interaction of numerous factors. Some interrelated factors and outcome of behaviour are discussed here.

Hormone, Environment and Sexual behaviour

Ethologists have remained interested in studying role of hormone and other factors in sexual behaviour. Daniel Lehrman (1964) and his collegues used three experimental group of ring doves to determine whether the presence of male or the nesting materials affects incubation behaviour of female doves. (1) Female and male kept in separate glass boxes. Females could see males. (2) Females housed with a normal male and nesting materials and (3) Females housed with a castrated male.

Female doves do not normally lay eggs if kept alone or with only females, but she begins to lay eggs soon after a male dove is introduced to her. This means that pituitary secretion in female is influenced by the presence of male. Simple experiments show that only the sight of a male dove is enough to cause ovulation in female dove. A male dove performs the typical courtship bow, even though separated behind a glass screen, is effective than a castrated (testis removed) male in the same cage. The hormones action at different stages of breeding cycle, vary in different birds. The external stimuli which operate as cues in the reproductive cycle also vary from species to species.

Hormone, Season, and Migration

How animals migrate begs an answer in terms of how they find their way and how they know where to go? The physiological answer has been worked out to meticulous details for some species. Migratory behaviour in animals is due to interaction between the environment and hormones. There are always immediate exogenous factors stimulating migration. The most regular and predictable seasonal change in the environment is the fluctuation of day length. Increased photoperiod during spring or decreased photoperiod during winter received by eye are converted to chemical messages by neu-

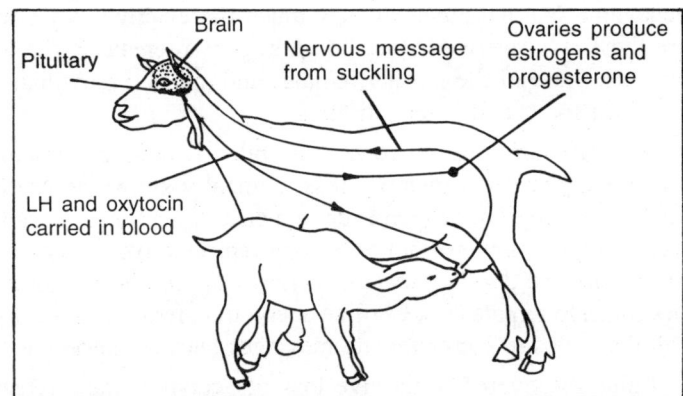

Fig. 3.24. Sucking by kids of goats causes secretion of luteinizing hormone (LH) stimulate the ovary to produce progesterone. These two hormones help in secretion of milk.

rosecretory cells, which act upon hypothalamus. The hypothalamus stimulate the pituitary gland to release gonadotrophic hormone.

Mechanical Stimulation, Hormone Secretion and Milking of Cattles

Sucking by kids of goats or cows causes secretion of luteinizing hormone (LH). Luteinizing hormone stimulates the ovary of mother to produce *estradiol* and *progesterone*. These two hormones are responsible for maintaining mammary glands in a state of readiness for milk secretion. During the pregnancy and birth of a baby there is rise in the level of prolactin in the body of mother. When the kid sucks the teat of mammary gland, the mechanical stimulation induces the hypothalamus to release oxytocin from the neurohypophysis. The rise in the level of oxytocin in the blood triggers milk secretion.

Gene, Environment and Hormone in Composing Aggressive Behaviour in Mice

Interaction of strain with early hormone treatment on perinatal androgenization and aggressive behaviour in inbred female mice was studied by Vale, Ray and Vale (1972). Neonatal androgen injection produced substantial increase in the aggressive behaviour of females whereas the males are nonaggressive. Male mice of heterozygous genotypes retained the ejaculatory action for a longer period following castration than did inbred animals.

Individual difference may arise due to genome, environment, or their interaction. Individual differences in copulatory behaviour in guinea pigs result from differences in the soma, probably in the central nervous system. Individual differences were restored after castration with a constant hormone level for all animals. Larson (1966) found similar results while working with rats.

Experience, Hormones and Behaviour

The inexperienced and experienced individuals for a behavioural act react differently in context of hormone action. Postcastration maintenance of copulatory behaviour in male cats is more prolonged if they had previous copulatory experience than if they are naive. The induction of sexual receptivity by the administration of *estradiole benzote* and *progesterone* to female mice becomes more effective as a function of the experience of the mice with such procedures.

PHEROMONE-ETHOLOGY

• Introduction • Discovery of pheromone and its role on behaviour • Importance of pheromones for Animal world • Pheromone producing glands and pheromone sensitive organs in animals • Classification of pheromones and their role on behaviour • Lee-Boot effect • Whitten effect • Bruce effect • Imprinting pheromones • Mimetic sex pheromone • Application of pheromones for the welfare of the mankind • Exercise.

INTRODUCTION

Pheromones are scents released by animals producing any kind of communication between conspecific. Karlson and Butenend (1959) proposed this term in context of sex attractant in insects. Pheromones released by the male individual stimulate the sex of female. Likewise pheromone released by the female, stimulate the sex of male. New millennium scientists have discovered sixth sense organ in human beings called Vomeronasal organ (V.N.O.) found in the nose of higher mammals. V.N.O. is found both in male and female and is sensitive to female and male sex pheromones. Sensory cells of V.N.O. remains attached with olfactory bulb of brain which carry smell up to hypothalamus of brain. David Verliner and his associates have synthesized an artificial chemical called P.D.D. (Pegna-4, 2 Dine-3-6-Dione). 1/100000000 part of 1 g. of P.D.D. cause sex stimulation in males. This chemical received by V.N.O of males increase the

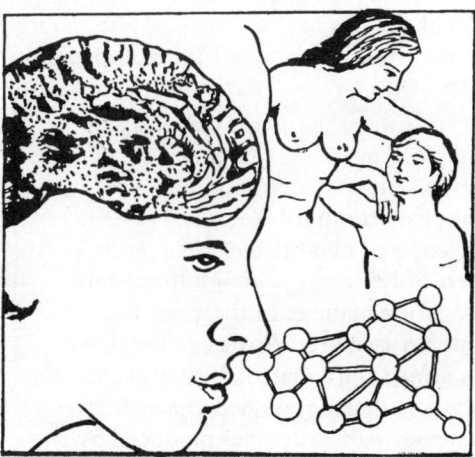

Fig. 3.25. VNO found in the human brain is the sixth sense organ concerned with sex.

waves in brain which is the indication of being tension free. This chemical is very costly and 1 mg. costs about 1 lac rupees. Pheromones are released in a very small quantity but exert great influence on behaviour. Dr. Adolf Butnend of Max Plank institute, Germany, obtained only 12 mg. female silkworm moth pheromone (Bombykol - $C_{16}H_{30}O$) from 2.5 lac female silkworm moth. American scientists could extract only 20 mg. pheromone (Gyplyor or Dispalur) from 5 lac female gypsy moth *(Pothytria americana).*

DISCOVERY OF PHEROMONE

Bonnet was the first man who questioned *why ants always move in a single line in orderly manner?* To get an answer, he performed an ordinary experiment. He placed heap of sugar at some distance from the colony of ants. Ants move *to and fro* in single line between colony and heap of sugar. Bonnet rubbed his finger across the path of ants and observed that ants stopped and searched about when they reached the rubbed place, waving their antennae in the air and tapping them on the ground. There was a gradual crowding of ants on both sides of the rubbed point, some coming from the heap of sugar

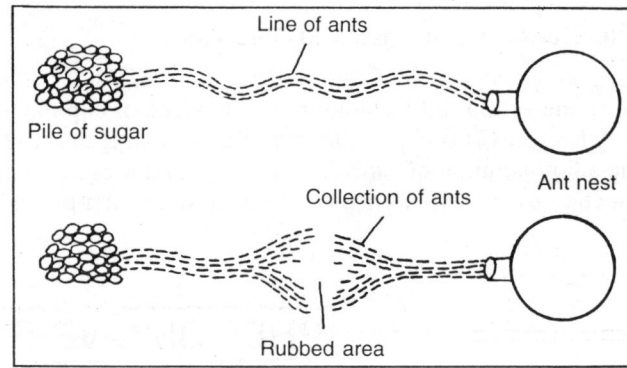

Fig. 3.26. Role of Pheromone in Ants : Bonnet's experiment with ants showing role of trail scent.

while others going towards food, until a few adventurous ants run on the rubbed place. Ants from both sides met, smelt each other and continued their journey. Bonnet assumed that it was actually a trail of chemical which ants could sense and follow.

Fabre worked with the chemical message in insects. He placed a female moth in a cage near a window and observed that within 15 hours numerous males of the same species came out the woods and collected around the cage. When he placed female moth in a tightly closed transparent glass container, where female could be seen but getting no odour, no male appeared. Fabre placed a few female moths in a container made-up of very fine wire mesh. In this case, male moths could not see females but could get essence of female. Maie moths gathered around wire mesh container. Fabre concluded that emission of a chemical (pheromone) by female moth through wire mesh attracted male moths for breeding.

The horse has in fact played a central role in the development of our knowledge of mammalian pheromones. Bernhard Zondeck (1934) discovered that mare excrete oestrogen in her urine which attract stallions for mating. In the past, horse thieves used to employ a cloth soaked in urine from a mare in heat to attract stallions that they wished to steal from a meadow. Pheromones produced by a bitch in heat attract all male dogs of the area in breeding season.

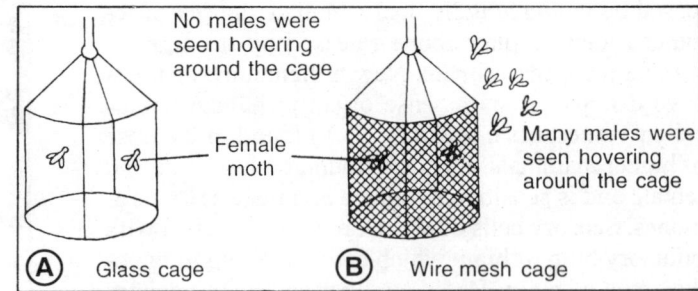

Fig. 3.27. Role of pheromone in Moths : Fabre's experiment with moth (A) Males could see the females but could not get her scent. (B) Male moth could see and get scent of female kept in wire mesh cage.

IMPORTANCE OF PHEROMONES FOR ANIMAL WORLD

Pheromones evoke specific behaviour which is very significant for survival and continuation of the species. For a race, it is important that an individual should not divert energy in *trial-and-error* learning to achieve the appropriate goal, specially in context of reproductive activities. In many species (especially insects) the female produces a pheromone attracting the opposite sex from distance away, to ensure mating. Aphrodisiac pheromone facilitate copulation after the two opposite sexes have come together.

PHEROMONES PRODUCING GLANDS AND PHEROMONE SENSITIVE ORGANS

Insects have been most extensively studied for their pheromone producing system. Pheromone producing glands of butterflies and moths remain associated with scales on wings called *androconia*. Female silkworm moth bear a pair of sacs on abdomen which emit a sex pheromone *bombykol*. Males find females with the help of this scent and mate with her successfully. Male Amauris bear a *scent patch* (scent cups) on each hind wings. Scent from these cups disperses by scent brushes associated with genitalia. An insect *Plaodia* bear scent glands which opens on either sides of the last abdominal segment. Mandibular gland of queen honeybee produces *queen substances* which keeps other females sterile. This helps in keeping large number of worker bees in the hive. *Nassanoff's gland* of honeybee present in between 6th and 7th abdominal segments secrete this pheromone. Ants bear many pheromone producing glands such as mandibular gland, labial gland, meta-pleural gland, pavan's gland, dufour's gland, anal gland etc.

Various structures are found in insects to perceive the scent of conspecific. These structures are present on antenna. These structures may be flat, cup shaped or in the form of short stubby hair. The pheromones released by a conspecific are perceived by these specialized structures and the messages are sent to elicit certain behaviour.

Among vertebrates, mammals have been most extensively studied for their pheromone producing exocrine glands and organs perceiving those pheromones.

The chief sources of mammalian pheromone are urine, faeces, saliva, and cutaneous glands. The most common use of urine and faeces is to identify *core area* – an area used and defended actively, *home range* – an area around core area actively used but not defended actively, *Territory* – an area around home range used frequently but not defended actively. Hippopotamus, Rhinoceros, Dogs, Foxes, Lion, Tigers, Leopard, Hyena etc. use their urine and/or faeces for identifying their pathways, feeding ground, sleeping sites and resting ground. Some mammals urinate or defaecate on rivals and defeated conspecifics. Slender loris monkeys and Copuchin (new world monkeys) soak their feet and hands in their urine and smear it on the foliage falling within its home range. Why do dogs urinate different places while walking? Dogs and many other mammals such as foxes, coyote slow loris use the urine to mark their territory (home range). After rainy season lions mark their territory by urinating on tree trunk.

Some mammals bear special exocrine glands (anal glands, salivary gland, mammary gland, miscellaneous glands) to release pheromones. Tiger produces *tigeramine* through urine for sex attraction. Male rabbits excites the female rabbit, spraying a stream of urine on her. This renders the female rabbit receptive to the male for mating.

CLASSIFICATION OF PHEROMONES AND THEIR ROLE ON BEHAVIOUR

On the basic of function, four types of pheromones are recognised.

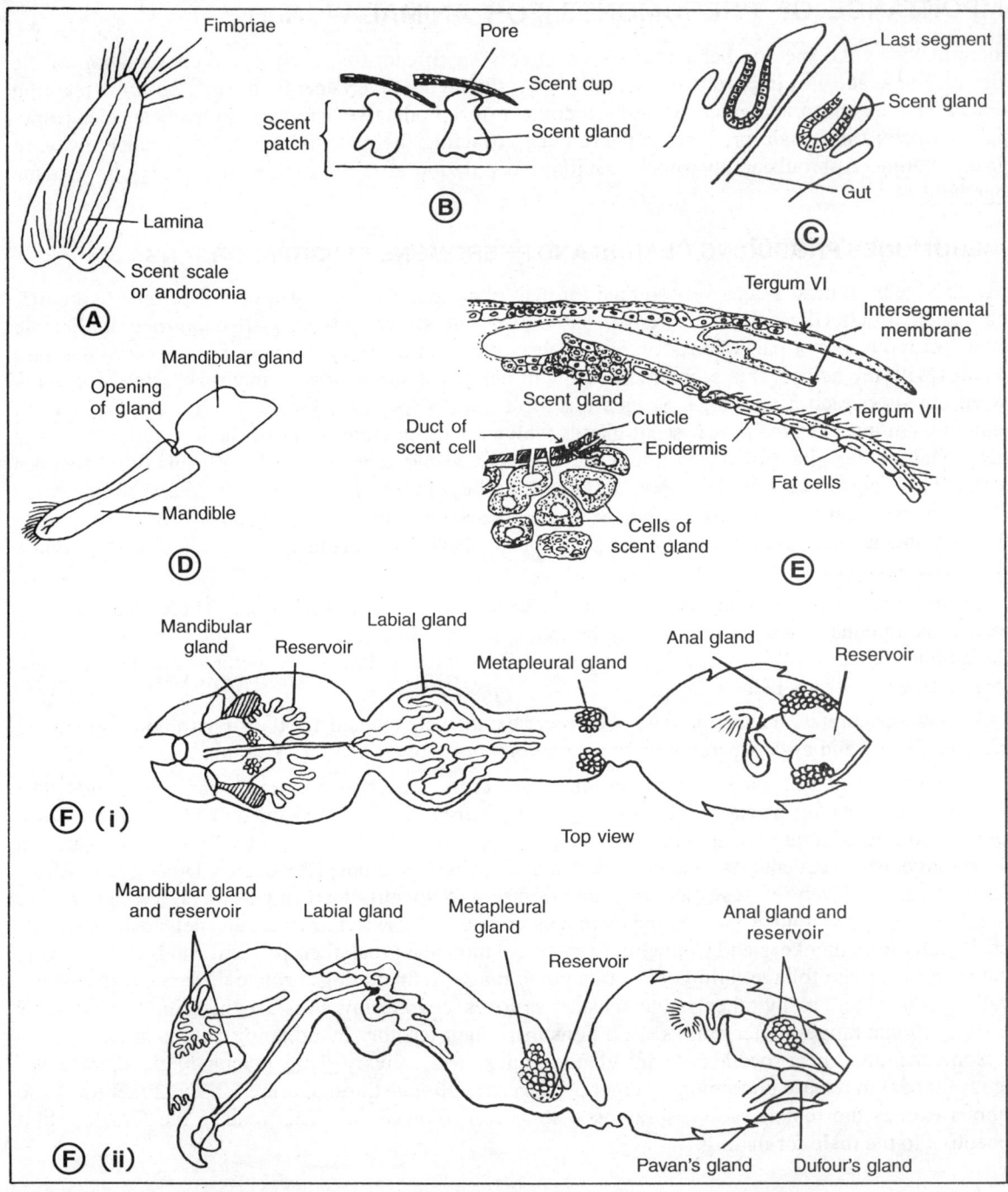

Fig. 3.28. (A-F) Scent Producing Glands in Insects : (A) Scent scales of butterflies and moths; (B) scent cups in males of Amaceris; (C) Invaginated scent glands in Plaodia; (D) Mandibular gland of honey bee; (E) Nassanoffs gland of honeybee (F_i) and (F_{ii}) top and side view of scent producing glands in ants.

I. Releaser or signalling pheromones
II. Primer pheromones.
III. Imprinting pheromones.
IV. Mimetic sex pheromone.

I. RELEASER PHEROMONES

These pheromones cause "Releaser" effect in animals by initiating an instinctive behaviour. Releaser pheromones have been studied in mammalian urine and foot pads where odours play an important role in attracting opposite sex. The pheromones help in recognition of oestrus females by males.

Sex-attractant/Trails and Alarm pheromones/released by insects are releaser pheromones. Insects depend on these pheromones for successful mate finding and reproduction. With the help of these pheromones opposite sex of insects are able to search its partner for copulation and further acts of reproduction.

Further classification of releaser pheromones may be done as (1) Sex-Attractant, (2) Alarm pheromones, (3) Feeding site attractant, (4) Defence attractant, (5) Trail pheromones, (6) Aphrodisiac pheromones, (7) Inhibitory pheromones and (8) Adverse effect pheromone etc.

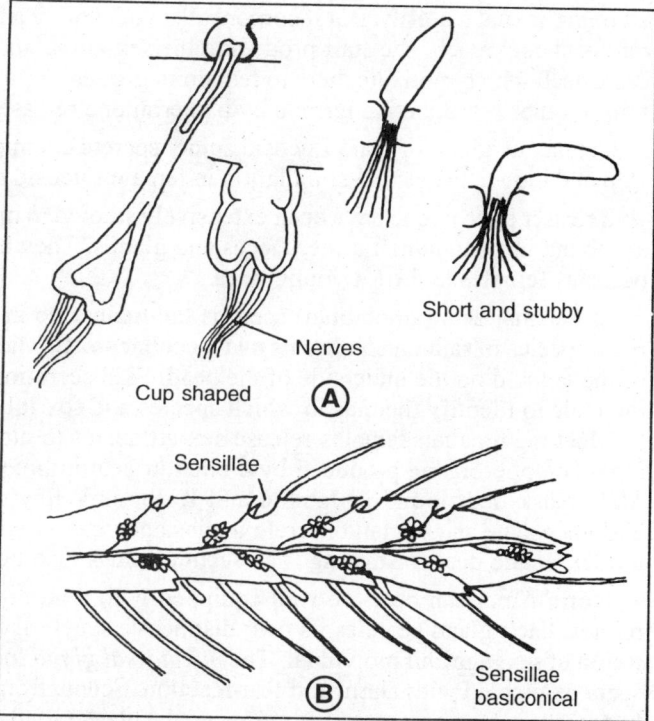

Fig. 3.29. Pheromone Sensing Organs : (A) Structure perceiving pheromones in insects. (B) Antenna of male Silkworm moth to receive pheromone.

1. SEX-ATTRACTANT

Female silkworm *(Bombyx mori)* releases a pheromone commonly called Bombykol ($C_6H_{30}O$-Trans-10-cis-12-hexadecadienol). Males of silkworm moth bear long antennae and each antennae bear more than 1000 *sensila* (Fig. 3.29). These sensila are like chemoreceptor and are specialized only to receive the smell of bombykol. This chemical is so effective that only one molecule is capable of stimulating one sensila. Male silkworm moth find females of their own species with the help of this pheromone finding organs. Once males reach near females, things become visual and other aphrodiasic pheromones including sex hormones act upon for further reproductive behaviour.

Queen honeybee *(Apis melifera)* attract males by a pheromone (9-oxodecenoic acid) produced in the mandibular glands, stimulating drone's olfactory receptors. This attraction occurs only from 20 to 30 meters above the ground. Having reached close to the queen with the help of sex attractant pheromone, the final approach is probably visual.

Female *Periplaneta americana* release a pheromone not named yet, (2, 2-dimethyl 3-isopropylidency cloropyl propionate) which act as sex-attractant for male cockroach. If *corpora allata* of female cockroach is removed just after moulting, the female cockroach fails to produce this pheromone after attaining sexual maturity. But if corpora allata of another adult female is transplanted to the corpora allata removed cockroach, she start producing the sex-attractant. Aggregation pheromone is also released by cockroach which motivate them to remain in groups. A pair of reproductive termite inhibits the production of other reproductive termite by a pheromone released by her anus.

Cutaneous gland of male Lucosid spider secrete chemical substances which is absorbed by female's skin and induce the sexual stimulation in female Lucosid spiders.

Releaser pheromone have been extensively studied in mammals including man. Releaser pheromones are found in mammalian urine, faeces and glands. They help in attracting opposite sex, recognition of oestrous females and own young ones.

In Salamanders (amphibian) scent is the main clue in recognition of opposite sex of own species. Each species of salamander has its own peculiar smell. Male Salamander bear Herdonic gland at the base of the tail and on the underside of the head. Skin secretion of females possesses the odour that enables the male to identify them as to which species and sex it belongs.

Most mammalian females release sex-attractant to attract males for courtship and copulation. Sex attractant pheromone produced by a bitch in heat in breeding season attract all male dogs of the area. Male musk deer found in Jammu and Kashmir Valley of India bear a musk gland in lower side of abdomen. The musk gland secrete a substance called *muskon*. It emit a strong and pleasant smell to attract female deer for mating. The scent of musk also helps in marking territory.

North American deer are well equipped with a number of *suboriferous glands* that secrete pheromones. Each gland secretes its own distinctive scent. Scent from the *tarsal gland* is for mutual recognition of sex, age and individual. The *metatarsal gland* located on the outside of the hind legs, secrete a scent associated with alarm and fear reaction. Scents from the gland in the forehead is used for making home range. During aggressive posturing the black tailed deer opens the orifice of the post *orbital gland* fully.

In human being, olfactory sensity for pheromone is comparable to that of the dog but this is suppressed in the adult life for psychosexual reasons (Dominic, 1978). Olfactory clues play an important role in an infantile psychosexual development. The change in the quality of the odours of human female are progesterone dependent and each stage of menstrual cycle has distinctive odour. McClintock suggested the existence of *copullins* in human female vaginal secretion which stimulates mounting and mating. Dr. Geoge Dodd identified human pheromone in male sweat. It is identified as X–anrostenol and it attracts the females during sexual interaction. A perfume called androm costs $275 for an ounce.

Pheromones help in maintaining mother child bond. By the sixth week the baby recognises mother by mother's body scent. Striking sexual differences have been observed in the ability of human to smell certain substances. Odour of *exaltolide* (synthetic lactone of 14 hydroxy tetradecenoic acid) is felt clearly by sexually matured ladies mostly at the time of ovulation.

A mother rat licks her nipples so that her blind pups can follow the scent to suck the milk. In mice, male urine contains releaser pheromones for attracting females or orgnising aggressive activities and communicating fear between individuals. In rats, a maternal phero-

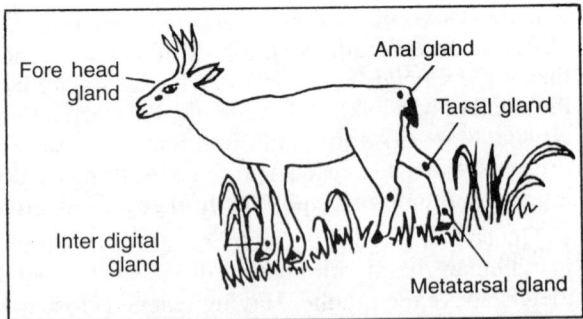

Fig. 3.30. Pheromone Producing Glands in black tailed deer : Black tailed deer bear different scent glands on different locations of body. Secretion and smell of each gland has some meaning.

mone is produced by the female for synchro-
nizing the mother and young relationship
(Leon, 1974). Vaginal secretions of sheep,
hamster and rhesus monkeys act as releaser
pheromones. In primates including human
beings vaginal secretions contain short chain
aliphatic acids called "copullins" whose function is perhaps releaser pheromone.

2. ALARM PHEROMONE

Termites discovering a crack in their termitarium emit an alarm scent that attract workers to repair the crack. Alarm pheromones
are also produced in ants in the form of *for-

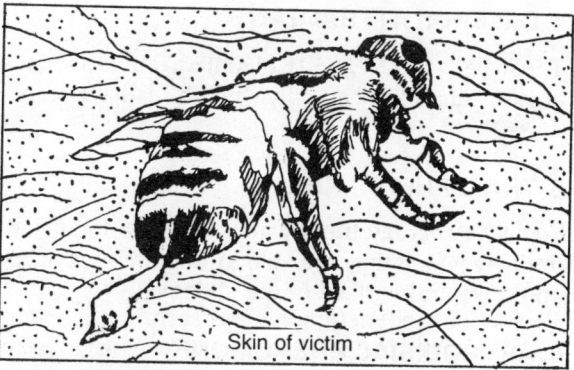

Fig. 3.31. A worker honeybee releasing alarm pheromone after stinging a person.

mic acid from the abdomen to protect themselves from enemies. Honeybees while stinging any person
releases alarm pheromones with poison and immediately moves to fellow members of the colony to
show her sting and flutter to aggravate the fellow members for attack. Alarm pheromones are produced
when social insect is threatened in some way. It involves attraction of the other workers or soldiers for
attack. The alarm pheromone of the bee *Trigona* is produced by the mandibular glands.

Fresh water and marine fishes produce alarm pheromones by flask shaped cells present in the skin,
whenever an intruder approaches a school of fish. Alarm pheromones are also produced in the skin cells
of a toad tadpole. Whenever the tadpole is injured, all other tadpoles in the medium move either to the
bottom or run away from the site of occurrence. If nerve leading to the olfactory organ in cut in the
tadpole then no alarm response is observed.

Alarm pheromones are produced by numerous mammals like antelope pole cat, tree shrews, monkey,
lemur etc. Antelope produce alarm pheromones from large glands conceded in the fur on the sacral
region of the body by contracting sacral muscles. Tree shrews of Asia bear special scent glands. Male
tree shrew release its urine on the branches of the trees and presses his throat gland against various
objects of the vicinity to mark the boundaries of his territory. Madagascar ring - tail lemur presses its tail
tip against the odourous glands present on the inner right and left forearms and the scented tail is moved
in the air to disperse the scent in the environment. They also rub the gland of the limbs against tree
branches to propogate the scent. The Indian black buck antelops mark the territory with scent, produced by the orbital gland of the body. The saliva of boar contains odourous steroids that is essential for
prolonged act of coitus.

3. FEEDING SITE ATTRACTANT

The bark beetles *Scolytidae* aggregate in large numbers on host trees. Invasion is directed by odour
of the host plant. Female *Dendroctonus* bores into its host plant and produces a pheromone called
exobrevicomin. This pheromone is released in the faeces and attract more beetles to invade the tree. The
males, on arrival, produce a closely related pheromone *frontalin*,which together with the volatile *myrcene*,
emitted from the host plant, enhance the effect of exobrevicomin so that more and more beetles may
arrive at the tree.

4. DEFENCE ATTRACTANT

The male *Lycus loripes* (Coleoptera) emits a scent which attract other fellow beetles. Lycus is distasteful beetle with yellow colour which birds have learnt to avoid. Predators avoid them because they are in mass.

5. TRAIL PHEROMONE

Social insects lay trails which facilitate food finding by other members of the colony. Ants lay scent trails by which they are able to find their way about. Termites produce a trail pheromone from a gland on the ventral surface of the abdomen.

6. APHRODISIAC PHEROMONE

The term Aphrodisiac pheromone is used with respect to pheromones which facilitate copulation after the two sexes having come together.

When a male *Danaus gillipus* overtakes a female he extrudes his hair pencils and dusts her with pheromone transfer particles. These particles carry the pheromone which stimulate via the olfactory sensilla of the antennae, and induces the female to land. The male then hovers over the female for some time and finally lands and copulates with her.

7. INHIBITORY PHEROMONE

Pheromones inhibiting the response to other pheromones produced by the same species are called inhibitory pheromones.

Verbenon reduces the response of Dendroctonus (beetle) to its attractant pheromones so that excessive aggregation of this species leading to overcrowding on the host plant is avoided.

8. ADVERSE EFFECT OF PHEROMONE

The pheromones produced by larvae of *Anagasta* induces the parasite *Venturia* to make probing movement with its ovipositor and so the chances of a larva being parasitised are increased (Corbet, 1971). Pheromones may advertise the presence of an insect to predators and potential parasites. The clerid beetle (*Thanasimus dubius*) is predator of Dendroctonus. It locates its host by responding to the pheromone *frontalin*.

Variation in response to releaser pheromone

Due to different environmental conditions and concentrations, pheromones may exert different types of behaviours in the recipient. Male moths which are normally nocturnal, do not respond to the sex attractant pheromones of females in daylight. The sex attractant pheromones of many moths induce unwind flight by the male when they are present in low concentrations. In high concentration the males attempt to copulate. A pheromone '*citral*' of a bee Trigona functions as trail pheromone in low concentration but it functions as alarm pheromone in high concentration.

II. PRIMER PHEROMONES

These pheromones induce a delayed response and prolonged stimulation mediated through the nervous system and endocine glands (mainly pituitary gland) and initiate a chain of physiological adjustment modifying the behavioural patterns. Queenbee substance ($C_{10}H_{16}O_3$) of honeybee and termites are primer pheromones. These pheromones attract worker to remain in aggregation in one hive: that help in maintaining social life. Worker bees of a colony licks this substance located in the head of queenbee. This also checks the ovarian cycle of worker bees. Members of one colony of honeybee also recognise their inmates by a specific odour.

LEE-BOOT EFFECTS

Van der Lee and L.M.Boot (1955) performed various experiment, related with influence of primer pheromones on behaviour on mice and came to the conclusion that if a few female mice are kept together in a cage during oestrous cycle then their regular oestrous - cycle is disturbed and delayed. The pheromone present in urine of female mice is perceived through V.N.O by them which disturbs regular oestrous-cycle. They called this phenomenon as Lee-Boct effect. Lee and Boot also observed that when 5 or 6 female mice were kept together there was an increase in the number of spontaneous pseudopregnancies, which could be prevented by removing olfactory bulbs (V.N.O) or isolating the female.

WHITTEN EFFECT

Whitten (1968) observed that sexual maturity in female mice is accelerated by the presence of an adult male mouse. The presence of an adult female mice retards it. The acceleration of sexual maturation observed in the presence of an adult male is due to odours (Primer pheromone) and tatctile stimulation.

BRUCE EFFECT

Helen Bruce (1961) a lady ethologist observed that odour (primer pheromone) of a strange male mouse checked the pregnancy of a newly conceived female mice. She called it Helen–Bruce effect. After copulation, female mice is sensitive to the presence of a stranger male up to a maximum of five days. After 5th day Helen - Bruce effect does not apply.

Odour of strange male suppresses the secretion of hormone prolactin. In absence of prolactin corpus luteum (ovarian) fails to develop and normal oestrous is restored. This occurs in following steps :–

Newly introduced male → Pheromone released through urine (aerial) → Received by female through V.N.O. → Hypothalamus → Inhibition of gonad stimulating hormone → Pineal gland → Lack of gonadotrophic hormone → Ovary → Bad effect on ovarian hormone → check the gestation.

III. IMPRINTING PHEROMONES

As the name suggests, such pheromones help in inducing the imprinting behaviour. Dominic (1978) studied in certain laboratory rodents, particularly mice, olfactory influence of the preweaning environment in their reproductive behaviour. Females of *Mus musculus domesticus* reared with their parents and reproductive behaviour was studied. When they become adult, it was found that, generally females mate males of strains different from their own. They display sexual preferences for males of their subspecies (*Mus musculus bactrianus*). Such a sexual preference and a version of the males of the two subspecies are not exhibited by females which are revised by their mothers alone. In the absence of male parent, not exposing to the odour of male parents, no inhibitory printing occurs in female young mice.

IV. MIMETIC SEX PHEROMONE

There are exceptional cases where one organism produce a mimetic sex pheromone. One of the most complex and bizarre mechanisms is the sexual impersonation of female *thynnine wasps* by certain *orchid species* (plant) of Australia. The flower parts mimic the shape, colourings and even the odour of the female wasp, and the impersonation is so convincing that the male thynnine wasp, track this odour to an orchid, and tries to copulate but in fact to pick up the petal. In the course of the attempt, the males body comes into contact with pollen bearing sacs, of the flower. The sticky pollinia adhere to the male and when male thynnine wasp finally gives up the futile task of trying to carry the "female" away, the pollen sac go with him. The pollen sac bearing thynnine wasp male tries the same act with another orchid flower and transfer pollen to the orchid flower, pollinating it rather than a female of his species. Further studies tells that the males learn, probably from the unrewarding consequences of grappling with orchid flowers, not to respond to odours coming from orchid plants. Thus, the male wasps habituate to stimuli, learning not to respond to cues that originally triggered copulatory attempts.

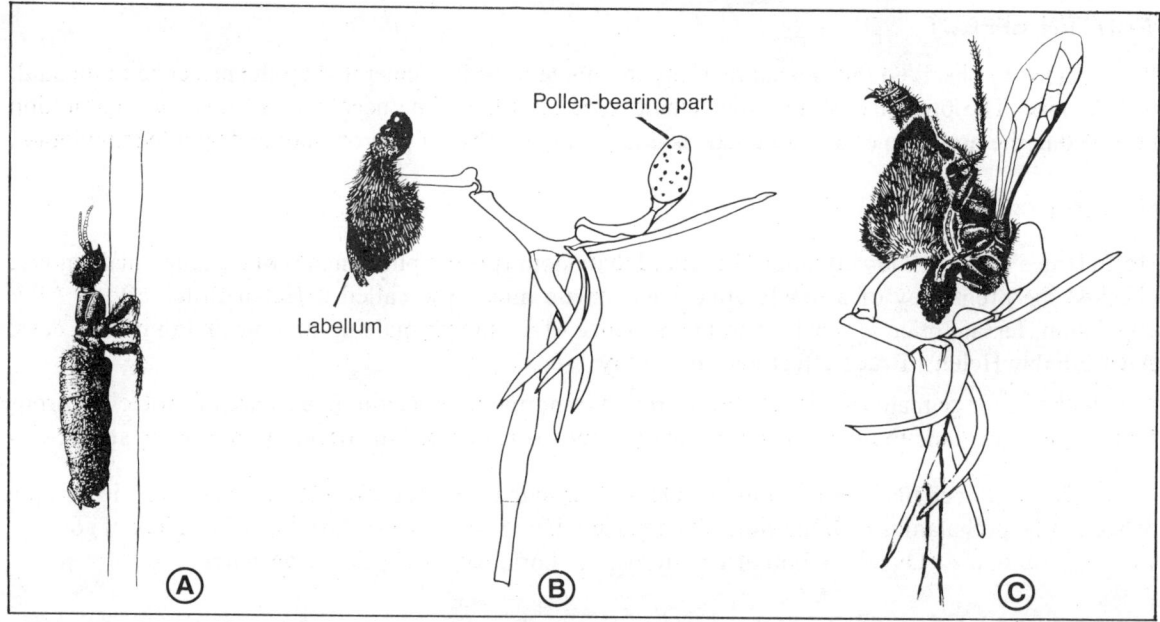

Fig. 3.32. Example of Mimetic Sex Pheromone (A) A wingless female thynnine wasp on her perch, where she releases a sex-pheromone that will attract males of her species; (B) An Australian orchid with a highly modified petal, the labellum that vaguely resembles and smells like a wingless, pheromone releasing female wasp; (C) Male thynnine wasp trying to mate with an Australian orchid flower.

In context of mimetic sex pheromone produced by orchid plants, question arises that this happened accidently in course of evolution of orchid plant or something else forced orchid plants to achieve pollination by this means. The question needs further research for answer.

APPLICATION OF PHEROMONES FOR THE WELFARE OF MANKIND

Pheromones are useful in captive breeding of pet and wild animals. It also helps in breed improvement of poultry, horses, cattles, dogs, pigs, goats and sheep. A sow in heat recognises a boar by the scent emitted by his saliva. For artificial insemination a person applies pressure on the back of sow (which is applied by mounting boar) and sprays artificial pheromone of boar. After then the sow allows the insertion of spiracle and semen through which artificial insemination is achieved.

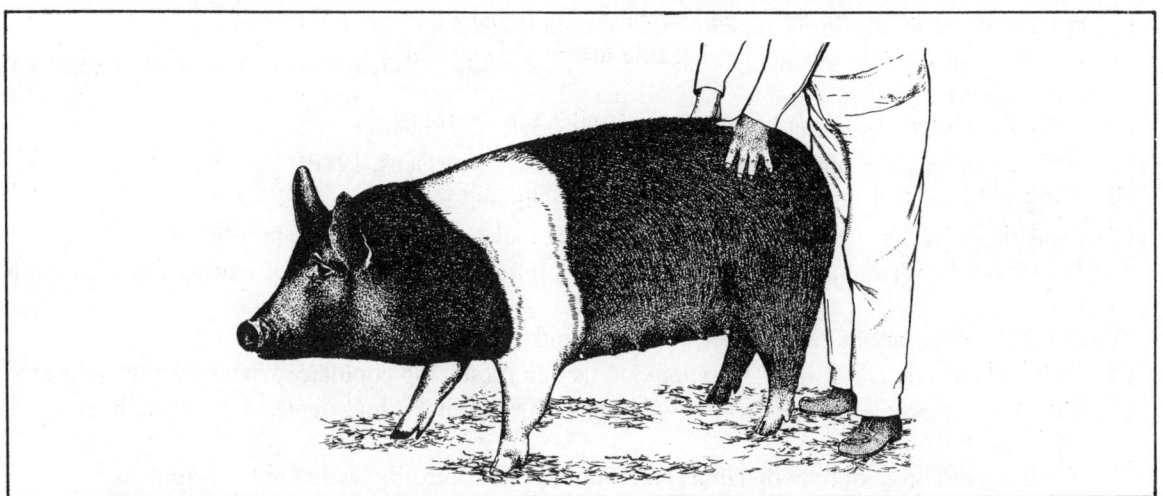

Fig. 3.33. Artificial insemination of sow using artificial pheromone and mount pressure.

With the help of pheromones, we can apply a eco-friendly way of controlling insect pests. Use of artificially synthesized sex - attractant pheromones, harmful insects like mosquitoes, flies, cockroaches etc. can be eliminated from our habitat. We can use aggregation pheromones which attract them to come together and make groups. Now mass killing of insects can be done by applying insecticide at a confined place. The battle between man and insects is going on and this method to control harmful insect pests is cheaper, safer and eco- friendly.

EXERCISE

1. What composes behaviour of animals ? Mention important factors composing animal behaviour. Explain the mechanism of their functioning.
2. Mention some examples, supporting the statement that genetic makeup of an individual determine behaviours.
3. Describe the case of cross of two different species of love birds to produce intermediate form in context of transporting nesting material.
4. Describe avoidance learning in mice in context of "gene environment interaction", determining behaviour.
5. Write in 50 lines the methods for studying "physiological and chemical routes from genes to behaviour"
6. Describe the role of genes in *chemotaxis* in the bacterium *e. coli* investigated by J. Adler.
7. Describe behaviour genes discovered in *Drosophila*.
8. Describe Hirsch and Kimling's investigation about *geotactic behaviour* of *Drosophila melanogaster*.
9. Describe polygenic inheritance of *calling songs behaviour* of crickets (*Teleogryllus commodus*).
10. Write a short note on "genetically induced behavioural disorders in human beings".

11. Write a short note on gene causing *Schizophrenia* and *Maniac depression* in man.

12. Write a short note on "Behavioural effect of hormone" in only 200 words.

13. What do you mean by Neuroendocrine control upon behaviour? Describe functions of hypothalamus in Vertebrates. (Civil services, 1989)

14. Discuss the relationship of the endocrine system to behaviour. (Civil services, 1987)

15. Discuss with suitable example, what role the pheromones play in animal behaviour ? (Civil services, 1986)

16. Write an account on insect pheromone. (Civil services, 1889)

17. Distinguish between pheromone and hormones. (Civil services, 1986)

18. Write short notes on Invertebrate endocrine system and behaviour.

19. Parasitic castration ? How Sacculina change the male sex of host crab into femaleness.

20. Describe a few interesting cases of Endocrines influencing behaviour of fishes, birds and mammals.

21. Describe important human endocrine system and its role on behaviour.

22. Write 50 lines on *Genotype - Hormone* interaction producing copulatory behaviour in chickens.

23. Give some examples of "different behaviours of same individual treated with same hormone in different seasons".

24. Write in brief "role of hypothalamus and pituitary" in controlling behaviour of animals.

25. Write short notes on Importance of pheromones in human life.

26. Define pheromone and give brief history of discovery of pheromone.

27. Describe different pheromone producing glands and pheromone receiving organs in insects.

28. Classify and describe pheromones in 200 lines only.

29. Describe mimetic sex pheromone in context of mating attempt of male thynnine wasps with orchid flower.

30. How pheromones can be used for welfare of mankind. Discuss in brief.

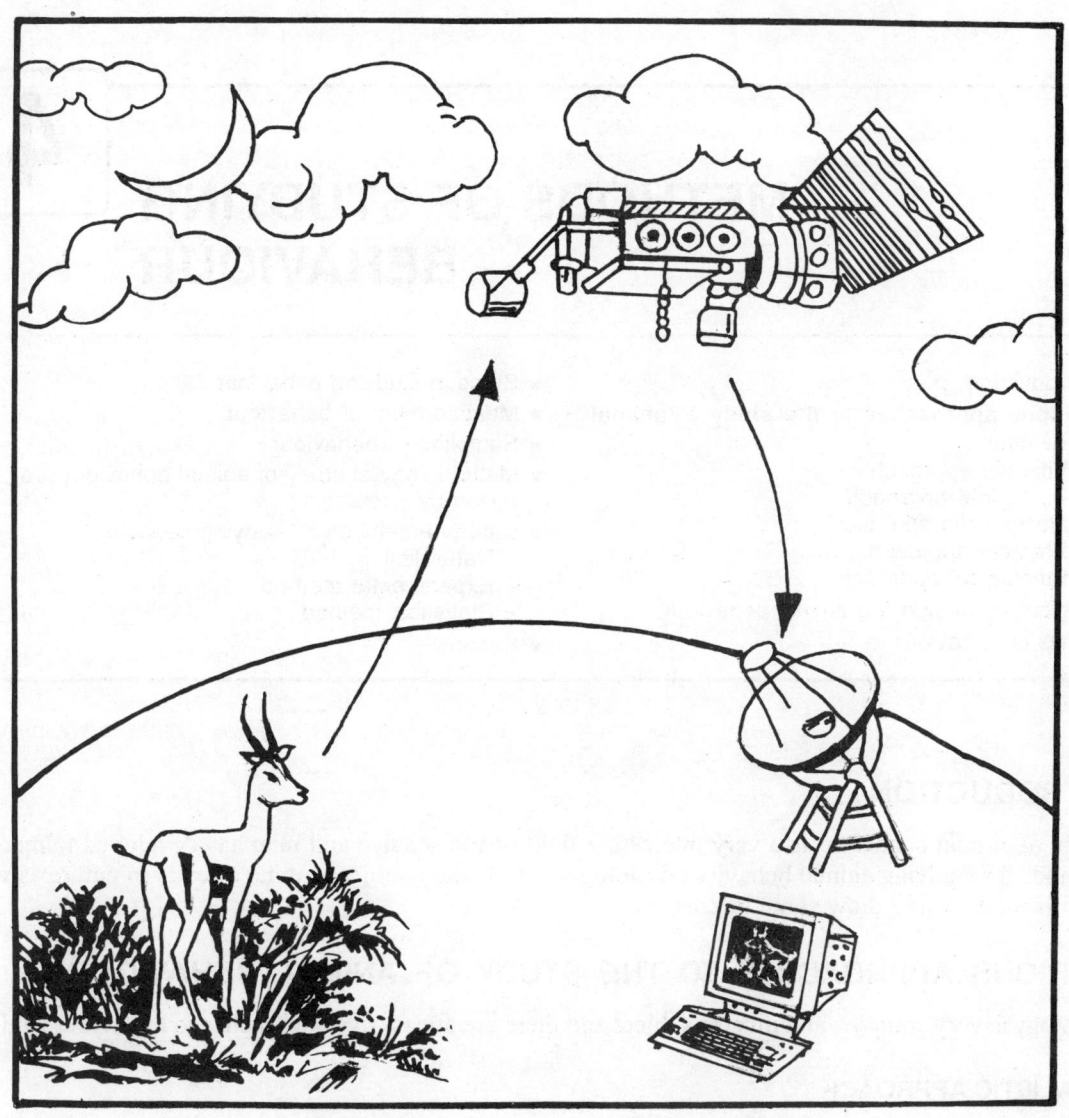

*S*tudy of animal behaviour is most challenging field of biology and man has developed numerous methods for doing so. Watching activities of animals and simply presenting the facts has been one of the old hobbies of man. Methods of study of animal behaviour by ethologists is different from casual watching. They observe animal behaviour with some purpose and test alternative explanations to draw some inferences. This chapter describes different methods of studying animal behaviour.

METHODS OF STUDYING BEHAVIOUR

INTRODUCTION

Study of animal behaviour is a very interesting field of life science and man has developed numerous methods for studying animal behaviour. Ethologists study their subject animal directly in nature as well as in laboratory and draw some inferences.

VARIOUS APPROACHES TO THE STUDY OF ANIMAL BEHAVIOUR

Ethology is very complex and diverse subject and there are atleast five approaches to behaviour studies.

VITALISTIC APPROACH

Behavioural activities of animals and its relation with the changes in the environment is vitalistic approach. It involves the total rejection of any study of the animal outside its natural environment. The technique has its foundations in natural history and has provided a wealth of valuable data.

ECOLOGICAL APPROACH

Relation between the behaviour of a species and other living beings along with non - biotic components of environment is ecological approach. Ecological approach proceed in two ways. It can focus either on a group of species or on a particular habitat. In focussing on the habitat, one would be interested in the parallel behavioural adaptations which are found in certain habitat. This suggests the divergent and convergent evolution of behaviour.

MECHANISTIC APPROACH

This approach is an experimental approach and involves the study of particular aspects of behaviour under controlled conditions in a laboratory. This technique is however, used extensively in psychology and was pioeered by Pavlov, Skinner, Kohler and Koffka. This approach may be criticised on the grounds of the artificiality of the experimental situation.

PHYSIOLOGICAL APPROACH

It involves the physiological basis of behaviour. Its branches – Ethogenetics, Neuroethology, Ethoendocrinology and Pheromone–ethology deals with the relation between genetics, nervous system, hormones, pheromones and behaviour respectively. We have studied in Chapter 3 that Genetics, Nervous System, Hormones, Pheromones etc. play vital role in composing behaviours in species.

ETHOLOGICAL APPROACH

This is the contemporary approach of behavioural investigations and an attempt to explain responses, observed in the field and in terms of the stimuli, eliciting the behaviour, it involves both of the techniques outlined above, and given by Lorenz, Frisch and Tinbergen.

DIFFICULTIES IN STUDYING ANIMAL BEHAVIOUR

1. Animals exhibit an extraordinary degree of diversity in their behaviour. Two species do not behave in the same manner and all individuals of one species do not behave in all respects exactly in the same manner. Moreover, the same individual do not respond exactly in the same way all the time. Therefore, it is difficult to formulate behaviour like physical science.
2. The study of more than one behaviour simultaneously is even more difficult.
3. We use our sense organs to interpret the behaviour of animals. The interpretation of inferences drawn by us may be wrong. Colour vision of honeybees is different from human vision. Our eye is not sensitive to Uv rays but honeybees are sensitive to it. Flowers that appear to us to be white in sunlight may have distinct patterns when viewed in Uv light. A dog is able to smell a variety of

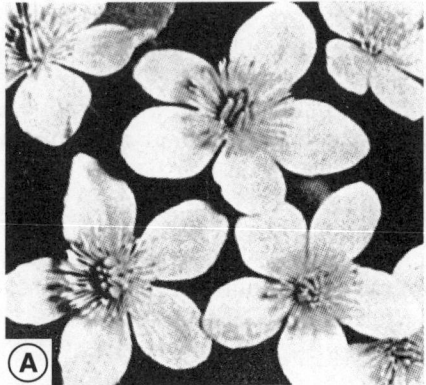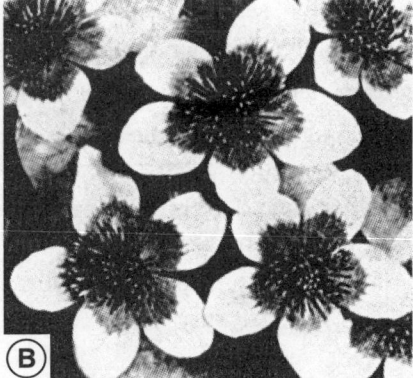

Fig. 4.1. Flowers look different in colour when seen in two different lights : (A) The picture records what the human eye can see and the flower has no nectar guide pattern. (B) The picture is the view which approximates to what a bee sees, photographed through an ultraviolet sensitive system, a striking colour pattern is revealed.

smells all meaning something to him but many of them may remain completely unrealized to the human olfactory organ. The dogs are able to hear sound waves of very low frequency (lower than 5 hertz) which is not possible to hear for us.

4. While studying animal behaviour man tends to put himself in the place of subject animal, thinking that the subject animal observes, perceives and feels in the same way as he does. We usually infer that a growling dog is angry, a chirping bird is happy, a purring cat is contented, a wide - eyed deer in frightened. But we do not know whether animals have way of expression exactly like human emotions. The interpretation of the behaviour of animals, as if they think in human terms is called *anthropomorphism*.

5. Ethologists studying animal behaviour in nature face hazards of encountering dangerous animals and plants, bad weather, variable food supply, monotony and above all life threat from poachers. Dian Fossy devoted her life studying behaviour of Gorillas in jungles of Africa. Fossy's concern and protectiveness about Gorilla population led to her murder by the poachers.

UNITS OF BEHAVIOUR

One behaviour includes a large number of short acts called units of behaviour. Territorial behaviour, courtship behaviour, mounting, copulation, post copulatory acts etc. combine together in hierarchical order to represent *sexual behaviour*. Here sexual behaviour is one behaviour and territorial, courtship, mounting, copulation etc. are units of sexual behaviour.

STEPS IN STUDYING BEHAVIOUR

Observation of animal behaviour is done stepwise. The important steps are :

1. Selection of behaviour pattern
2. Objectives of study
3. Synopsis of research
4. Chalking out of the unit of behaviour
5. Deciding an appropriate methodology
6. Reconnaissance observation
7. Taking notes i.e. making ethogram.

While recording behaviour, *states*, *events* and *bouts* are noted down specifically.

State : An on going behaviour, like a peacock pheasant dancing, a pigeon flying, a bird making a nest are called state. This kind of behaviour can be timed with a watch.

Event : Change of state is event. For example, a dove taking off or landing. Events generally occur so rapidly that they can only be counted.

Bout : A repetitive occurrence of the same behaviour is called bout. For example, pecking of grains by pigeons.

MEASUREMENT OF BEHAVIOUR

Measurement of the behaviour is the assignment of numbers to animal's behaviour. In general there are four scales of measurement.

1. NOMINAL SCALE

On a nominal scale numbers are used as labels and no ranking is possible. Each number functions as a label attached to an animal. For example, pregnant women in a nursing home could be labelled 1, 2, and 3 corresponding to the classification – normal, diabetic and hypertensive.

2. ORDINAL SCALE

Scores can be assigned to the observations in such a way that the rankings obtained are meaningful, for example, in a survey on effect of hormone on sexual behaviour result may be ranked according to the scale:

(i) Poor i.e. no effect
(ii) Fairly effective i.e. slight effect
(iii) Good effect i.e. elicit desired response
(iv) Very good effect i.e. elicit response in no time
(v) Very strong i.e. elicit response strongly and in no time.

3. INTERVAL SCALE

It measures the property of number called additivity. Here the numbers assigned to animals tell us that the animals labelled by them are distinct from each other. They also tell us how much different one animal is from the other in respect of the measured characteristic. All arithmetical and statistical operations fitting the nominal and ordinal scales can be applicable to the interval scale.

4. RATIO SCALE

A ratio scale is so called, because the ratio between the numbers assigned to the points on the scale signify the ratio of the measured values of the objects to whom the numbers are assigned. As the ratio scale shares with the interval scale the properties of additivity and equality of intervals can be applied arithmetically and statistically. Scales of measurement of behaviour have been summarized in the Table 4.1.

Table 4.1 Different scales of measurement of behaviour

Scale	Measurement requirements	Behaviour pattern
Nominal	Mutually exclusive and totally inclusive category	Presence or absence of aggressiveness, emotion etc.
Ordinal	A unidimensional scale	Possessing peak order maternal behaviour etc.
Interval	A unidimensional scale	Possessing intelligence and learning
Ratio	A unidimensional scale	Possessing physiological scale of loudness – brightness – pitch

SAMPLING OF BEHAVIOUR

Behaviour can be studied in different levels. Accepted levels are *species, population, family, dyad, individuals, body parts, muscles, neurones* etc. The ethologist must observe two things : (1) He/she must decide at what level work will be conducted and how the study will integrate into what is already known at the levels. (2) Ethologists should prepare a written description in accurate, complete, clear and concise method. Set of comprehensive descriptions of the characteristic behaviour patterns of a species population/individual prepared consistently is called *ethogram*.

Table 4.2. Ethogram prepared on some units of sexual and reproductive behaviour of rat

1. *Primary contact & encouragement for contact (courtship)*: Nasal–nasal, Nasal–anus (movement in circle).
2. *Sexual* : Male follow opposite sex, climbing of male, embrace female with the help of fore limbs, penetrate male genitalia into female genitalia, discharge semen. Female raise the tail, show lordosis, catch hold of neck of male. After copulation and separation clean genitalia.
3. *Agonistic (aggressive) for territory* : Threat, attack, follow, escape, turn, separate, bite, physical combat, defend by keeping back in front of the enemy.
4. *Social behaviour* : Sand bathing, tunnel marking, contact on ventral and lateral surface, rub anal part on the wall of tunnel.

METHODOLOGY OF STUDY OF ANIMAL BEHAVIOUR PROPOSED BY ALTMANN

Most widely accepted methodology of study of animal behaviour was proposed by **Altmann** (1974) in which following points are important: (1) Ad libitum (2) Focal animal (3) Scan or instantaneous sampling (4) All occurrences (5) Sequence sampling and (6) One – zero.

1. **Ad libitum :** One selects a species of animal and lives with them in their habitate for a required period and behaviour of interest is noted.

2. **Focal animal sampling :** Selected individual of interest gets the highest priority for recording its behaviour. If an ethologist is interested in studying mother and infant relationship in rhesus monkey in nature, then he/she identifies some female rhesus monkeys wearing infants individually by using body cues. Now ethogram is prepared in a definite time or period.

Different methods are adopted to identify individual member. Individual member of a species bear identifiable individual marks. With the help of natural individual marks, behaviour of deer, lion, porpoises etc. have been studied. The age and sex of the individual also help in identification. In absence of natural marks, animals are captured and marked either by colour/ number/plates tagged on convenient part of body. Physical alterations such as cutting feathers, horns, tails, ear etc. or making scars on body, help in identification. After marking, animals are set free and observed by various methods.

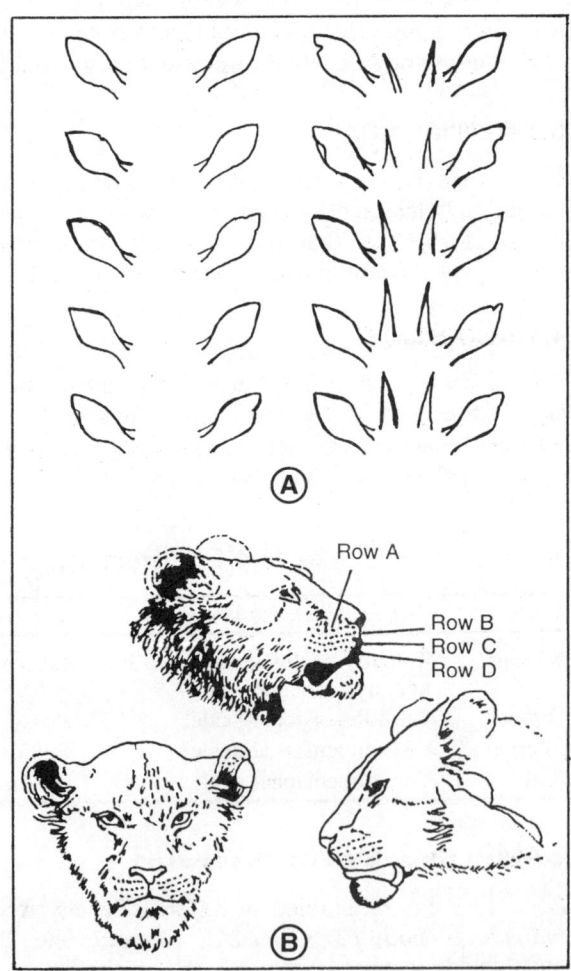

Fig. 4.2. Identification of different individuals : (A) In deer group on the basis of pinna. (B) By arrangement of their vibrissae in lions.

3. **Scan sampling** : Several individuals of a species are observed one after the other in quick succession in pre-determined time interval. Their behavioural acts are noted on a well designed checklist. One of the important uses of this method is to estimate the percentage of time the individuals of a group spent in various prejudiced activities. Suppose, one wants to know how do members of a Hanuman langur group make foraging programme in respect of time in a day/week or month? Then, three criteria have to be decide. (1) Activities we are interested in (2) Time duration for scan, depending upon the size group (3) Duration of interval.

4. **All occurrence sampling** : Only one behaviour is taken into account and recording of all concerned units is done carefully. While studying the interaction between two species of animals one can note what kind of interactions was there, agonistic or amicable? If agonistic then whether it was chase, overthrow, threat or something else? All occurrence of selected behaviour is possible if three factors exist. These factors are (i) Observation conditions are adequate (ii) the behaviours have been carefully defined so that they are easily recognised (iii) the behaviours do not occur more often than the observers can note them.

5. **Sequence Sampling** : The attention is focussed on a chain of behaviour of an individual. For example, courtship displays by male grebes, nest building by a male weaver bird etc. In sequence sampling observation is done right from the beginning to the end of the behaviour.

6. **One - zero sampling** : Only the two extreme end of a behaviour is studied. Whether behaviour occurs (one) or not (zero) during sampling. This method has five features :
   (i) In each sample period the occurrence or no occurrence is scored.
   (ii) Behaviour of one or two individuals is recorded in each sample period.
   (iii) Occurrence refers to either an event or a state.
   (iv) The sample periods are generally short.
   (v) Results are presented as frequencies (number of sample periods in which it occurred divided by total number of sample periods).

DIFFERENT METHODS OF STUDYING BEHAVIOUR

Usually following three methods are used by ethologists for the study of animal behaviour : I. Naturalistic, II. Experimental, and III. Statistical.

I. NATURALISTIC

Systematic observation of activities of animals in wild is naturalistic study. Numerous ethologists devoted their lives and accumulated valuable informations on animal behaviour by staying with wild animals in their habitat. J.V.L. Goodall spend more than 40 years in the forests of Tanzania in Comb National Parks to study different behaviours of chimpanzees *(Pan)*. A young Japanese named Takayoshi Kano (1973) dared to enter in Africa's most remote and dangerous jungle to know behaviour of a ape called Bonobo. This ape is our evolutionary cousins about whom we were unaware till 1973. Dian Fossy devoted her life studying different behaviours of Gorillas in jungles of Africa. She used to spend so much time with them that she was virtually accepted as one of the members of their population. George B. Schaller spend about 3000 hours in studying behaviour of African lions and wrote excellent books on their behaviour. I. Devore carried out exhaustive observations on baboons. Done and his colleagues used 7,334 meter cinema film to study courtship behaviour of golden eye ducks.

Some precautionary measures is a must while studying animals in wild.

1. Observation of behaviour of wild animals in their habitat should be done without any interference. To solve or minimise the effect of outside factor interference atleast two types of precautions

must be taken. (a) Observer should hide himself in bushes or caves or watch from towers. (b) Make animals used with observer during observation so that their behaviour may not be influenced and modified.

Observer makes small hole in their hinding place so as to fit binocular, lens of camera, telescope, video camera. etc. through which activities of animals are observed and recorded.

Another problem is to locate wild animals. Many instruments are used in locating wild animals for studying their behaviour. Atleast four methods are used to locate and study behaviour of wild animals.

(a) *Foot print* : Animal (especially mammals) is located individually by its foot print. Tigers are identified by their peg marks.

(b) *Radio-telemetry* : Radio transmitter have been used for locating wild animals. A mini radiotransmitter is fitted in the suitable part of animal. For this purpose, first of all, tranquilizer is injected in the body of individual animal with the help of shot gun. A mini radiotransmitter is fitted in the body of the tranquilized animal. Now the animal is set free in the forest or sea. The observer keeps a receiver which is tuned with the transmitter. With the help of receiver, observer follow the animal and observe its behaviour. Radio tracking system has been made completely automatic by transferring time and directional information in a computer.

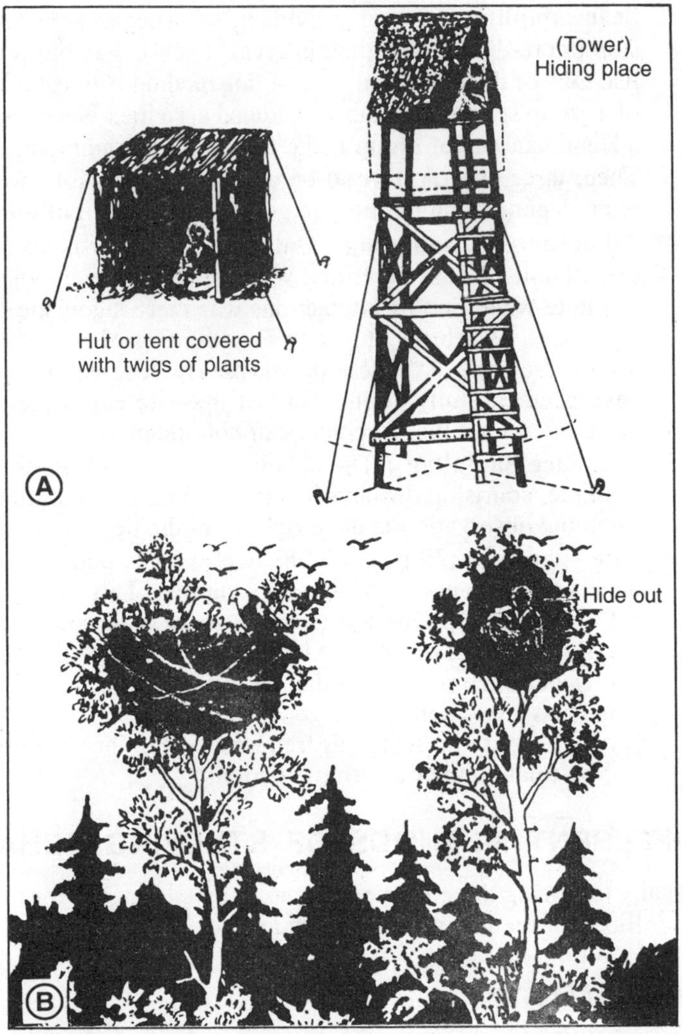

Fig. 4.3. Study of wild animals : (A) Tower for observation of behaviour of wild animals. (B) Study of Birds : To study behaviour of birds a hide out made on tree.

(c) *Satellite telemetry* : This system consists of two polar orbiting stations– United States National Oceanic and Atmospheric Administration Satellites with numerous earth based receiving stations and data processing center. Satellites collect and process data from radio fitted animals from earth.

Satellite telemetry system has successfully tracked elephants, musk ox, polar bears, dugong and many other species (O'shea and Kochman, 1990). The signals which are given out from

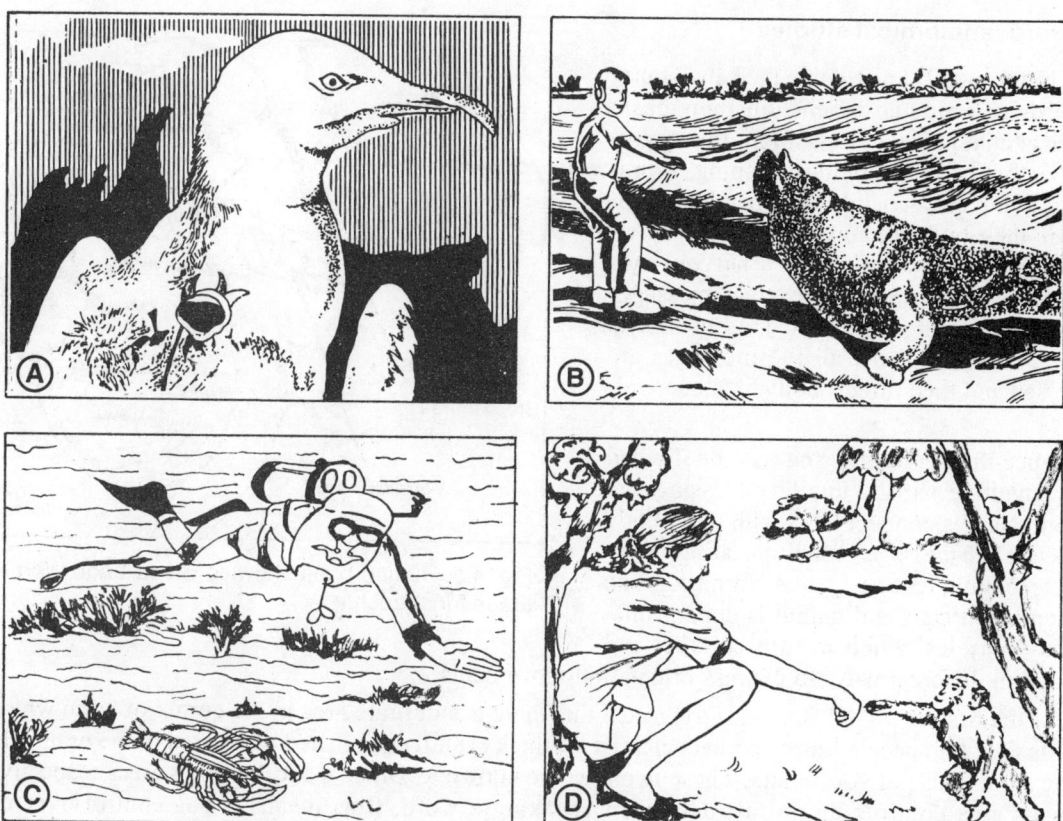

Fig. 4.4. Radio Transmitter for tracking animal: (A) A herring gull fitted with a ratio - transmitter for observation of foraging behaviour. (B) A scientist recording the voice of a sea lion on sea shore. (C) A scientist tracking the lobster for knowing the path of their migration. (D) Jane Goodall making friendship with a baby chimpanzee.

radio are received by satellite, which directs them to the earth to be received by a dish linked to computer for analysis of its activities.

(d) *Modern electronic gadgets* : Many modern equipments are used for studying animal behaviour in wild. These equipments are tape recorder, video photography, cinematography, recording polygraph etc.

Computer application is a new method for recording rhythms in animals developed by Prof. R.P. Reize and Mr. Rangarajan Kumar Swamy. Subbaraj and Chandra Shekharan studied the behaviour of 32 mice through computer application in circadian rhythm research.

II. EXPERIMENTAL METHODS

The study of behaviour in laboratory by experiments is carried out by utilizing following three methods.

1. Neuro-anatomical studies.
2. Neuro-physiological studies.
3. Neuro-chemical studies.

1. Neuro–anatomical studies

This is universally known that the behavioural patterns of animals depend on their basic physical anatomical composition. In any animal, activities like running, jumping, swimming, flying etc. depends on appendages present in their body. In animal, all these activities are mainly controlled by a nervous system. In short, this system receives messages from surrounding, and also gets messages from within the body, all the messages are analysed and then directs body to act accordingly.

Hence the nervous system can be divided into cognitive parts – input, processing and output. Nerves connect CNS with other body parts just like message - communicating cables in telecommunication system. Input is done by sensory organs and output is done primarily by muscles which in turn contract and expand in different ways to express orientation movements.

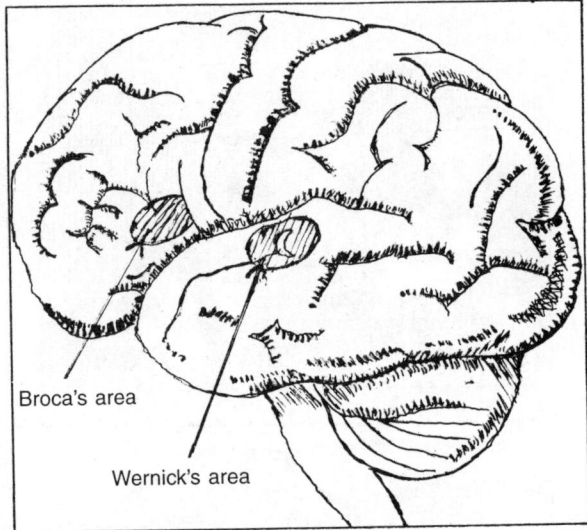

Fig. 4.5. Human brain showing Broca's and Wernick's areas for speech.

For the first time Paul Broca (1861) stated that there is a definite area in the cortex of brain which is responsible for speech. Later another scientist Wernick (1880) established other area in the brain which is the store house of vocabulary. These two area are known as Broca's and Wernic's areas respectively. Broca's area controls the infrastructure for speaking a word, (this means it has control over neck muscles and larynx) and Wernick's area is word retriever or dictionary. A lesion in Broca's area causes stammering in speech and there is difficulty in understanding the words spoken by such a person though the person would talk sensibly. If there is lesion in Wernick's area then the person can talk clearly but the speech is not coherent.

Many centers in the brain responsible for particular behavioural types have been identified. In an experiment, rhesus monkeys were subjected to choose between object of varying shapes and were rewarded by banana for picking up the triangular one. Monkeys with their visual cortex removed could no longer perform this test. It suggests that visual cortex is the part involved in learning to discriminate between various shapes.

The median hypothalamus and ductal grey matter of the midbrain are controlling centres of aggression and defect in cats. Discovery of different nuclei of hypothalamus and their role in controlling vital activities like feeding, drinking, sleep, aggression, mating etc. were made using neuroanatomical techniques.

2. Neuro-physiological studies

Several methods of studying physiology of nervous system at its unit level i.e. physiology of neurones has given a new direction to ethology. The proper study of neuronal physiology began from 1942 but this kind of study was performed by a physiologist Malpighii in the 17th century. The Italian scientist Galvani (1793) discovered that the muscles and nerves produce electricity. This finding laid the foundation of electrophysiology. The discovery that the messages in nervous tissue travel in the form of electric current led to a finer neurophysiological method to study behaviour. Following method are applied to study neurophysiological activities.

(A) Recording of Bioelectric Events

Since the beginning of 19th century practice of recording the electrical potential of active nerves with the aid of implanted electrodes is going on. For the measurement of electric current and voltage, very fine electrodes of glass are inserted into neurones. The diameter of those electrodes is about 0.1 to 0.5 m. Electric current released by neurone is very low and hence it is measured in millivolts i.e. 1/1000 by special amplifier. Electrical impulse released by neurones are recorded by oscilloscope for visual analysis. These techniques has now become a routine tool of neurophysiologists and neuroethologists. Study of electrical activity in different parts of brain is possible with the help of stereotaxic machine. The first successful recording of brain waves from the skull of man was done by Berger in 1929. He named this technique as EEG – Electro Encephalogram. R.W. Hess (1930) got success in recording brain waves in cats. His research was honoured with Nobel Prize in the year 1945.

Neurophysiological experiments are carried in two different ways.

(a) The first one involves *recording of the normal electrical impulses* in brain and correlating them with behaviour.

(b) The second method is *Stimulation, Ablation* and *Lesioning* of some points of brain of animals and studying its effect on behaviour.

(a) Recording of the normal electrical impulses

Four types of electrical brain waves have been recorded in the brain of human being : (i) *Alpha waves* (α-waves); (ii) Beta waves (β-waves); (iii) Theta waves (θ-waves); and (iv) *Delta waves* (δ-waves).

(i) **Alpha waves** (α–waves) : Produced from parietal and occipital lobes. These waves are produced when the person is at rest with eyes closed. At this time man is awaken, remaining in peaceful relaxed mood.

(ii) **Beta waves** (β–waves) : These waves are produced from frontal lobe when brain is stimulated by sensory input or mental activity. These waves occur at the time of thought and in normal daily alertness.

(iii) **Theta waves** (θ–waves) : These waves are produced from temporal and occipital lobes when man is under emotional stress. Theta waves are associated with earliest stage of sleep, hallucination and creativity.

(iv) **Delta waves** (δ–waves) : These waves are produced during deep sleep.

(b) Stimulation, Ablation and Lesioning

Complex behaviour patterns can be produced by *electrical stimulation* of certain parts of the central nervous system. Many controlling loci

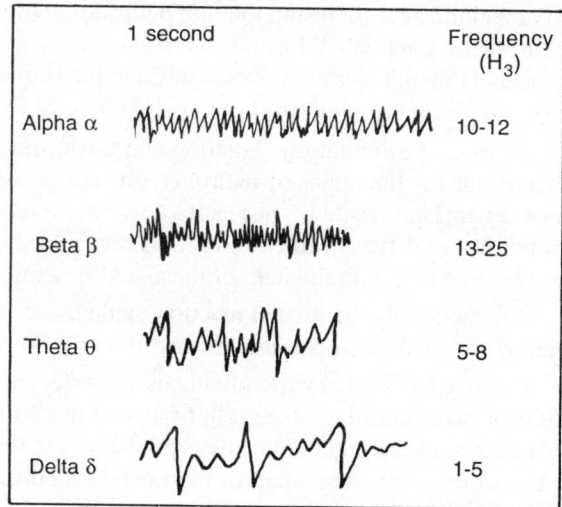

Fig. 4.6. Electrical Impulses and Behaviour : Recording of the normal electrical impulses in brain and correlating them with behaviour.

are identified in birds and mammals (rats, cats, dogs, etc) including human beings by technique of electrical stimulation. In this process different regions of CNS is stimulated by electrode implantation and relation between the area stimulated and the behaviour observed is established. In the electrical stimulation of attack behaviour, the rooster is stimulated by electrodes implanted in a particular part of its brain. Rooster starts to move towards the keeper and as stimulation is continued it attacks. J. Flynn (1929) elicited prey catching behaviour in a cat by stimulating a particular locus in the diencephalon.

A. Zukerman (1965) was able to develop behaviours like fleeing, courtship and threat by electrical stimulation in different regions of a pigeon's brain. E. Von Holst and Von Saint Paul (1960) could elicit sleeping behaviour in cock by stimulating the brain stem. Holst and Paul gave an interesting finding that when two separate areas of the brain responsible for contrast behavioural patterns are stimulated simultaneously, a very different responses take place. T. Brown (1967) identified two separate loci in a cat's brain that induced growl and flee. Simultaneous stimulation of these two loci produced aggressive behaviour. Suppose two areas in brain A and B are stimulated then the following variation might occur:

(i) Superposition of both patterns ($A + B$)

(ii) Average ($A + B/2$)

(iii) Alternate ($B, A, B,$ or A, B, A)

(iv) Disappearance ($A + B = 0$) and

(v) Suppression of one of the patterns (A or B).

To know the relationship between particular neural structure and behaviour, method of *ablation* and *lesioning* of brain parts was in practice in 19th century. But in the beginning of 20th century these techniques were dropped as these were crude methods. Later different finer methods came into existence. Now-a-days laser beams is used for lesion purpose which is safer and less injurious to experimental animal.

In ablation certain regions of the brain are destroyed and their function is deduced from the abnormal behaviour it causes in the animal. The *ablation* (removal of tissue) or *lesion* (pathological changes in tissue) may be done by surgery but small lesions are produced by passing electric current or by neurotoxic kainite acid. In lesion method neurones are inhibited or destroyed while in the stimulation method neurones are activated. Lesions were made by aspiration (suction of small part of brain with a machine) in which thin needles are inserted through the skull and small part of brain is sucked out. Lesions are also made by freezing small portions with cryogeny.

Process of Stimulation, Ablation and Lesioning is useful only for recording superficial neural stimulation but for the study of neurones present in deep sheet of brain some advanced and sophisticated instruments are needed. These are known as *stereotaxic instruments*. With the help of these instruments condition of different internal parts is received. Stereotaxic maps of brain of many animals have been made available with the help of these instruments.

After studying the mental reaction made by stimulation, the animal is killed and its brain and areas of nervous system are operated out and then the fine sections are cut and studied under microscope.

Lashley performed experiments on the effect of brain lesions on learning. He investigated the retention of maze learning in rat, after parts of the cortex had been removed. In one of his experiments he used a maze with eight blind alleys on the way to the goal box. All the rats were trained to their maximum performance and then a part of their cerebral cortex was removed equally and symmetrically from both hemisheres. When the rats had recovered from the operation, they were re-tested in the maze and their errors scored over a number of re-learning trials. The lesions amounting to score 10% of the cortex have little effect but beyond these errors, begin to rise.

Now the brain is being explored for its various functions using *tomographic techniques*. Tomographic techniques include any method that produces images of cross-section of the body reconstructed by a computer programme. This is most widely used technique with reference to behaviour and is known as PET (Position Emission Tomography). It has been discovered that there is more blood supply to the part of the brain which is actively controlling behaviour at that time. For this the person is given a special solution of sugar. This sugar is tagged with a radioisotope brewed in a small, low energy eyclotron, by tracing the radioactive substance. An expert doctor can pinpoint areas of normal and/or abnormal activities. The PET scanner detects the rate at which different parts of the brain use up this special test solution of sugar. A computer is attached to the PET scanner showing activity of brain in different colours on a TV screen.

Different spots were obtained in different areas of brain in a PET experiment performed on a person. When the person was allowed only to see, dark spot appeared at the back of the brain (Fig 4.7a) indicating that eyes of the object were open and the visual cortex was active. When the person was allowed to see and hear, a dark spot appeared on the left side of the brain (Fig. 4.7b) indicating that the spoken language was analysed by the left hemisphere. The dark spots in front indicated that the words heard brought the brain imagination and planning into action, Which is a function of frontal lobe. When the person was allowed to see and listen music, along with imagination and planning, music appreciation center on the right temporal lobe of the brain also activated. (Fig. 4.7c). When the person listened to music from one ear, friend from other ear and was also allowed to see. The PET scan showed dark spots at all sides (Fig. 4.7d).

III. STATISTICAL METHOD

Behavioural studies in the usual case yield time series data. Data may be collected from a complete record of the events at fixed interval of time or data may be collected on the sequence of activities without a time base on focal animal or their groups.

Statistical data help to draw inference concerning, conditions, durations, intervals and latency of behavioural acts. If the events in a time series are independent of one another there will be no significant correlation among the time of their occurrences. Auto correlation coefficient may be used to determine the existence of such correlations.

Table 4.3. Advantages and Disadvantages of Naturalistic, Experimental and Statistical analysis of behavioural traits of organisms

Methods	Advantages	Disadvantages
Naturalistic	Best way to acquire knowledge concerning natural behaviour patterns, both individual and social variables may be isolated for future experimental analysis	Lack of control may lead to ambiguity in interpretation
Experimental	Rigid control over environmental events. Ability to manipulate variables in systematic manner. Excellent for isolation of relevant antedecent conditions (causes).	Artificial or laboratory condition may affect generality off findings
Statistical analysis	Excellent for population. Relationship among many measures can be determined by correlation techniques. Does not imply causation	Lack of controls leads to difficulty in interpretations (correlation)

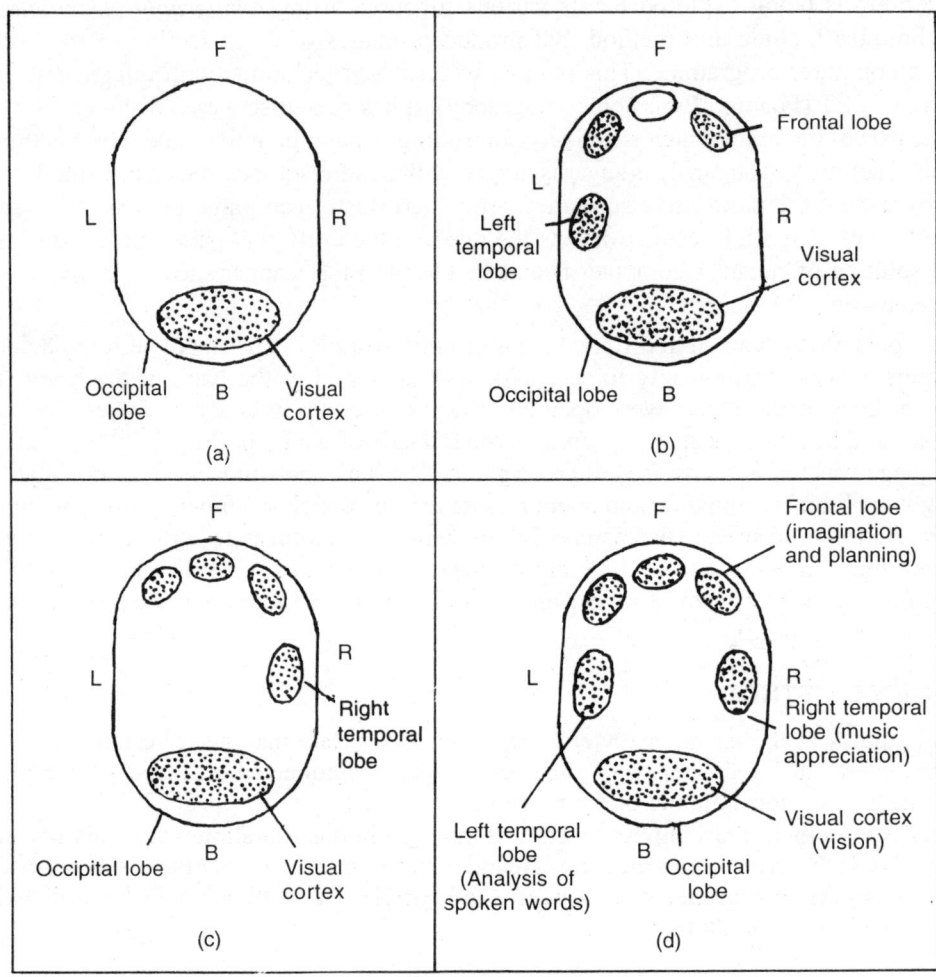

Fig. 4.7. Position Emission Tomography : Diagrammatic representation of PET scan photographs (a, b, c, d) performed on a human brain.

Descriptive statistical data are used to help to draw inference concerning condition which brought about change in statistical value, e.g.. it is known that density of animals may be related to geographical conditions (latitude, longitude, altitude), climate and other ecological aspects. Suppose we had data showing relative population densities of a species for a period of 10 years and a systematic shift out of one region into another was observed. We might be able to relate this shift to certain ecological factors and thus be able to predict that when certain aspects of the ecology changed there would be a movement out of a particular region.

Cluster analysis is particularly well suited for ethological purposes. Cluster analysis proceeds through computing similarity measures between behaviour types and grouping the entities by application of one of several algorithms available for the purpose. Cluster analysis is helpful in identifying common casual factors in behaviour.

Statistical data help us to describe certain behavioural events in terms of average, variability, correlation, etc.

Many significant results may be gained from multivariate data through principle component and factor analysis. The purpose is to examine variation within a population.

Multivariate analysis of variance and discriminant analysis technique provides powerful qualitative tools to examine the pattern in inter group behavioural phenomena.

EXERCISE

1. Mention important difficulties in studying behaviour of animals. Why is anthropomorphism a dangerous in interpreting the behaviour of animals.
2. Write short notes on Naturalistic, Experimental and Statistical methods of studying behaviour.
3. What are modern methods of studying animal behaviour ? Give example in brief a few old and new basic methods of studying animal behaviour.
4. Define unit of behaviour, components of behaviour, ethogram, scales of measurement of behaviour.
5. Describe observation of animal behaviour without interference, identification of individual animals, methods of locating animals in jungle.
6. Describe steps in studying behaviour and measurement of behaviour.
7. Give an account of sampling of behaviour.
8. Describe Neuroanatomical studies of animal behaviour in 100 lines only.
9. Describe different neurophysiological studies of animal behaviour.
10. Write short notes on Stimulation, Ablation and Lesioning of CNS parts and behaviour.
11. Describe independent and dependent variables under experimental methods.
12. Describe application of computer in studying behaviour.
13. Give a brief idea of various approaches to the study of animal behaviour.
14. Write about techniques given by Altman (1974) to study animal beahviour.
15. Describe different methods of studying behaviour.

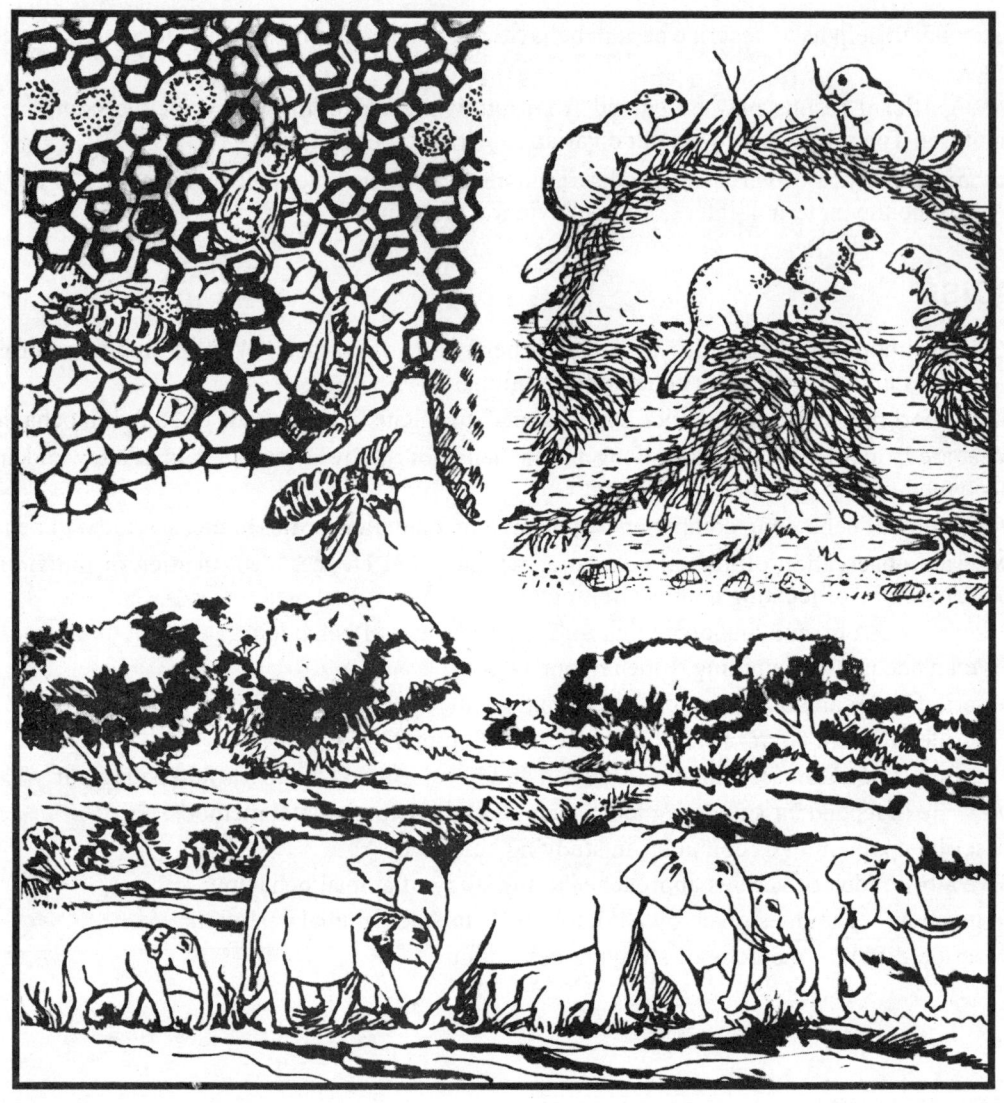

We have been taught from our childhood that the man is a social animal, but many of us might not be knowing that many other animals are also social. Tiny insects like honeybees, ants, wasps and termites are highly social. Insect society is 30 to 50 crore years old and their society is real paradise, where each member ceaselessly keeps on contributing for the welfare of the society without any personal greed, nepotism, lust or jealousy. Social life of insects, birds and mammals has attracted behaviourists and a good amount of literature is available on this topic. This chapter deals with interesting aspects of social behaviour of important social animal species.

ANIMAL SOCIETY   5

INTRODUCTION

The grouping of individuals of the same species for positive interaction between them is called society. In a society many individuals of a species live together in an integrated manner so that each contributes in some specialized way to the welfare of the society. Studies on social organization of animals began in an organized manner with the work of W.C.Allen (1938) and his students. Since then, serious studies in this field have accelerated rapidly and numerous ethologists provided valuable informations about different aspects of the social behaviour and social organization of different species of animals.

AGGREGATION AND SOCIETY

Chance gathering produced solely by external factors is called aggregation. Aggregation due to external factors breaks as soon as the prevailing factor disappears. School of fishes, herd of wildebeests and zebra are aggregation (not true society) and are also called as survival group. "Permanent union of individuals of same species living together by mutual positive interactions between them is called society." Alverdes considered societies to be genuine communities which exist by virtue of some particular social instinct. According to Tinbergen "positive interaction between one individual with other members of the same species in a society is known as social behaviour." The study of social behaviour is called sociobiology.

PROPERTIES OF SOCIAL GROUPS

Eisenberg, Wilson, Brown and Grier proposed some characteristics of social groups in their respective studies.

1. INVOLVEMENT OF MANY INDIVIDUALS

One of the most important characteristics of social behaviour involves the number of individuals of the same species that actively remain together in a group. A true society involves adults, subadults, juveniles, infants of different age and sex classes.

2. RECIPROCAL COMMUNICATION

Communication between conspecific through different ways is one of the essential elements for keeping the members of a society together.

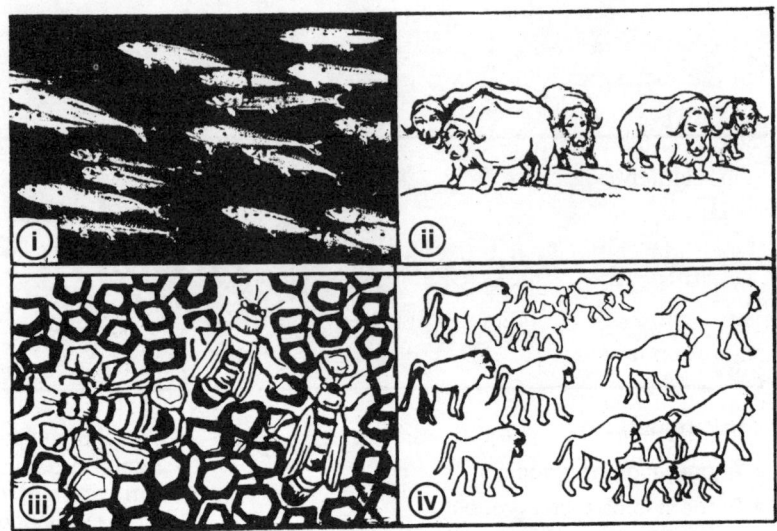

Fig. 5.1. Aggregation and society : (i) A school of fish (Mackerel) in aggregation called as survival group (ii) A herd of wild buffalo is also survival group. (iii) A colony of honeybee *(Apis florea)* representing true society. (iv) A group of baboon is a social group.

3. DIVISION OF LABOUR

Different members of a society perform different works. Division of labour is well marked in social insects and social mammals.

4. COHESION

The individuals constituting a society tend to remain in close proximity to one another. Countless ants, termites and bees (sometimes more than 50,000 honeybees) are found in one hive. Members in a troop of baboons while moving tend to remain in close proximity. The adult and dominant males (ADM) remain in the center close to females, while adult subdominant males (ASM) take dangerous positions at front.

5. PERMANENCE AND IMPERMEABILITY

Individuals making up a society tend to remain in its original form. Organized societies resist entry of outsiders.

6. OVERLAP OF GENERATION

Overlap of generation means "families of a few generations living together". In a highly developed social group there may be two or three generations that remain together throughout the entire year. In a herd of elephant there may be mother, daughter and grand daughters.

7. ALTRUISM

This is the way in which some members of a society spend time and energy in caring for other members of the society. Extreme altruism occurs all the time in colonies of termites, ants, some bees and wasps. Colonies containing thousands of workers cannot reproduce but instead sacrifice themselves in many ways for the welfare of other individuals of the society. An altruistic act increases the personal fitness of the recipient while it decreases the individual fitness of the donor. Altruistic behaviour had not previously been explained by the theory of natural selection.

Origin and existence of sterile castes among honeybees and termites poses a difficult problem for natural selection, as such individuals are not maximizing their own reproductive potential, instead, they work for the benefit of the colony. An interesting case of altruism in baboon is observed. The leader of the troop marches ahead of the team and encounters enemy first. It may be killed during encounter and then the other baboon takes the charge standing in second line of defence.

Parental care is a form of altruism. Parents invest in their offspring at the expense of their own survival and chances of future reproduction. The role of the sexes in parental care varies from species to species. Monkeys, apes and human beings exhibit many kinds of altruistic behaviour. Care of young is done not only by their parents but also by other members of the group called *aunt behaviour*.

In context of "altruism in primates" the example concerns "consorting", which is a habit of males. Many species live in multi–male groups. A male stays close to a female during the receptive phase of her oestrous cycle, and defends her from the advances of other males. It is an adaptation developed due to male competition component of sexual selection. In the olive baboon *(Papio anubis),* Craig Packer observed a rare phenomenon. Two male baboon occasionally co-operate to fight off a third male. Obviously, two will be stronger than one, which makes the advantage of co-operation. The advantage, however, is only for the one male that copulates with the female. Only one male is gainer, while the other male also had taken the risk of life in the fight, but gets no benefit. He has behaved altruistically. When another female in the troop comes into oestrus the role of the same two males is reversed. Male who had previously been "solicited" into co-operating to defend a female (but did not copulate with her), now copulates with this female. It is an example of "reciprocal altruism". Reciprocal altruism is found in species that form stable groups with individual recognistion.

Practice of donating blood and organs in humans appears to be case of altruism. The loss of blood carries a possible fitness cost to the donor and providing a fitness benefit to the recipient. The striking thing about the exchange is that the donor and recipient are not related and indeed are very unlikely ever to meet. Many human behaviours, like blood donating, organ donation (eye donation, kidney donation) child adoption etc. are very recent cultural phenomena in human society.

SOCIAL DIVERSITY

Animal kingdom can be divided into four pinnacles for studying social behaviour conveniently.

   I. Colonial lower invertebrates

  II. Colonial insects

 III. Non Mammal vertebrates : Fish, Amphibia, Reptile and Birds

 IV. Social Organization of Mammals

COLONIAL LOWER INVERTEBRATES

Aggregation of individuals for mutual benefit and interdependence are developed in some invertebrate species. Members of order Siphonophora, class Hydrozoa of the phylum Coelenterata (or Cnidaria) exhibit polymorphism which is a striking example of a colonial system. Individuals are physically united in colonies and specialize as non - reproductive or reproductive zooids.

Except class insecta of phylum Arthropoda true social system lack in other invertebrates. Many ethologists may not consider members of order Siphonophora (Obelia, Physalia – Portuguese man of war) as an example of social system because the entire colony comes from a single fertilized egg (zygote). The different zooids are formed by budding asexually. Here division of labour of several organ system have become so specialized that each organ system is working as an individual making a colonial system.

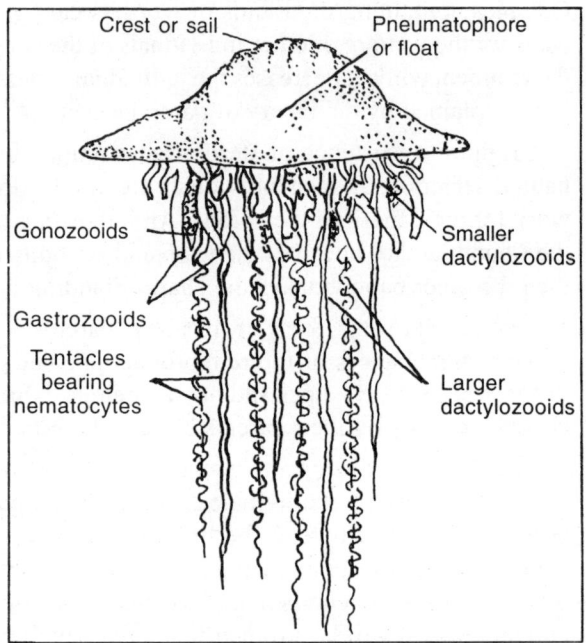

Fig. 5.2. Colonial System in Siphonophora : Physalia exhibiting colonial system. This can be treated as society or not is a matter of debate.

COLONIAL INSECTS

• Introduction • Social behaviour among members of order : • I. Hymenoptera - Honeybee - Wasp and Ants • II. Isoptera - Termites • Characteristics of social insects • Human and insect societies.

INTRODUCTION

Insect society is a wonder world, for more organised and functional in many ways in comparison to any other society. It is real paradise, where each member ceaselessly keeps on contributing for the welfare of the society and race continuity without any personal greed, lust or jealousy. Most species of honeybees, ants and wasps of order Hymenoptera and termites of order Isoptera of phylum Arthropoda are perfectly social.

SOCIAL BEHAVIOUR OF HONEYBEE

Nearly 500 species of bees are social. Social honeybee make a permanent house, made up of sheets of wax. In the spring, a honeybee colony that has grown sufficiently large will split in two, with the old queen and half her workers remain in old hive. Remaining workers along with a daughter, who will become a new queen make a new colony. Over the next few days, scout workers fly out in a mass around their queen workers make chambers in the ground, in cliff, and in hollow trees. There are often many such sites within range of the waiting swarm, but only some motivate a worker to perform a dance back at the swarm, a dance that communicates information about the distance, direction, and quality of the potential new home. Other workers attend to a dancing scout and may be sufficiently stimulated to fly out to the spot themselves. If it is attractive to them, they too will dance and send still more workers to the area. Eventually most scouts will be advertising one location, and then the swarm leaves its temporary perch and flies to the most popular nest site.

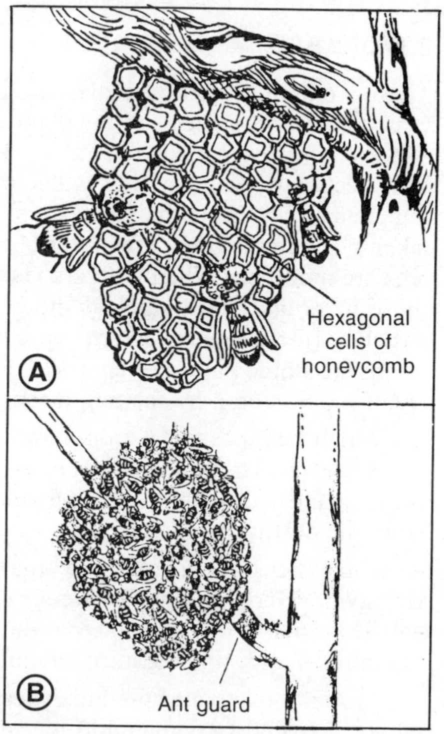

The worker bees produce wax for the formation of the new hive and are known as BUILDERS. New hive is made hanging vertically from rock, buildings or branches of trees. The house of honeybees is termed as hive or comb. It consists of thousands of hexagonal chambers of cells made up of wax secreted by the builder's abdomen. The resins and gums secreted by plants are also used for construction and repair of the hive.

The young are kept in the lower and central cells in the hive which are the "Brood cells". In *Apis dorsata* brood cells are similar in shape and size but in other species brood cells are of three types viz., worker cell for workers, drone cells for drones and queen cell for the queen. The queen cell is used once only while rest are used a number of times. There are no cells for lodging the adults. They generally keep moving about on the surface of the hive. The cells are mainly intended for the storage of honey and pollen specially in the upper portion of the comb. Colony of honeybee consists of three castes – Queen, drone, and workers.

Fig. 5.3. (A) A colony of honeybee. (B) Chemical Application to Protect colony : Defensive mechanism of honeybee by ant attack. Asian honeybees (Apis florea) coat the approaches to their exposed nest with a sticky ant trap.

1. QUEEN

Queen is a fertile female. Only one queen is found in a colony. The size of the queen is largest among other castes of bees. Queen can be easily identified by its long abdomen, strong legs and short wings. The queen has a ovipositor on the tip of the abdomen. It is the egg laying organ. The contribution of queen for its society is to lay eggs.

2. DRONE

Males are called drones. Drones are haploid fertile males. The size of drone is smaller than queen but larger than sterile females i.e. workers. They copulate with the queen and fertilize her eggs.

3. WORKERS

These are diploid sterile females and are smallest in size. Their sterility is due to three reasons — diet effect, queen substance and the pheromone. Their numbers in colony is the highest. They do all works of the colony, except egg laying. Workers inherit behaviour of doing all the works of the colony (such as collection of pollen grains, water and nectar from flowers, cleaning and defending the colony, nursing embryo etc.) from their ancestors. It is an inborn instinctive behaviour. Numerous adaptations have taken place in the body of worker bee to perform various functions of the comb. Its body is hairy and legs are modified. When workers visit a garden of flower and sit on a flower, pollen grains adhere to these hairs and other parts of the body. Worker clean off pollen grains with the help of a special structure (the cleaners) present on each forelegs. Pollen brushes are present on every leg and pollen grains are stored in the pollen basket present on the outer surface of tibia on hind legs. Nectar and water is collected in crop by sucking through mouth parts.

Worker bees possess *Nasonov scent gland* in their abdominal region. A pheromone is released from this gland which attracts other bees. This is also helpful in marking the food and water sources by foraging individual and providing guidance to other bees to return back to correct home. It also helps to mark the nesting site an essential factor for maintaining cohesion among bees.

Worker bees bear a defensive organ at the tip of abdomen. This defensive organ is modified ovipositor having a large poisonous storage sac and a sting. Poisonous storage sac contain a poisonous chemical. This chemical is injected into the body of enemy through sting. Worker bees attack collectively to the intruder and sting the intruder collectively.

An Asian relative of the honeybee, *Apis florea,* builds an exposed honeycomb on a branch of tree where it would be vulnerable to ant predators. Worker bees coat the branch on which the nest is supported with rings of a chemical substance so sticky that ants cannot enter to the colony.

NUPTIAL FLIGHT

Most interesting part in the life cycle of honeybee is its way of mating. Mating takes place during a flight called nuptial flight. Virgin queen takes a flight followed by males. A few males only succeed in mating. Queen and other males return to their comb. But now worker bees allow only the queen and all males are driven away and they die in nature. Polyandry is relatively rare in insects where a single female mates with several males. But polyandry is common phenomenon in honeybee. Queen honeybee mates with several drones in succession during her nuptial flight.

COMMUNICATION AMONG HONEYBEES

Honeybees with their complex behaviour and social organization have always fascinated human observers. This tiny insect detect polarised light, memorises the details of their environment, learn and communicate about food source among members of comb.

Karl von Frisch after 20 years of experimental work could reveal that worker bees communicate information about the location of food source through the movements on definite path called "bee dance". The dance is performed on the hive. Frisch revealed this in the year 1967 and got Nobel prize for this contribution in the year 1973. The information given by scout bees to the members of her colony by dance is called as "language of the bees'. In other words, the dance displays of bees encode fairly specific information about the distance and direction to good foraging sites.

If the forager bees has found a rich new food source, a distance within 50 meters from the hive, she performs roughly a circular path called "Round dance". She moves in circles alternately to the left and to the right, turning first one way and then the other way. Other workers follow her in round dance and are then stimulated to set out on foraging flights.

If the food source is more than 50 meters from the hive a forager performs a "Waggle dance". In waggle dance she moves in a narrow semicircle, turns along its diameter, making a figure of '8'. This waggle dance conveys information about both the direction and the distance of the food source.

A foraging bee on the way to a discovered food source notes the angle between the food source, hive and sun. During a waggle dance she transposes this information onto the surface of the comb. If the bee walks vertical waggling strait up the comb, the feeding place will be found by flying directly towards the sun. If the honeybee walks horizontal and waggling straight down the comb, the food is located directly away from

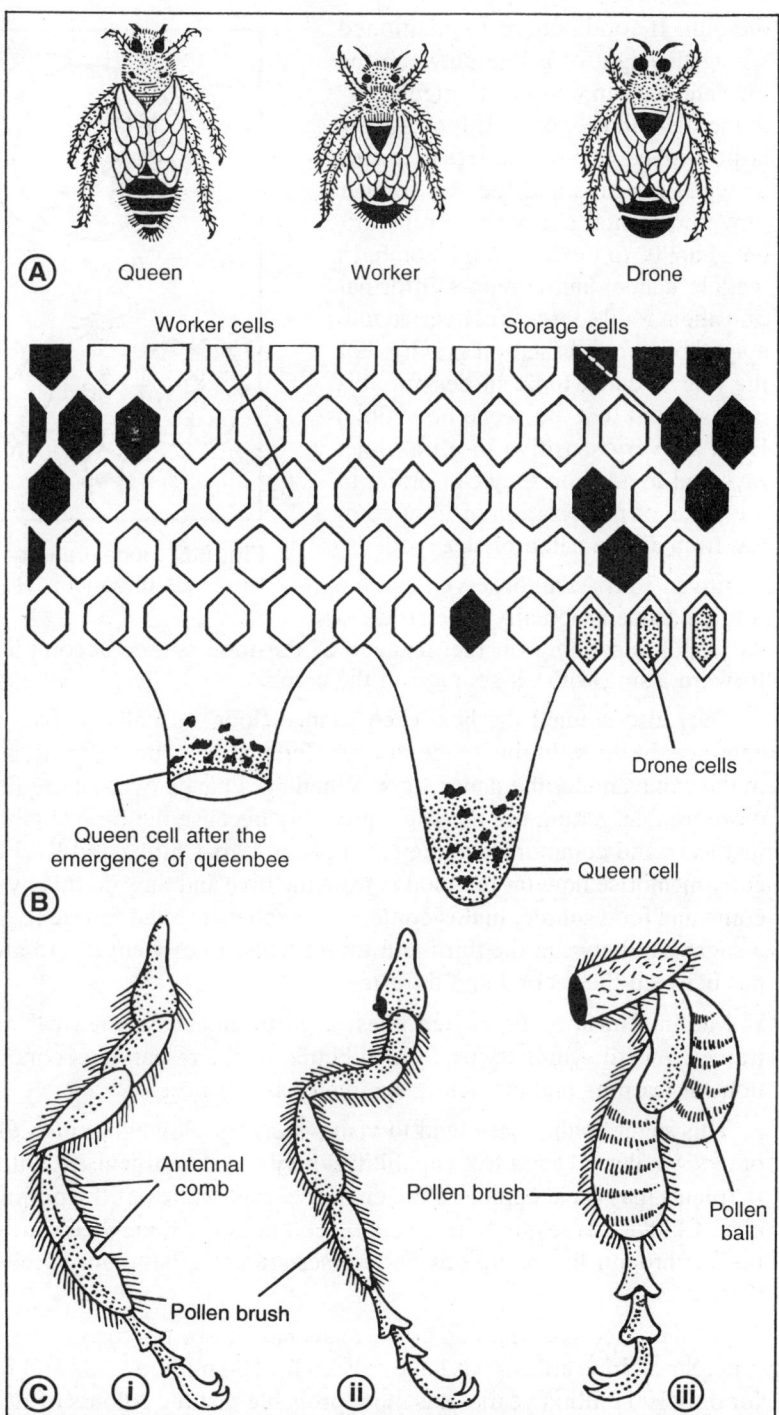

Fig. 5.4. (A) Different castes of honeybee : (i) Queen, (ii) Drone, and (iii) Worker; (B) A part of honeycomb; (C) Adaptations in legs of worker bee for carrying pollen grains.

the sun. If food source is positioned 90° to the right of a line between the hive and the sun waggle oriented at 90° to the right on the comb. If food source is positioned 90° to the left of a line between the hive and the sun forager move horizontal and waggle runs oriented at 90° to the left on the comb. In waggle dance, sun-compass information about food source is converted into a symbolic code based on gravity. For the waggle dance to be successful, it is not essential that the scene be visible. Bees are very sensitive to ultra violet rays and in addison they can orient to the plane of polarization of light coming from a blue patch of sky.

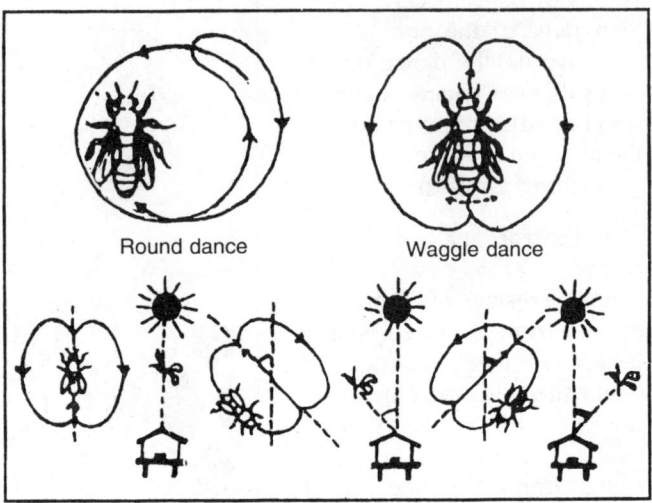

Fig. 5.5. Honeybees communicate about food site through two kinds of dances: Round dance and Waggle dance.

Jurgen Tautz et al. observed that the waggle dance is actually "one stride" - its length depending on the distance of the food source accomplished by the waggling bee moving forward, using with all six legs on the comb.

They also studied the honeybee "dance floor", usually a space within 10 centimeters of the nest entrance. In the wild this space in over empty combs, but in artificial hives there are likely to be larvae in the combs under the dance floor. When bees dance over larvae filled combs, the other workers have more trouble getting the message, probably because the proper vibrations are dampened. Bees do not just learn and communicate, they also count. Lars Chittka and Karl Geiger determined that bees apparently memorise how far the food is from the hive and they do this by counting landmarks in between the comb and food source. In this context researchers erected four tents in a line as landmark in a field, with a sugar bait between the third and fourth tents. Bees went to 3rd and 4th tent though sugar syrup was put between the second and third tents.

Martin Giurfa et al. trained bees to go to either symmetrical or asymmetrical patterns. The bees trained toward symmetry performed better, so the researchers concluded that "bees have a predisposition for learning and extracting symmetry as a feature.

This suggests that bees tend to visit symmetric flowers (which often have more pollen). Giurfa and others wonder if "cognitive capabilities may occur in organisms with rather small nervous system," and if "plants may have exploited the cognitive capabilities of the pollinators during the evolution of flowers." Chittka has studied the visual receptors in the honeybee's arthropod relatives. The more "ancestral" arthropod like scorpions and horseshoe crabs have only green and ultraviolet photoreceptors in their eyes.

All the insects, spider and crustaceans have three photoreceptor pigments, for green, ultraviolet and blue. Since these arthropods have existed for 500 million years and flowering plants came into existence for only 100 million years - it is more probable that the colours of flowers evolved to attract insects than that insect like bees evolved an interest in the colours of flowers. Stingless bees of the tropics offer a rich source of information on diverse communication systems.

The possible ancestral pattern

Workers of some species of *Trigona* (stingless bees) perform unstructured excited movements coupled with a high pitched "humming" when they return to the nest with high - quality nectar. This behaviour arouses hive mates, who request food samples from the "dancer" and detect the odour of the source on the dancer's body. With this information, they leave the nest and search for similar odours.

A modified pattern

Workers of other species of *Trigona* makes a substantial find marks on the area with pheromone produced by its mandibular glands. As the bee returns to the hive, it continues to chew on grasses and rocks every few meters. At the hive entrance there may be a group of bees waiting to be recruited. The forager leads these individuals back along the trail it has marked.

A still more modified pattern

A number of stingless bees in genus *Melipona* separate distance and direction information, unlike *Trigona* bees. A dancing forager communicates about distance to a food source by producing pulses of sound; the longer the pulse of sound, the farther away the food is. In order to transmit directional information, the recruiter leaves the nest with a number of followers and performs a short zigzag flight that is oriented toward the source of nectar. The lead bee returns and repeats the flight a number of times before flying straight off to the nectar site with the novice bees in close pursuit.

Sons and daughter on desire

The queen is capable of choosing sex of her offspring. If she desires to produce sons, she closes the spermathecal duct and prevents sperm from reaching the oviduct so that only unfertilized eggs are laid. Unfertilized eggs develop parthenogenetically into males. If she desires to produce daughters, she lets some sperm flow from the spermatheca into the oviduct so that fertilized eggs are laid. Fertilized eggs developed into females.

Food determining fertility and sterility

First 2-3 days all larvae are fed with a special food called "*Royal jelly*". After that all larvae are fed with coarser food called '*bee bread*'. Only one larva is fed with "Royal jelly" throughout its development. This larva develop into queen bees. Larvae fed with bee bread develop into workers.

The queen normally produces one or more chemical substances, called pheromones, that are meant to suppress the femaleness of workers and prevent them from developing their ovaries and laying eggs. This suggests that queen controls the workers for well being of the society and the workers have to behave in altruistic manner.

SOCIAL BEHAVIOUR OF WASP

Wasps show transition from the non social to the social life. In the course of evolution transition from solitary to social life, species would have gone through different stages.
1. Nesting together without much interaction.
2. Nesting together with interaction and some division of labour.

3. Nesting together with one morphologically specialized queen or a small number of such queens, who alone can reproduce. Wasps nest together, cooperate in nest building and brood care, and show some division of labour. But there is no morphologically differentiated queen. Most workers, can become queens if the opportunity presents itself. Besides, almost any female member of the colony can start a nest and bring up her offspring by herself without participating in social life. Thus wasps live in a primitive society. There are only two social aspects in context of social behaviour of wasps :

(i) the relationship between workers and grubs, and

(ii) the division of labour amongst their co-workers.

One Indian species of wasps *Polistes herbreus* (Fabricius) are social. The adult are smaller and yellowish in colour. The most prominent social wasp is *Vespa orientalis*. It is brownish and larger than yellow wasp. *Vespa magnifica* is largest social wasp and it is dark brown in colour.

Wasps prepare their nests over walls, ceilings, and trees near human habitats. Nests of French wasps (*Polistes*) and Indian wasps (*Ropalidia*) have some hexagonal chambers in which embryos are reared. Wasps remain active in summer and hibernate in winter.

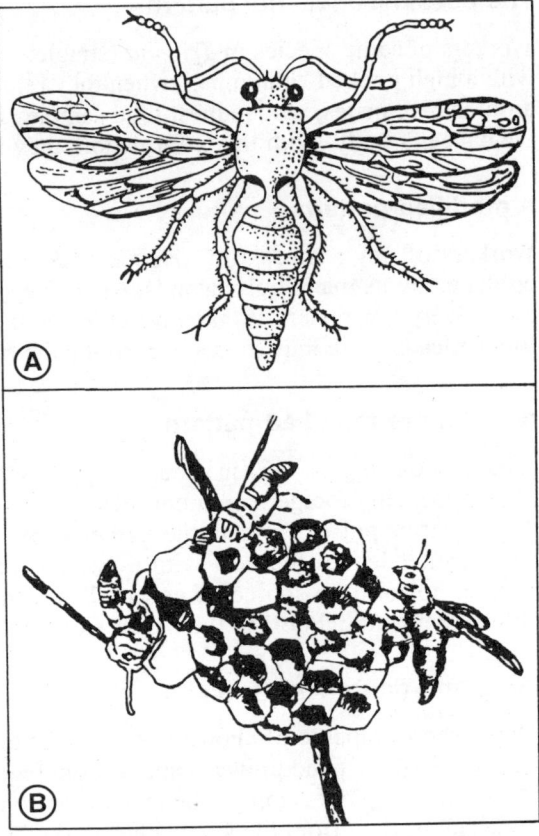

Fig. 5.6. Social wasp : (A) An Indian social wasp *Vespa orientalis*. (B) A nest or French wasps (*Polistes*).

NEST OF WASP

Ropalidia marginata and *R. cyathiformis*, two species of wasps found in southern India are primitively social. These wasps build their nest from paper which they themselves manufacture from cellulose fibres scraped from plants. The size of the nest is very small, rarely exceeding 500 hexagonal cells. Except for the brood, the wasps move on the surface of nest and not in it. The number of wasps in a colony rarely exceeding 100. This makes it easy to mark every individual wasp and make detailed observations on its behaviour, its interactions with other members of the colony, and its contribution to the welfare of the colony.

Castes

Wasp colonies do not have a well – differentiated queen. All wasps in a colony look alike. But only one female in *R. marginata* and few females in *R. cyathiformis* functions as queen in a colony. The wasps in a colony fight and the winner becomes the next queen. She may be queen for sometime only because she is often challenged and driven away by one of the others, who then becomes the next queen. The individuals who are not queens at any given time act as workers. They do not reproduce but perform all the works of the nest (build the nest, forage for food, care for the brood and defend the colony).

New nest is organized by one female or a group of females. If it is a single – foundress colony, the foundress acts as queen and manages all by herself to bring her eggs to adulthood. In a species of wasp in which solitary female must leave her nest unguarded when foraging, the foundresses apply ant repellent to the stalk of the nest.

In a multiple – foundress nest, one of the foundresses assumes the role of queen while the others assume the role of workers. *R. marginata* queens mate with a minimum of 3 males and simultaneously use sperm from different males and produce a mixture of full and half sisters among their daughters.

The queen lays eggs in the cells of the nest. When the eggs hatch into larvae they are fed on a diet of spiders, hemipteran bugs, and caterpillars and occasionally some nectar, by the queen herself in single - foundress nests and by workers in multiple - foundress nests under normal conditions. Some of the workers (foragers) search food and building material. Other workers specialize in staying home and working on the nest and on the brood. Among these, some are more aggressive toward other members of the colony, and these are called *fighters*. The remaining wasps work on the

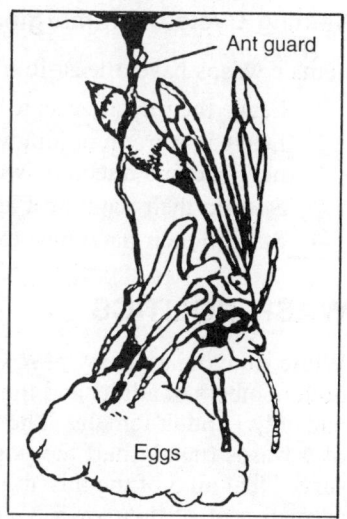

Fig. 5.7. Ant Repellent : Paper wasp rub the pedicel of their nest with a chemical "ant repellent".

nest quietly and spend much time just sitting and grooming themselves, and these are called *sitters,* Larvae pupate in the same cell. Pupa metamorphose into an adult. The entire process of maturing from an egg into an adult wasp may take about 2 months.

If the wasp emerging from the pupa is a *R. marginata* male, it will stay on the nest for about a week and then leave to lead a wandering life, mate with some foraging female wasp, and die. *R. cyathiformis* males spend their whole life in the colony except for brief periods when they leave the nest apparently to mate with wasps from the colonies. Mating never take place on the nest. If the emerging wasp is a female, she have atleast four different options. She may leave to start a new nest all by herself. She may leave with a group of females to do so, or she may join females from other colonies to start a new nest. She may remain on the nest and assume the role of a worker in the colony of her birth. She may remain on the nest, work for some time, and eventually drive away the queen and take charge as the next queen in the colony of her birth. Such a power struggle may also take place between the co-foundresses in a new colony, so that one foundress may replace another even before producing any offspring.

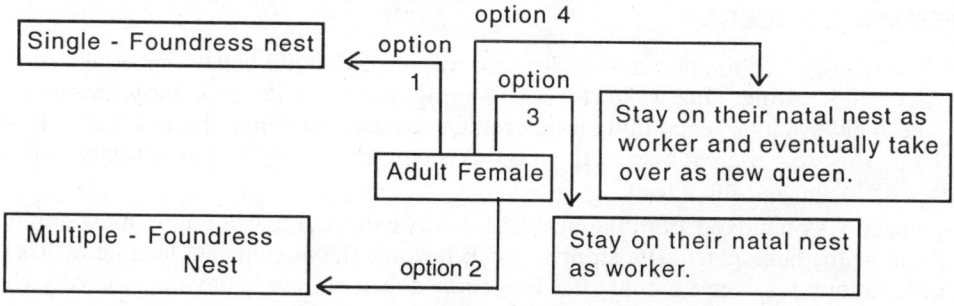

Nesting Cycle of R. marginata

Female wasps have atleast four different options :

1. Leave their natal nests to initiate single-foundress nest;
2. Leave in a group or join with female of other colony to initiate multiple-foundress nests where she may become queen or worker;
3. Stay on their natal nest as workers; and
4. Stay on their natal nest to eventually take over as new queen.

WASP POLITICS

While studying a colony of *R. cyathiformis* Gadagkar (1981-82) found that there was a steep decline in both numbers of adults and the number of brood being reared. On the evening of may 31, 1982 colony had only 11 adult females. The very next morning only six females remained on the nest. Disappearance of 5 wasps (nearly half the population) overnight was a very remarkable happening. Latter on he observed that all 5 of the missing wasps (individually marked with spots of different-coloured point) had a small nest of their own. Gadagkar inferred that these 5 wasps had deserted their original colony, perhaps revolting against the authority of the queen, and had decided to start their own new nest. He also observed that one of the particularly aggressive individuals on the original nest, had become the queen on the new nest. One aggressive wasp had led the revolt and fled away with her followers. Further observations revealed that colony fission turned out to be good for both the Rebels and the *Loyalists*. Both colonies grew rapidly. Thus the fission of colony increased the fitness of both the *Rebels* and *Loyalists*.

Now so many questions raised in the mind of Gadagker. How did Rebels mange to get together and leave at the same time and reach the same site to start a new nest? Was it a snap decision or had revolt been brewing for some time ? Was there some form of group politics even before leaving the parent nest fission? To get an answer to these questions Gadagkar along with his colleagues measured behavioural co-ordination within and between subgroups (Rebels and subgroups) using a mathematical index called Yule's association coefficient. Further question arised in their mind, whether there was more co-ordination within subgroups than between subgroups. For instance, did wasps within a subgroups synchronize their trips away from the nest and did loyalists and Rebels avoid each other? It was found that the Rebels had high positive association coefficients among themselves. Similarly, the loyalists among themselves also had a positive association coefficient, although this was not as high as the value among the Rebels. In contrast, Rebels and Loyalists had a negative association with each other. Conclusion may also be drawn that the wasps had differentiated into two subgroups well before the fission. Loyalists and Rebels behaved as two co-ordinated subgroups and avoided each other. It is interesting to note that Indian politicians play the same type of game while defecting from their party.

WASPS FORM ALLIANCES

In early 1985 Gadagkar had another nest under observation. He found behaviour of two of the wasps, in a colony, very interesting. One wasp (**R**) was very aggressive and particularly, towards a specific wasp (**B**). Queen always intervened in their quarrel. Queen used to climb on the fighting **R** and **B** and separated them. This was of great help to **B**, who was no match for (**R**). **B** was not only trying to avoid **R** but also trying to appease the queen.

One day queen was removed from the nest and it was expected that the next most dominant individual **R** would be the next queen. But surprisingly **B** become the next queen, in spite of **R's** presence. **R** stayed in the colony for over a month after **B** become queen but her behaviour was very erratic. She did not participate in any nest activity. She occasionally take some food from one of the foragers. Why was **R** so much more aggressive towards **B** than towards other individual? Why was the queen so "considerate" of **B**? Was there some kind of alliance between **B** and the queen? If so, did it have any influence on **B's** becoming the next queen after removal of the original queen, even though **R** was higher in the dominance hierarchy? These questions need further study.

WORKER WASPS CHOOSE THEIR QUEEN

An interesting case of worker's choice in queen selection was observed by Gadagkar (1985) during a queen–removal experiment with R. *cyathiformis*. There was two contenders, **B** and **O**, to replace the existing queen. Both "**O**" and "**B**" were more or less equally dominant. After removal of the original queen **B** took over the place of the queen and **O** promptly left the colony. **B** was apparently not a very good queen. All the other wasps stopped foraging and began to simply sit on the nest. It was like human tool down strike. **B** began to cannibalize on existing eggs to make room for her to lay her own, since no wasp would build new cells for her. Eventually other wasps began cannibalizing on brood too and there was chances of colony being abandoned. One interesting happening was going on there that "**O**" occasionally came back to the nest, as if to check on how **B** was doing. She never spent the night on the nest but would only visit occasionally. Within 11 days "**O**" returned to the nest and **B** left. Now the behaviour of the rest of the wasps was dramatically altered. They began to work. They built new cells for their new queen **O** to lay eggs in. **B** also visited the nest time to time, as if to see how her rival, **O** was doing. After a few days **B** rejoined the nest. She faces a great deal of hostility from the resident wasps. **B** had to spend nearly whole day being subordinated by several residents before she was accepted back into the colony. Why did the wasps not co-operate with **B** when she first took over as the queen? If she was not good enough to be a queen, why did she succeed in the first place, especially in the presence of **O**? Need to answered. Wasps are capable of recognizing individuals and they can modify their attitude based on the recognition.

SOCIAL BEHAVIOUR OF ANTS

The ants are among the most highly evolved social insects. Like honeybee and termites they also have a very complex social organization. About 90% ant species are social. Six species of Indian ants are :

  (i) *Monomorium* : Large and black ants living in cervices of walls, trees, trunks etc.
 (ii) *Componotus* : Common back, house ants.
(iii) *Solenopsis* : Small and red, house ants.
 (iv) *Dorylus* : Winged ants which appear around light after rains.
  (v) *Aenictus* : Common and gregarious army ants.
 (vi) *Oecophylla* : Red, tree ants.
(vii) *Formica* : Make mound nest.

Nest formation

The new colony is founded by a single newly fertilized queen. Some species do not construct nests. They simply take abode in cervices, holes under stones, or logs. Some species temporarily occupy nests of other ants, a relationship termed *plesiobiosis*. Most species make their own nest. The nests or formicaries are of different types located in different places. Ants make subterranean nests excavating galleries and chambers in the grounds, used as nurseries for brood, granaries for storing food. Many species make mound nests. Such mound nests are well exhibited by species of Formica. *Formica rufa* make mounds of 60–160 cm. in diameter. Some species construct suspended nests made of earth cartoon (Saliva mixed with Vegetable matter) or silk hanging from trees in tropics and containing anastomosing galleries and chamber.

African weaver ants (*Oecophylla longinoda*) and Asian weaver ant (*Oecophylla smaragdina*) construct large conspicuous nests on tree by weaving together several leaves with silk. They obtain this silk from their own larvae. The colony of weaver ants consists of a single queen and two kinds of workers, the larger major workers who forage, construct the nest, and take care of the queen, and the smaller minor workers who care for the eggs and young larvae. The adult worker cannot produce silk. The silk is produced by

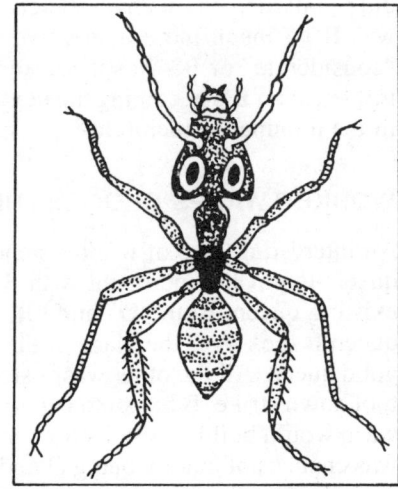

Fig. 5.8. Black Indian Ant : *Monomorium indicum.*

the larvae. It is well known to us that in most insect species the larvae use their silk to spin cocoon inside which the pupae undergo metamorphosis. The major weaver ant workers who need silk, hold larvae together during nest construction to obtain silk from these larvae. While some major workers maneuver and hold leaves together, other major workers hold larvae in their mandibles and weave them across the leaf. This makes the larvae release strands of silk from silk glands underneath their mouth. Male larvae have smaller silk gland and contribute less silk for nest construction or cocoon.

DIFFERENT FORMS OF ANTS

The ants show an extreme case of polymorphism. According to Imms (1948) at least 29 distinct types of morphologically different individuals are known. The main castes are queens, workers and males.

1. QUEEN OR GYNES

These are the fertile females. Queen is largest is size in comparison to other castes of their species. The antennae and legs are relatively shorter and stouter and the mandibles are well developed. Some species are winged while some species are wingless. Usually large individuals are termed *macrogynes*, and dwarf ones, *microgynes*. Unlike honeybees, a colony of ants contains several queens.

An egg laying worker, gynaecoid, occurs in colony. She becomes normal queen if queen is lost due to any reason. Rarely there occur some peculiar individuals, called gynandromorphs. They bear external secondary sexual characters of both male and female.

2. WORKERS OR ERGATES

Sterile females are called workers or ergates. Ergates are smallest in size. They are characterized by a reduced thorax, and small eye. Workers are mostly dimophic. The larger workers are called the *macregates* and dwaft individuals *micregates*. Macregates are called the pahelwans of the insect world for their ability to lift too much weights. They also have amazing sense of direction. Soldiers are modified workers (sterile female). They are without wings, with distinct heads and powerful mandibles. They protect the nest from enemies. Besides protection they serve to crush the seeds and other hard food for inmates.

Number of *army ants* in a colony is very huge containing up to 22 million individuals. While on march they eat up everything edible in their path. Army ants (*Eciton*) have three types of workers. *Small workers* perform the task of feeding the developing broods. *Intermediate size* of workers act as foragers or scout ants. These search the site of food. Largest size of workers are soldiers defending their colony. Some soldiers attack the colony of other insects and capture the young larvae and pupae of other insects using them as food. Sometimes soldiers of ants bring home the larvae and pupae of other ant colonies. These captured larvae and pupae after hatching are used as slaves.

3. MALES OR ANERS

These are small, fertile, winged individuals, they bear proportionately smaller head, reduced mandibles, longer antennae, well developed reproductive organs and genitalia. The larger individuals are called the macraners and the smaller one micraners.

Life-cycle

Mating occurs in nuptial flight. The queen lays eggs of about 0.5 mm size. The eggs hatch into larvae. The body of larva is legless and cylindrical. The queen feeds them with her saliva until the pupa stage. In a short time they change into the perfect insects. The earlier generations are of wingless worker which soon take over the charge of the colony, feeding and attending the queen and the brood. The winged males and females are produced later. Usually the ant colonies are perennial and continue to grow in size for many years. The population of nest of ant vary from a few thousand up to 5,00,000.

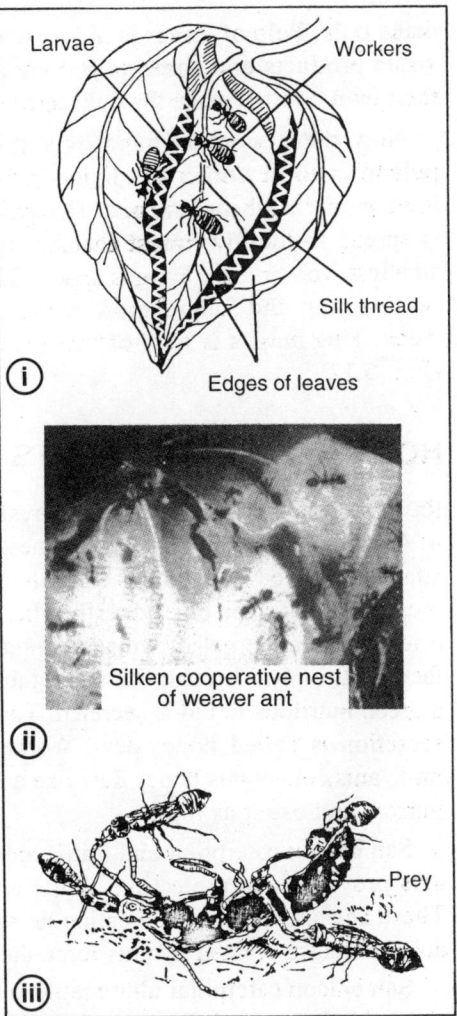

Fig. 5.9. Nest of Leaf : (i) The Indian Weaver ant *Oecophylla smaragdina* making nest of leaves. (ii) Silken co-operative nest of Weaver ant (*Oecophylla longinoda*) (iii) Co-operative prey capture by ants: A group of weaver ants carry a much larger insect, which they have killed.

FARMER ANTS

You will wonder to know that in South American rain forests "fungus gardening species" of ants are cultivator like human beings. These ants are gardening fungus since last 50 crore years. It means all ants are not scavenger. These ants do gardening of fungus in 180 meter radius in its burrow.

These ants cut small pieces of leaves of plants of rain forest and carry them to their nest. They hand over these pieces of leaves to other workers. These worker ants clean these pieces of leaves and cut them in very mini pieces. These fine pieces of leaves are chewed and masticated by worker ants and make pulp. Pulp of leaves is mixed with waste products and some secretions of their own body to make the pulp fertile.

Now these workers hand over this pulp to smallest worker ants living in the lowermost chamber of the nest. This pulp is spread in the lowermost chamber by smallest worker ants. Fungus spores fall on this pulp and fungus grow within a week. This fungus is food of these ants (Fig. 5.12).

HONEY COLLECTOR ANTS

Rattle ants are found in tropical forests of Australia. They make suspended nests attached with leaves of plants. Sah baloon is caterpillar of small blue butterfly. These caterpillar bear a small tube on dorsal surface of its body. Through this small tube a green nutritous liquid is secreted. This secretion is called honey dew. Worker

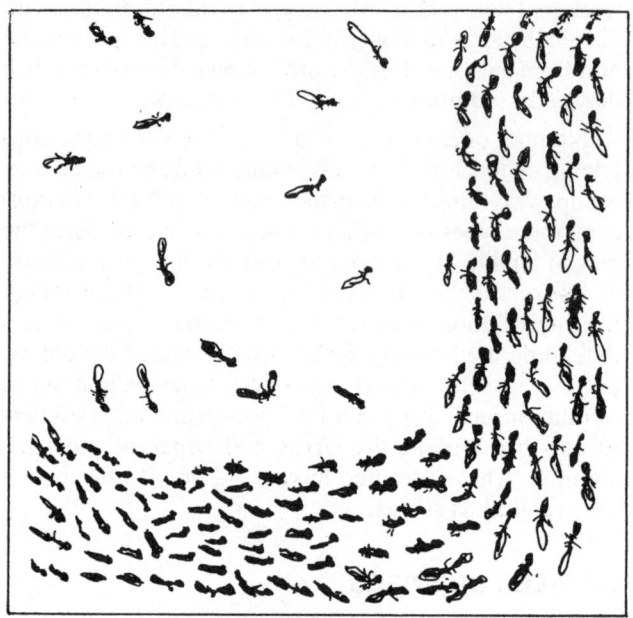

Fig. 5.10. The Amazonian army ants form a long column which moves along devouring everything in its path.

rattle ants collect this honey dew like dairy workers. Ants collect and store honey dew in store house of burrow and use it as food.

Sah baloon caterpillar and Rattle ants live symbiotically. Catterpillars provide them honey dew and ants provide them protection. Rattle ants protect these catterpillars from spiders and other enemies. These ants are capable of creating noise by to and fro movement of dry leaves and hence called rattle ant. The noise created by ants force the predator of caterpillar to withdraw.

Sah baloon caterpillar allure rattle ants to remain next door neighbour. They hypnotise ants by emitting a kind of sound. Singing caterpillars are also there. They call ants by singing song. The song of these caterpillar is not audible to human ear. The song is not like vibration in air but vibration on the solid stem of plant. Ants receive this vibration with the help of a receptor organ present on their legs. These songs can be heard with the help of microphone.

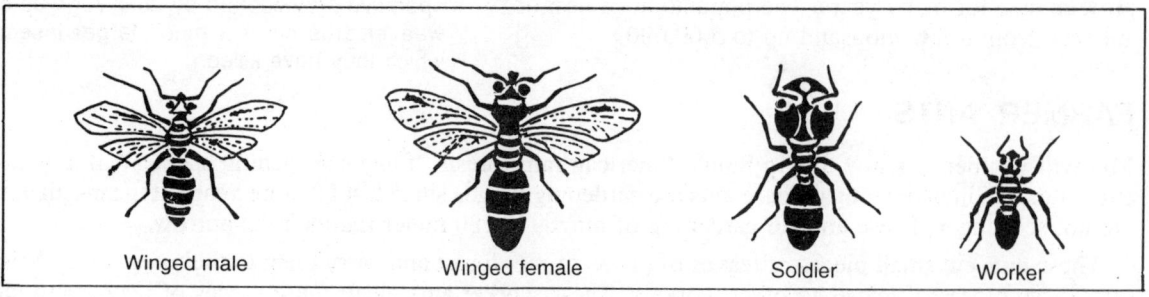

Winged male   Winged female   Soldier   Worker

Fig. 5.11. Different castes of ants.

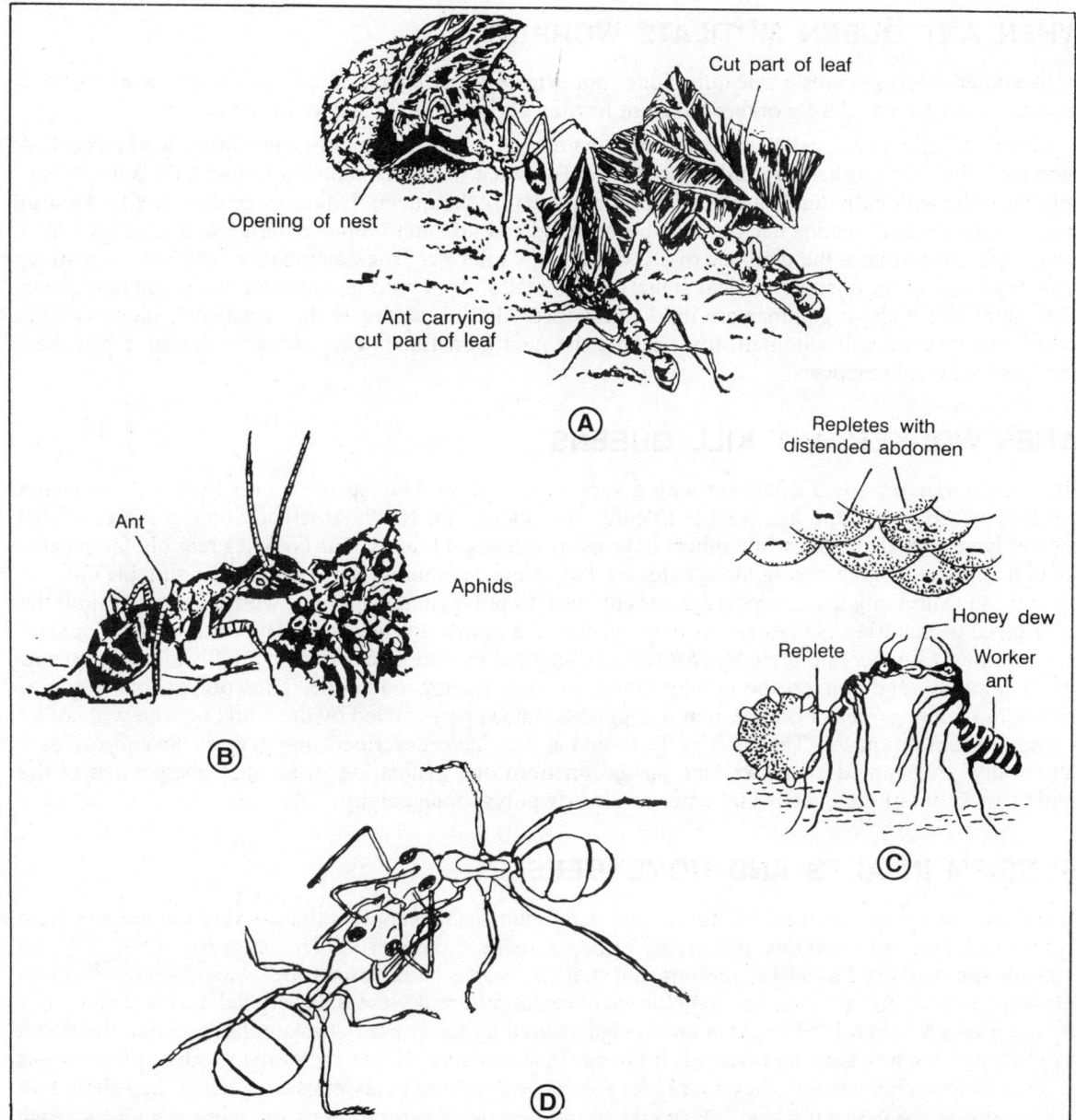

Fig. 5.12. Farmer ants : (A) Cultivator ants cutting leaves in small pieces, carrying these pieces to their nest to cultivate fungi on it. (B) Many ant species collect honey-dew from aphids and (C) increase the secretion of this substance by caressing the aphids with their antennae. (D) Food sharing between workers of the ant, *Formica rufa*. The worker on the left is receiving food from that on the right which has regurgitated of a drop of liquid from its crop and offers it between the outstretched mandibles.

Some ant species collect honey dew from herds of little insects called aphids. In yet another species workers form living "honey pots", as they hang upside down from the roof of their nest, their abdomen hugely distend with honey.

WHEN ANT QUEEN MUTILATE WORKER

Unlike other species of ants a true queen does not exist in *Diacamman*. It appears that the workers have learned to reproduce. Here workers have not lost the ability to mate and store sperm.

Christian Peeters et al. called such queens as gamergates. The gamergates have little wing buds called gemmae, while the worker do not have gemmae. But what makes *Diacamma* remarkable is what happens after the ants individuals are physically mutilated by the queen. If the queen dies, the first ant to emerge subsequently retains her gemmae because there is no one to remove her gemmae, and she then systematically mutilates the gemmae of all who emerge after her. The gemmae are required for mating, probably because they send chemical signals to the males. Ants with gemmae are dominant and queen like, while ants without gemmae are mild and worker like. If gamergate dies accidently the next individual to emmerge will automatically become the next gamergate. The workers who have had their gemmae mutilated reappear.

WHEN WORKER ANT KILL QUEENS

Fire ants (*Solenopsis*) is a small ant with a very painful sting. One species *Solenopsis invicta* occurs naturally in Argentina and has been accidently introduced into North America. Some colonies of this species have a single queen while others have many queens. Monogynous colonies rear big fat queens, suitable for starting new monogynous colonies. Polygynous colonies rear small queens, suitable only for entering and surviving in other polygynous colonies. In polygynous colonies, workers seem to limit the food given to maturing queens and if they encounter a really strong queen (By virtue of their genetic make up), they kill her and there by ensure that a single dominate queen does not bully all other queens into submission and convert the colony into a virtually monogynous one. Thus polygynous colonies cannot turn monogamous because their polygynous state is perpetuated by the workers, who will not let a single queen dominate. That is why Ross and Keller have described polygyny in *Solenopsis* as a "culturally" transmitted character, one passed on from one generation to another irrespective of the genetic make up of the queens that enter an already polygynous colony.

BOSSISM IN ANTS AND HONEYBEES

In ants and honeybee colonies, the queen emit pheromones, that suppress the workers and prevent them from developing their ovaries and laying eggs i.e. make them sterile. This suggests that the queen controls the workers for selfish reasons and that the workers are forced to behave in an apparently altruistic manner. Recently Keller and Nonacs have put different view. They argued queen pheromones are not meant to control the workers but as signals used by the workers to voluntarily curtail their own reproduction because they are better off if the queen reproduces. Hence they use the queen pheromones as a signal to decide whether they should let the queen continue to lay eggs or whether they should do so themselves. So who's the boss ? From the point of view of natural selection, there is no boss ; each individual attempting to maintain society.

SOCIAL BEHAVIOUR OF TERMITES

Only one member of order *Isoptera* 'Termite' exhibit social habit very similar to ants, bees and wasps. Termite is commonly known as "Dimak" or "White ants". Although termed white ants, they are not ants. They are distinguished from ants by the absence of a constriction or peduncle between the thorax and the abdomen. Ants have unequal wings (anterior pair is larger), whereas the termites have equal wings. Termites live on wood and are nocturnal, whereas the ants live on sweet chemicals and animal's matter and are diurnal. *Microtermes obesi* and *Odontotermes obesus* are two common species of termites found in India.

NEST OF TERMITE

The primitive species of termites feed upon wood and excavate galleries in wooden structure. Some species construct carion nest of masticated wood. Carion nest are ovoid or rounded. The nest may attain the size of a football and placed up the trees. You may wonder to hear that termites are the most efficient engineers and that the entrance to their mounds always faces north. They build excellent natural air conditioning systems, which modern day architects are at pains to figure out. Many species burrow in the ground and constructs a nest or *termitarium*. They consist numerous tunnels and chambers, and may be entirely subterranean or with a mound above the surfaces. Such termitaria may be a few meters high and 9 meters in basal diameter. The termitaria are made up of sand particles cemented together by saliva and faecal matter of termites. On drying the material becomes hard like cement. The natives of the Congo clear the termitaria of termites and use them as dwelling huts.

MEMBERS OF COLONY

The colony of termites is well managed by division of labour as termites exhibit polymorphism. Colony comprises two major castes (A) Fertile caste and (B) Sterile caste.

(A) **Fertile caste :** The fertile caste is of the following three forms :

  (i) **Long winged adults or Colonizing Adults :** Winged adults are produced in good number in rainy season and are actually winged males and female. Male and female individuals go on nuptial flight and copulate in the sky. After fertilization the female may have a new colony separately. Males have well developed eyes and wings. Long winged adults are of two types.

   (a) **Queen :** The queen of *M. obesi* is 5 to 7.5 cm. in length. The sole function of the queen is egg laying. She lays about 70,000 to 80,000 eggs in 24 hours. The life span of a queen is recorded to be 5 to 10 years. The queen lives in royal chamber of the nest and feeds royal jelly. The queen is well served by the workers.

   (b) **King :** The king is the father of the colony living with the queen in the royal chamber. It is developed from an unfertilized egg by feeding on nutritive diet. It fertilizes the queen repeatedly to produce fertilized eggs for the hatching of the winged males, females and workers. Life of the king is shorter than the queen. So the king is replaced by a new one.

  Both true kings and queens have two pairs of wings in the beginning but wings are ultimately discarded and only their truncated base remains present.

  (ii) **Short-winged adults (Brachypterous) :** These are supplementary or substitute or neotenic king and queens. Body is less pigmented. The two pairs of wing are short, vestigial and pad - like.

  (iii) **Wingless form (Apterous) :** These are worker-like substitute kings and queens which occur in the more primitive species. The body is without pigmentation. There are no traces of wings.

(B) **Sterile castes :** These are wingless forms with rudimentary reproductive organs. This is of three types :

  (i) **Workers :** The workers are numerous and they perform all the duties of the colony except reproduction. The body has little or no pigmentation. The workers are commonly dimorphic, but sometimes trimorphic comprising small, intermediates and large individuals.

(ii) **Soldiers :** The soldier are highly specialized. They are concerned with the defence of the colony against predators. They are pigmented and large - headed individuals with projected prominent mandibles. In some species three grades of soldiers - small, medium and large are present.

(iii) **Nasutes :** In higher genera *(Eutermes)* the mandibulate soldiers are replaced by snouted forms called the nasutes. These are relatively shorter individuals with vestigial mandibles. Their head is prolonged into a rostrum, bearing the opening of a large frontal gland at its apex. The sticky secretion of the gland is inflicted upon their enemies in warfare and is used to dissolve hard substances, like concrete which fall in the way of the workers when building nest.

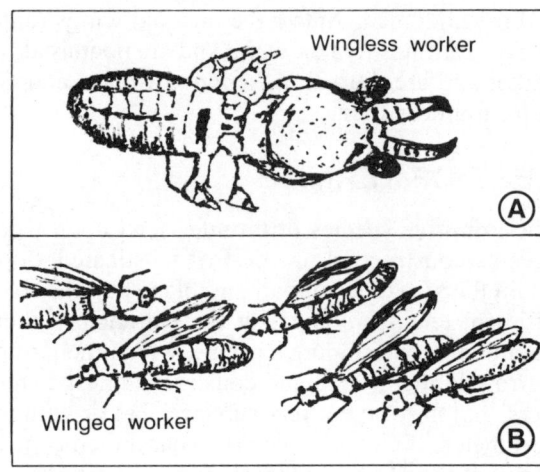

Fig. 5.13. (A) Wingless worker; (B) Termite Worker.

LIFE HISTORY

1. Swarming and Mating

During rainy season, the winged forms (queen and king) take a flight known as swarming. After a brief flight, these winged forms land on the ground and shed their wings. The flight is not a true nuptial flight, but only a dispersal flight since mating does not take place in the air. Mating takes place after they have descended to the ground, but before shedding their wings. Unlike honeybee, mating is further repeated at irregular intervals. The king cohabiting with the queen for whole life.

2. Founding new colonies

Each colony is founded by a royal couple. Together they excavate a small burrow or cavity in the ground, called the nuptial chamber. The first laid eggs, by the young couple develop into workers. The workers assume the duties of nest.

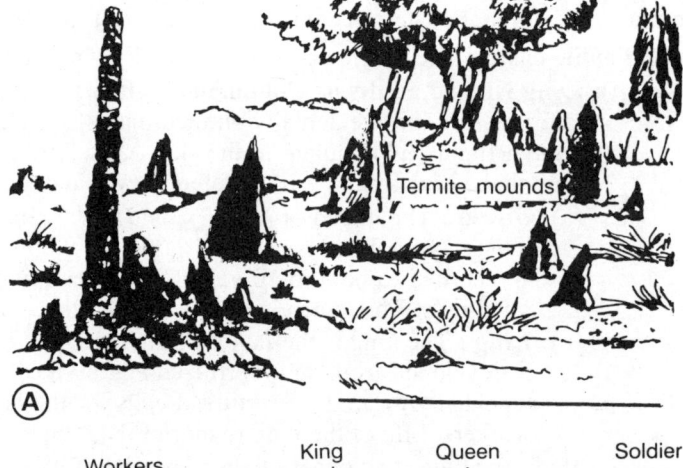
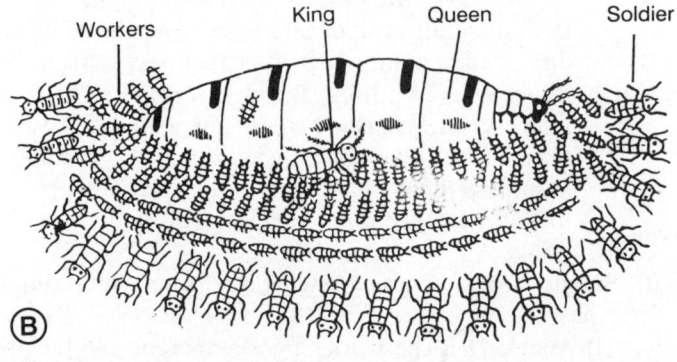

Fig. 5.14. Nest of termite: (A) Mounds and (B) termitarium of termites.

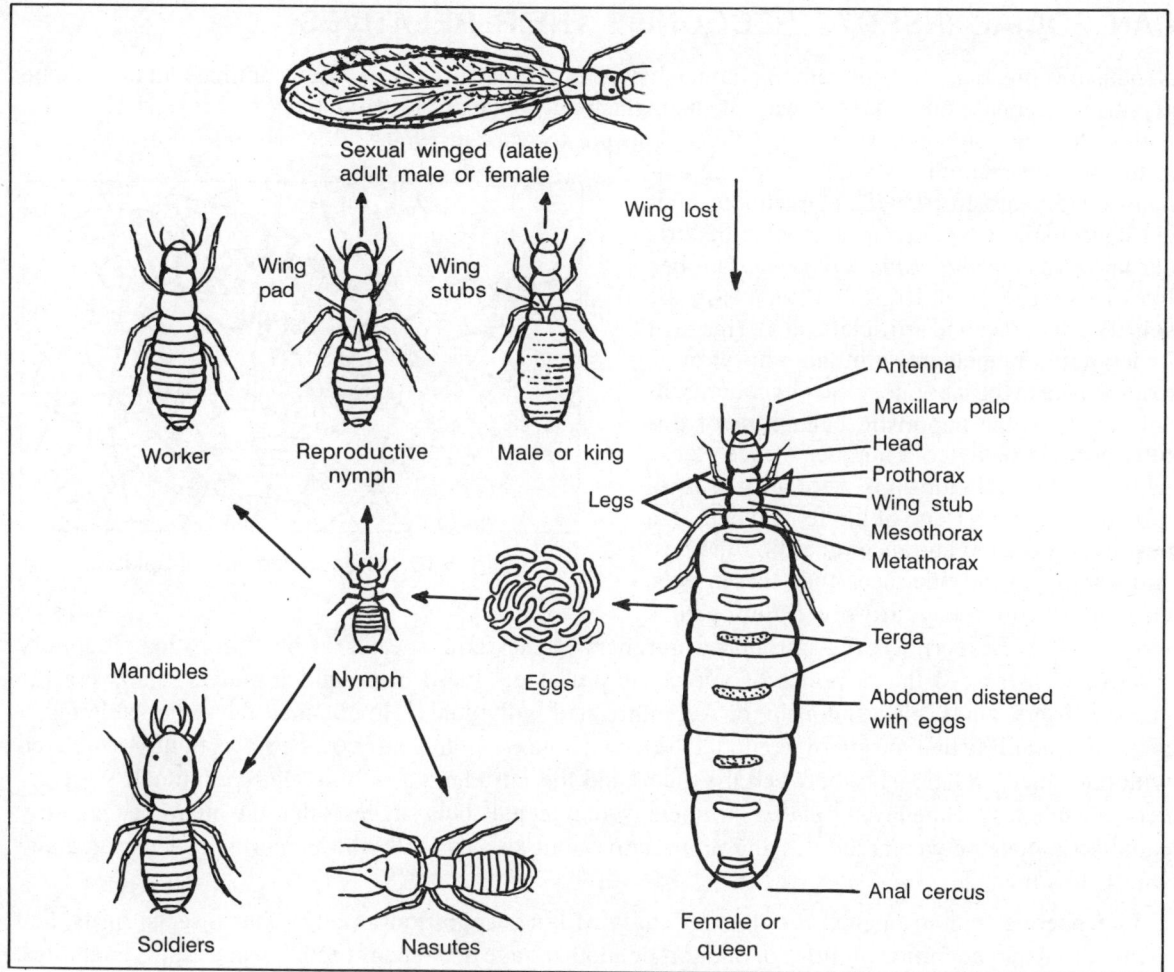

Fig. 5.15. Different Forms and Life Cycle of termite.

SOCIAL BEHAVIOUR OF SPIDERS

Most spiders are solitary. There are, however, a few species that have communal web construction and co-operative prey capture system. They also defend their young collectively. A few species of spiders show parental care in which the young remain on the web and are fed by their mother. In some species the young spider build their own small webs next to their mother's web. The highest stage in the evolution of the web construction is that several spiders may run out of subdue a large prey.

The nature of social systems of spiders strongly suggest that this evolved via the familial route among orb-weaving spiders, sociality appears to have evolved via the para social route. The beginning of sociality was probably clumping of webs in unusually favorable sites. This led in a few cases to the joining of webs and construction of a communal retreat.

CAN SOCIAL INSECTS RECOGNISE THEIR RELATIVES

Nepotism is practiced not only among human beings but is also practiced among animals. In order to be nepotistic, animals must have a way of distinguishing between close relatives and distant relatives. Although Hamilton's inclusive fitness theory was put forward in 1964, but no serious effort was made to test the kin recognition abilities among animals for 15 years. In 1979, Les Greenberg studied nepostistic behaviour in a species of little bee known as *Lasioglossum zephyrum*. This bee lives in a maze of underground tunnels in the soil. The bees taken to artificial habitat (maze of underground tunnels made in laboratory) quite readily mate in the laboratory. So Greenberg was able to study the nepotistic behaviour of this little bee. He obtained a number of bee stocks whose genetic relationships were all known to him. It is typical for one of the female bees in a nest to sit near the entrance, guarding the nest and warding off intruder bees and other insects. Greenberg put the guard's efficiency to a

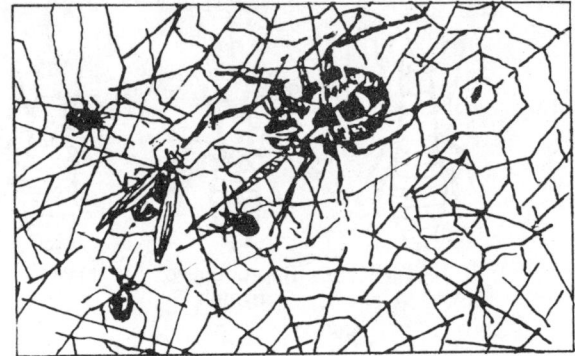

Fig. 5.16. Co-operative nest of Spiders.

severe test. He experimentally introduced intruders of the same species of bees from his laboratory stocks and measured the response of guard. He presented guard bees with intruders who were the guard's sisters, aunts, nieces, cousin, or were unrelated individuals. He obtained the remarkable result that the probability that the guard would let the intruder pass her and enter the nest was tightly correlated with the genetic relationship between the guard and the intruder. Closely related individuals were accepted while less related or unrelated intruders were rejected. This suggests that the guard bee not only can discriminate between relatives and non relatives but also can tell who is more closely related and who is less related.

Greenberg's finding opened the door of study of kin recognition among other insects, birds, and mammals. Kin recognition abilities of one sort or another have now been studied in marine invertebrates, mites, sweat bees, honeybees, several species of ants and wasps, termites, fishes, frogs and toads, iguanas, several species of birds, and a variety of mammals. In most cases, kin recognition is achieved by smell or body odour. We might think of every individual carrying on its body a relatively distinct odour label and in its brain an odour template. If the labels and templates are genetically determined then they will vary between related individuals in a graded manner so that identical twins have identical labels and templates, siblings have slightly different labels and templates, nieces and nephews have more different ones, and cousins still more different ones, and so on.

The source of colony specific odours is not completely known ; but probably it develops from the diet of the colony, as individuals frequently regurgitate food to one another, and minor differences in the diets of different colonies would give them characteristics of different odour. Kalmus and Ribbands (1972) moved two hives of honey bees from a typical honeybee environment to an isolated moor which had only one species of flower. The level of fighting between the individuals of two hives decreased, perhaps because they increasingly came to recognise each other as members of the same hive. Likewise, when parts of hive were isolated and fed on different diets the level of fighting within a hive increased. The learning of odour of hive perhaps takes place during a sensitive phase of imprinting.

Another question arises that whether honeybees and other social insects can distinguish closely and distantly related individuals from within their own colonies? For instance, honeybee queens mate with several males, store sperm from all of them, and use such mixed sperm to produce several different patrilines of daughters at any given time. Daughter belonging to different patrilines are half sisters. Inclusive fitness theory predicts that honeybee workers will give better and preferential care to their full-sister larvae (with whom they share 75% of their genes) than to their half sister larvae (with whom they share only 25% of their genes). The current state of our understanding of whether worker honeybees are so nepotistic as to prefer full-sister larvae over their half-sister larvae for queen rearing can be stated as "Motive is determined by genetic make up". It is advantageous to a bee to invest her reproductive effort in a larva three times as closely related to herself as alternative larvae. Bees can tell the difference between related and unrelated larvae and differential treatment of larvae will influence which became queens. Half - sister versus full-sister discrimination is actually an important element in queen rearing by colonies under natural swarming conditions.

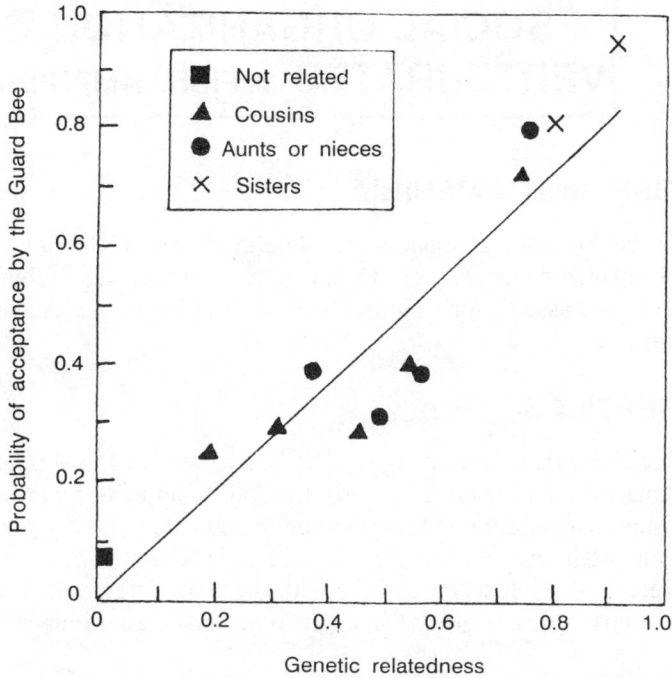

Fig. 5.17. Casteism in Insects : Kin recognition in a sweat bee *Lasioglossum zephyrum*. Guard bees were presented with intruder bees whom they had never encountered before. The probability of acceptance into the nest of the intruder bee by the guard bee was significantly positively co-related with the average genetic relatedness between guard bee and the intruder bee.

HUMAN AND INSECT SOCIETIES

Unfortunately, people often believe that the highly complex society of human being represent a crowning achievement of evolution. It is quite mistaken impression that human society is superior to primitive society of insects. Human society is supposed to be a social system based on differences in family origin, rank, wealth etc. It is based on learning, abstract intelligence and communication by language. Moreover human society is complex giving higher emphasis on the faculty of reasoning, on the contrary the society of tiny creatures like honeybee, ants, wasps, termites etc. is fully guided by instinct and their own way of communication i.e. pheromone system. This is the key to the continuation of their race for more than 3 crore years. Success of human society is mainly measured in terms of the individuals as well as the community, but the insect society success is measured in terms of the colony (society) and not the individual.

SOCIAL ORGANIZATION OF NON-MAMMAL VERTEBRATES : FISH, AMPHIBIA, REPTILES AND BIRDS

FISH AND AMPHIBIA

Except birds social organization of non-mammal Vertebrates viz., fishes, amphibians and reptiles is very disorganized type. Not even single species of fishe, amphibia and reptile is truly social. School of fishes and close association of individuals of amphibian species may be a common occurrence but they do not form society.

REPTILES

Social organization among reptiles is also confined to simple short time interactions between male and female during breeding seasons. Crocodiles and alligators watch their eggs and after emergence of the young, they are trained for swimming and catching they prey. Nile crocodiles have a novel method of foraging in group. They form a semicircle where a water channel enters. They also face the inflow of water and catch fishes coming with the water stream. It would not have been possible for just one or two crocodiles to block the water to get sufficient number of fish.

BIRDS

Many species of birds are social. Bird's society consist families or flocks. A permanent flocking arrangement is found in Herons, Quills, English sparrow, Cliff swallows etc. Love of companionship bind them into a family flock of social group.

Family flocks of birds may be of feeding, sleeping, nesting or migrating groups. Family of cliff swallow travel together during migration. In the winter time feeding flocks are found around the bases of western mountains which chickadees, kinglets, juncos etc. occur. The chickadees are noise creators and serve as liaison to hold them together.

Herons often forms interspecific breeding colonies around great salt lake. The blue Herons start assembling and are joined successively by night herons, snow egrets and glossy ibies. Pelicans and gulls nesting together on island of great salt lake is a very common feature. One or two pairs make nest among mixed big colony. Example skuas among penguins.

Roulroul *(Rollulus roulroul)* of western India and Mourning dove *(Zenaidura macroura)* lives in pairs and outside the nesting period in smaller groups of families. Nicobar Pigeon *(Coloenas nicobarica)* is found from Nicobar east to the Philippines. Out of the breeding season it occurs in small flocks which fly from one island to another in search of food. Thus it is a colonial nester. The flocks often remain together even during the nesting period, building several nests of small twigs on one tree. During the nesting period the red and green macaws *(Ara chloroptera)* live in pairs. Out of the breeding season, the macaws occur in flocks that range through the trees in search of food. Young Blue - fronted Amazon Parrot *(Amazona aestiva)* roam in families or together with groups of other fledglings. Ring Necked Parakeet *(Psittacula krameri)* lives on the margins of forests, where it ventures in small flocks into fields in search of grain. The Roseate cockatoo is a gregarious bird that roams the countryside in flocks, separating into pairs only for the nesting period.

In colonial bird species social behaviour seems to be involved in the tight synchronization of every aspects of reproduction. This is true of the pink flamingo.

Penguins are only found in the southern hemisphere. They are essentially social and gregarious creatures. During winter, they gather is flocks on the icy shores of Antarctica. Some observers have estimated that up to half a million of these penguins may gather on the 200 hectare area of Adelie land. Most cormorant species nest in colonies.

There are a number of different weaver bird species which construct nests suspended from trees using dried grass. The south-west African social weavers, which are close relatives of the European sparrow, build enormous communal nests containing a large number of individual pairs, each with their own nest entrance.

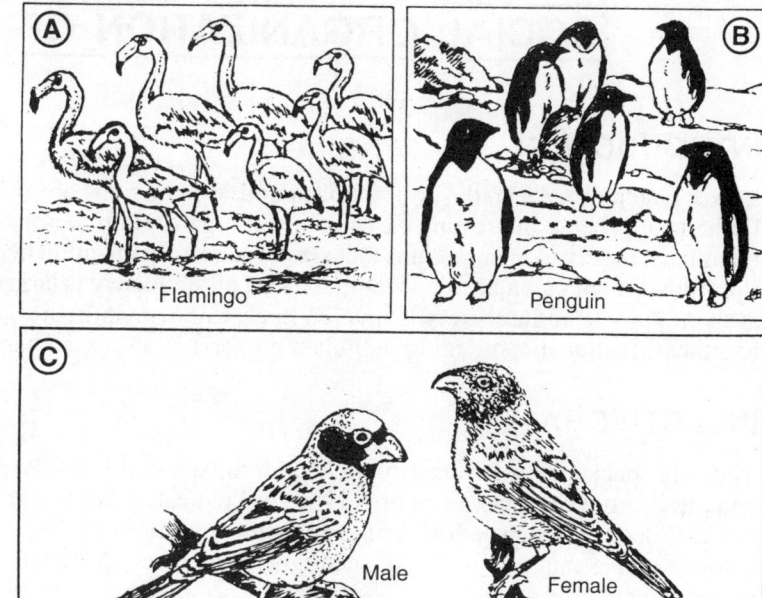

Fig. 5.18. Social birds : (A) Flock of Pink Flamingo. (B) Adelie Penguins. (C) Quelea.

THE ALARM CALLS IN BIRDS

If one of the members of a flock of birds foraging through the forest spots a predator (hawk) sailing through the trees, it may utter a thin whistled "seet" call. This alerts other birds to danger, and the flock may hide under the cover of a thick hedge or tree.

ROOSTING

Many birds of a species arrive at a high place (tree, tight rope or building) in the evening and rest collectively in night. Munia sleep in a row, on a perch, and each bird likes to have a bird on either side of it, in order to keep herself warm and safe. No one likes to be at the end of the row. So after three or four birds have perched ready to sleep, the next bird comes along and tries to force its way into the middle. If it is unsuccessful, unwillingly goes to the end of the row and pushes with all its might against its neighbours and the bird at the other end of the row also pushes. Sometimes one of the birds in the middle is so squashed that it is pushed off its perch and then has to take an outside place or sleep standing on the backs of the other birds.

Another amusing thing about these munias is the way they sing to one another. The munias sit in a row and then suddenly one of them draws itself up to its full height and sings a sweet little song. As soon as it is over, another munia takes his cue and breaks into a song likewise. Thus they have regular little concerts.

SOCIAL ORGANIZATION OF MAMMALS

INTRODUCTION

Lower mammals especially Prototherians and Metatherians are solitary but many species of subclass Eutheria are social. Interesting cases of social organization in non- human mammals is discussed here. It has been observed in eutherians that size of social organization depends on the length of parental care. If the duration of parental care is long, the size of the society is larger and if the duration of parental care is short, the size of the society is smaller. In case of many primates, including man generations may live together. Mentionable orders of sub-class eutheria is discussed here.

INSECTIVORA

The only species of order insectivora known to be social is the *Streaked tenrec*. It is colonial, living in complex burrow systems. Eisenbrg (1981) has indicated that this species is polygynous, with a colonial harem. Social communication in *Streaked tenrec* is largely by vocalization and scent signals. Communication includes mutual sniffing of scent glands on meeting. Territorial marking with faeces is common in this insectivora.

RODENTIA

Rabbits are colonial and live in multimale/multifemale colonies. Pikas is colonial in which a male's

territory may include one or more females. Belding's squirrels live in multimale/multifemales colonies made up of territorial female-bonded clans. Some rodents may have variable social organization depending on the nature of their environment and population density. The house mouse *(Mus musculus)* ranges from being solitary to forming multimale/multifemale colonies. *Heterocephalus glaber* possesses reproductive female and three other castes, non-workers, occasional workers and frequent workers. Female members of these castes appear to be sterile and the male mate with the fertile female.

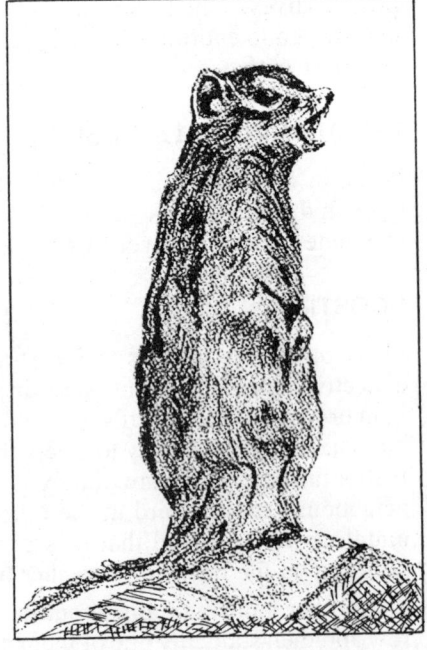

Belding's ground squirrels form breeding colonies with many burrows scattered over the Sierra Nevada Meadows. Male Belding's ground squirrels, emigrate from place where they were born and establish new home burrows about 400 meters. Therefore, the females in an area tend to be related to one another, where as the males are not. Moreover, dominant adult males leave an area after copulating with the receptive females there and so they are not in close contact with their "wives" and offsprings. The kin selection hypothesis predicts that females should give more alarm calls than males, because the risk to a female caller might be compensated by the improved chances of survival of her nearby relatives.

Fig. 5.19. A Belding's ground squirrel giving an alarm call.

Belding's ground squirrels produce a different alarm call, a special staccato whistle, (with each note detached) when it spot a prediatory mammal and a high whistle when an aerial predator sails overhead. Other squirrels stop what they are doing when they hear the call and either scan the environment for enemy or duck into their burrows.

Now the question arises, "is this a case of co-operation or, altruism ?" Squirrel giving an alarm call would risk his life for non relatives, not a strategic move in evolutionary terms. Altruism would be favoured natural selection either if it is directed towards genetic relatives or if it is reciprocated by the beneficiaries.

Paul Sherman had 1866 squirrels marked for individual identification and spend 3082 hours observing them, during which he witnessed 102 occasions when the squirrels encountered predators. The aim of Sherman's study was to discriminate between six competing explanations of the possible functions of squirrel alarm calls :

1. Distracting the predator's attention,
2. Reducing the likelihood of future attacks by the same predator,
3. Discouraging the predator by indicating that it has been spotted,
4. Warning others likely to reciprocate,
5. Warning as a group as a whole, and
6. Warning genetic relatives.

Sherman found no evidence that warning calls distracted the attention of predators or reduced the likelyhood of the future attacks, nor did he find any evidence that warning calls discouraged predators from pursuing the caller. In fact, callers were often chased and pursued and even killed by predators. That rules out the first three hypotheses. Hypotheses 4 and 5 were more difficult to falsify. Thus the only hypothesis that was supported was hypothesis 6, that alarm calls serve to warn relatives of impending danger. Alarm calls can be fovoured by natural selection even if they reduce the fitness of the caller if they also benefit genetic relatives.

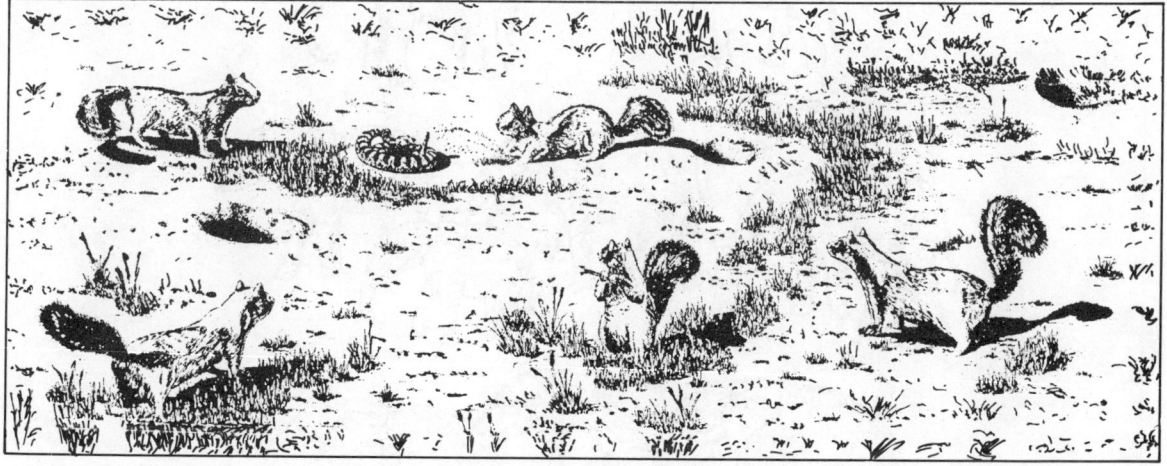

Fig. 5.20. Colonial California ground squirrels, have evolved mobbing behaviour. One squirrel kicks sand at a rattle snake, while other give a variety of alarm calls.

Sherman found that females give more alarm calls when they spot a predator than males. An even more interesting finding was the discovery that females help relatives as well as neighbours. This support that both the parental care and altruism hypothesis may apply to alarm calling by female Belding's ground squirrels.

In other species of ground squirrel, with a similar organization males do give alarm calls, but they do so only before leaving their mother's home area. Adult males and juvenile males that have left their relatives behind emigrated to a new area remain quiet when a predator approaches. The selective nature of alarm calling in ground squirrels is a beautiful example of the close match between the interact of the genes and behaviour.

PROBOSCIDEA (Pachyderms)

Elephants have always captured the hearts of humans. Their size, their majesty, their docility, their intelligence and affection fascinate us. There is no person who is not fascinated by elephants, be it Haathi of Rudyard Kipling's Jungle Book, or the baby elephant walk in Hatari. The TV documentary of the National Geographic Channel on the effortless swimming of Sri Lankan elephants under water is stunning.

Rob Slotow and Gus Van Oyte have studied elephant societies in detail. The societal behaviour of elephants is both family- and community-based and pecking order-prone. A herd of elephants is composed of an adult female and her young of different ages. Usually one of the oldest female in the group lead the herd. Members of one herd stay and feed together, caring for the young of one another. Herd take special care to orphan kids. Adult males form a separate herd and move separately, a bit away from the family herds. Herds of elephants are matriarchal i.e. females remain in their natal herd to breed while males are driven out at puberty. Hierarchy is maintained among the members of male herd, fighting over

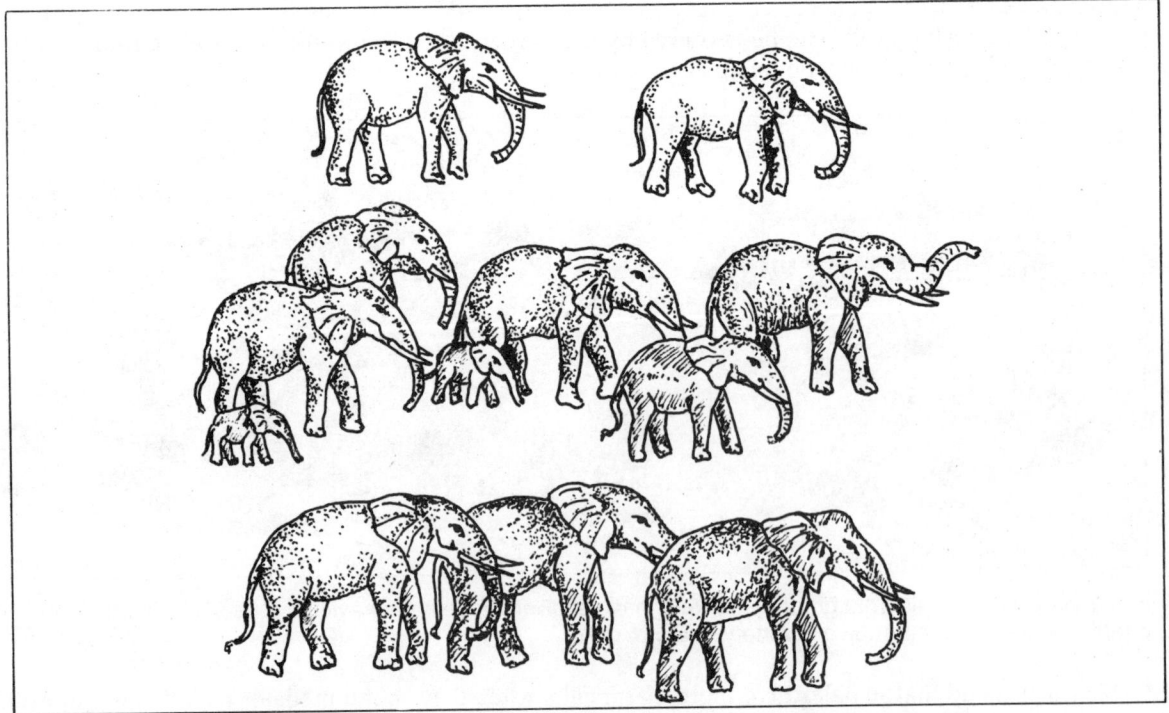

Fig. 5.21. Elephant Society : A herd of elephant. (Matriarchal society).

resources such as food, water and camp sites, Generally the bigger the elephant, the higher he rises in status dominating. When a male African elephant leaves the nursery herd he may join other males in a bull group. Bull groups are temporary aggregation but there is evidence that the bulls in an area know one other and have hierarchical organization. Height ranking males have intermitted periods of heightened sexual activity known as *'musth'*. Coming into *musth* can change the social structure because *musth* makes an elephant more aggressive. Since a community of elephants prefer to establish rank order through symbolic play acting than actual fighting and hurting, the *musth* automatically becomes dominant to those that are not in *musth*. When experiencing such a physiological rush, he leaves the bull herd and seeks receptive female partners in oestrus.

Females from groups, on meeting, show elaborate greeting ceremonies. They raise their trunk and greet each other with vocalization. Catti Payan, has found out that elephants communicate among themselves through infrasonic sound signals. There are many types of infrasonic sound signals out of which 31, which are produced by elephants have already been recognised.

In a herd of elephants, oldest female elephant, who is the head of the group, can talk to her group with infrasonic sound signal even from 8 km away. She communicate to their group members about dangers through the infrasonic sound signals. Different types of sound signals are applied for different type of informations. Catti Payan discovered that female elephant communicate to male elephants through infrasonic sound system "that I am receptive" during reproductive period. Female elephant becomes receptive only for 2 or 3 days once after 2 years. For this short period infrasonic sound signal is the only and best means of sending invitation to male elephants.

CARNIVORA

Among the cat family (cat, leopard, cheetah, tiger and lion) only cat and lion show matriarchal type of society in which central core of family is composed of interrelated females. Males are solitary and get entry into family only at mating time.

LION

The family of lion is called pride. Lions live in prides consisting of several adult females, subadult male and immature cubs. The success in hunting comes from co-ordinating their effort so that several members of the pride simultaneously attack the prey from different directions. The kill is then shared but not necessarily in a peaceful, equitable manner. The males, who usually contribute the least to the hunt use their muscle energy to gain major share and first access to the flesh. The females eat next usually in the order of their social

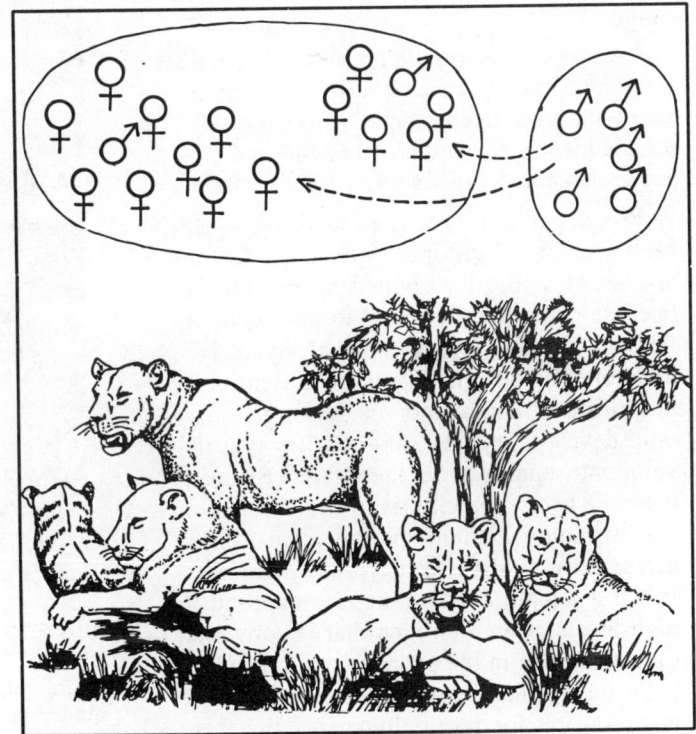

Fig. 5.22. Society of Lion : A pride of lion. Matriarchal arrangement in lion family.

status in the pride. Subadults and cubs have to be contented with left overs and may occasionally die of starvation. The conflict evident in the process of food sharing should not be mistaken from seeing the contrast between the tiger's solitary habit and the lion's social bent. Co-operation and conflict are inseparable components of any social group of animals.

HYENA

Spotted hyenas are highly social animals that live in permanent bands often containing several members. Clan members do many things together. They hunt big game (zebra, wild Ass etc.) co-operatively like wild dogs and protect the kill from other animals.

Competition for dominance in the group is most important because dominant females (alpha female) and their offspring gain more food than subordinate ones. The sons of alpha females "inherit" their mother's high dominance status. When fully mature, these male offspring emigrate to another clan of hyenas. If the son of a dominant female becomes the top male in his new clan, he will enjoy exceptional reproductive success because only the dominant male mates.

Hyena is the only species in the entire order carnivora whose females have a mimetic penis (pseudopenis). In fact it is difficult for a human to determine the sex of a hyena without being able to inspect genitalia at very close range.

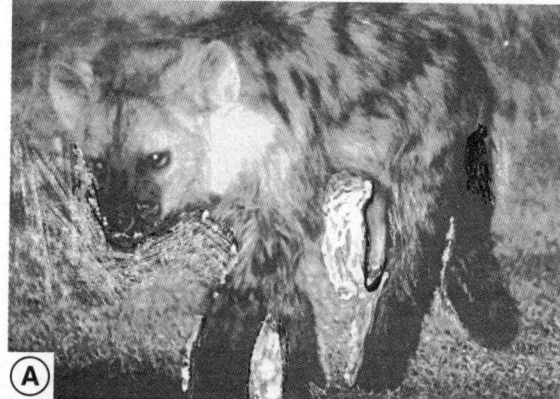

Pseudopenis is used in the spotted hyena's frequent "greeting ceremonies" to communicate with other hyenas. The observation that female hyenas have a mimetic penis and engage in elaborate "penis" sniffing rituals is funny.

Pseudopenis of female spotted hyena is a highly enlarged clitoris. Now the question arises : How did the spotted hyenas clitoris become penis like. It is due to hormonal effect and clitoris used as a special signal. Testosterone has key effects on the masculinization of mammalian embryos. During embryonic development the same tissues that develop into a penis under the influence of testosterone become a clitoris in the absence of the hormone. Female spotted hyenas must differ hormonally from typical mammals. When a female hyena alike, are exposed to high levels of an androgen that is converted to testosterone in the placenta and passed on to the developing foetuses. The male hormone is responsible for developing male traits, thereby masculinizing young females, producing an enlarged and penis like clitoris (pseudo-

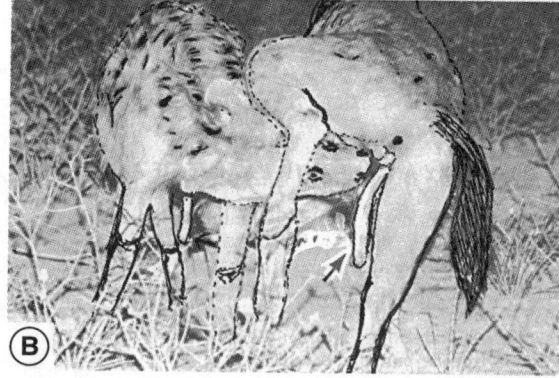

Fig. 5.23. Female Genitalia and Social Cohesion in Hyena : Pseudopenis of female spotted hyena. (A) A female with an erect pseudopenis walks toward another individual. (B) The greeting ceremony of female spotted hyenas. Here one female has pushed her head under the leg of the other to inspect the pseudopenis (arrow) of her companion.

penis). Supporting examples exist even in humans. A few pregnant women injected with testosterone at regular intervals (under medical supervision and desired doze of testosterone) the women giving birth to children having a greatly enlarged, penis like clitoris upon birth. A child with reduced penis, the mother was injected with dozes of testosterone at the time of pregnancy.

Though the enlarged clitoris (pseudopenis) is useful for social signal in female spotted hyenas but she has to pay its cost while giving birth to her pups. Because the female's reproductive tract terminates in the clitoris, her babies must pass through the clitoris in order to be born. Imagine a human male giving birth through his penis. The process of delivery in case of female spotted hyena is very difficult. Those who have seen a hyena giving birth in person or on film will never forget it.

CHIROPTERA

Many species of order chiroptera (Bats - *Pteropus* and flying fox) are colonial. Two types of social organization have been recognized in bats namely monogamy harems bisexual groups and polygamy harems. Harems of a species of bat *Phyllostomus discolor* consists of maximum 15 females per male. The south American colonial bat *Phyllostomus hastatus* roosts in cave. One male bat may have harem of 100 females.

RECIPROCAL ALTRUISM IN BATS

Gerald Wilkinson studied reciprocal altruism in vampire bats in Costa Rica. Vampire bats live in groups of 8-10 females, some of whom are sister and some are unrelated to each other. These associate with each other for 2 to 11 years and indulge in reciprocal altruism. Vampire bats fly out at night to feed on the blood of cattle and horses and then return to their roosting sites to spend the day. All bat do not succeed in feeding on all nights. Bats that fail to feed on three consecutive nights will die of starvation. Wilkinson observed that hungry bats beg food from well fed ones and will usually be offered some blood. Bats receiving blood are more likely to donate blood when they themselves are well fed and are harassed by hungry bats. The bats groom each other on their stomachs to know which one is well fed and who is hungry. They can remember the individuals to whom they have donated blood in the past. Usually they give blood to those who had obliged her in the past.

Australian gray-headed flying fox *(Pteropus giganteus)* is a colonial bat. Indian flying fox forms bisexual societies. There is a male hierarchy which confers breeding success on high ranking individuals. At parturition, female flying fox become segregated and form all-female nursery groups.

CETACEA

True society is not found in aquatic mammals. But some aquatic mammals such as whales, dolphin, common seal, gray seal etc. form disorganized society. Hump backed whale live in groups of 500 individuals during breeding period in the area of Bermuda and Hawaii. Mother calf bondage is strong for parental care. A mobile harem structure is found in the killer whale where an adult male with numerous female and young move in a synchronized manner. Common porpoise [a short-snouted genus *(Phocaena)* of dolphin family 1.25 to 3.75 meters long] live in larger groups. Other species of porpoise may form male and nursery herds. There is no evidence of social organization among dolphin (plantania) but common dolphin, spotted dolphin and spinner dolphin travel in large herds. Dolphin and whales communicate with their inmates through ultrasonic sound signals. Dolphin greet one another by "name" using signature whistles to keep track of one another in dark muddy waters and across distances. Dolphins have a clear and consistent vocabulary and are able to identify one another as individuals. Each dolphin develops a very specific signature signal and they always use the same call. Some people call it a name.

But because the dolphins seem to develop their own signature whistle the call are more like internet screen names.

Biologist Vincent Janik of the University of st. Andrews in Scotland studied the language of wild bottle nose dolphin. He recorded 1,719 whitles using 6 hydophones and a computer based method for finding individual dolphin as they made the calls. Each dolphin makes its own, distinctive whistle, other dolphin will imitate that whistle, presumably to contact and keep in touch with that particular dolphin. It is like keeping in acoustic contact. It is something that we know from birds and humans, too like monkeys and other primates. Dolphin use distinctive calls when they have found food. This one is a low-pitched "bray". "It really sounds like a donkey-bray". The others would rush in. So does it qualify as language ?. "Janik is not sure about it" but it is certainly a complex communications system. Now Janik is engaged in finding if mother dolphins and their calves use the distinctive signature calls.

Gregarious groups are found in fur seals and sea lions. The common seal has a small harem of maximum 10 females. The grey seal are sea bottom dancer but breeds on rocky coasts and has a harem of 1-10 females.

SIRENIA

Aquatic herbivours – The sea-cows or Manatees *(Trichccus)* and Dugong *(Dugons dugons)* are gregarious but the social tie is between mother and their children only. Its gestation period is about 11 months. Usually one young is produced at birth and is carried on the back of the mother till maturity. Female of Florida Manatees make a harem of males when she is in heat. Maximum number of male Manatees is 17. This herd is called "oestrus herd" members of which may have an aggregated rank order first to move into dry land to establish territory which they fiercely defend. The female join the male harem after one month of territory formation.

PRIMATE

Many species of primate such as *Mačacca mulatta* (monkey), *Semnopithecus*

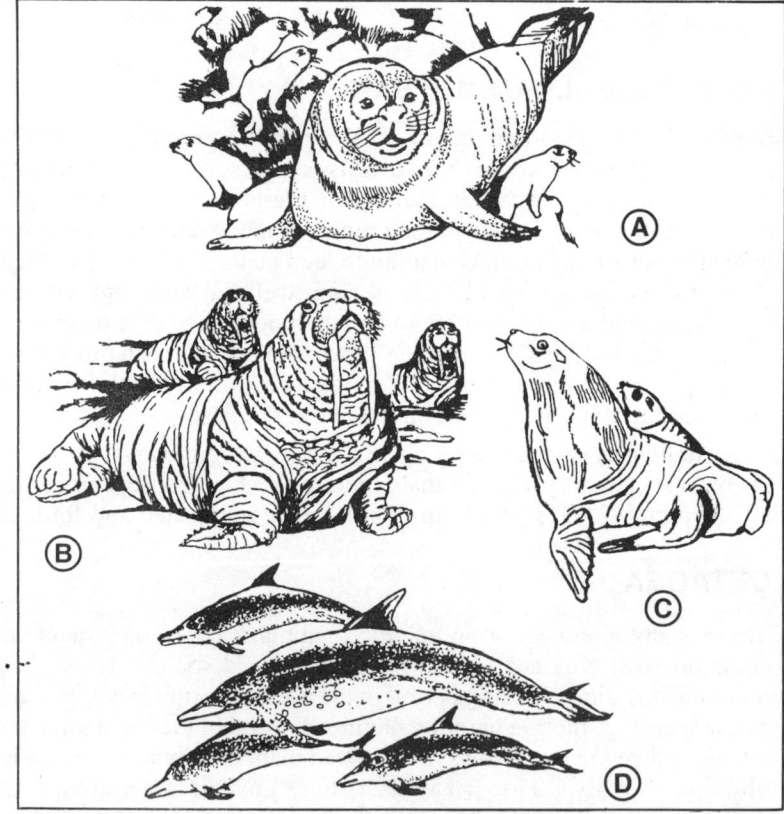

Fig. 5.24. Social Aquatic Mammals : (A) Fur seals. (B) Walruses. (C) Sea lion: Sea lions look much like their relatives the seals but most sea lions have small external ear. Their hind limbs can move forward to act like stubby legs, enabling them to lift their bodies off the ground. They form a well organized society. (D) Dolphin live in herd and learn ballet dance quickly.

(langur), *Simia* or *Pango* (Orangutan), *Pan* (Chimpanzee), *Bonobos* (pygmy chimpanzee), Gorilla and *Homo sapiens* are highly social. Member of this order are mentally developed. Individuals of most primate group exhibit four interesting social behaviours.

(i) **Allogrooming :** Members os the society clean hairs of each other and remove ectoparasites, especially lice. Usually subordinate clean the hair of master. Suppose a member (A) wants his hair to be removed from lice then he/she will put his body before any other member (B). He/she (A) will repeat this act if the other member (B) do not show any interest in allogrooming. Failure to elicit this/her behaviour to the other member (B) he/she (A) will start cleaning the hair of other member (B). This will initiate the tendency of allogrooming in the member (B) and it starts removing the hair of member (A).

Allogrooming is an important social activity. Grooming seems to have a function note only in the removal of ectoparasites but also as a "social cement" in the reaffirmation of social bonds. Usually grooming takes place between close relatives.

(ii) **Roosting :** The process of settling down at a place in night is called roosting. Members of a society come to a definite place and take rest collectively. In most primates roosting is an important social activity. This acts as reaffirmation of social bond daily.

(iii) **Mounting :** Members of one society mount on others time to time. This behaviour is related to copulatory behaviour. Here sex-differentiation cannot be done. Mounting behaviour was frequent in primitive man.

(iv) **Huddling :** Primates (Prosimians, monkeys and apes) embrace each other and take deep sleep at night, huddled together if it is cold.

The social behaviour of primates can be classified as follows :

1. MULTIMALE BISEXUAL SOCIAL GROUP

Gorilla, African baboon and monkeys (rhesus monkey, squirrel monkey, wooly monkey, spider monkey, Bearded Saki, Vakaris) show multimale bisexual social organization. Each social group has several males in which one is master or alpha male, and several females. Bonded females remain with their infants. In fact there are many small groups living together and forming a bigger group. One big group may have more than 200 individuals. Two major groups within multimale bisexual grouping are there : Those which do not divide in smaller feeding groups e.g. Gorillas and those which divide daily into smaller feeding group e.g. Baboons and Macaques.

(A) Gorilla

Schaller and his colleagues had to spend an entire year with the gorillas. More recently, another American naturalist, Dian Fossey, has conducted an extensive study of the mountain gorilla, spending five years observing the behaviour of this species in jungle. This young woman succeeded in winning the confidence of the gorillas by imitating their gestures and their sounds so that she became accepted as one of them. The observations conducted by George Schaller and Dian Fossey are packed with interesting facts. For example, the home range of a group of mountain gorilla, which will normally contain between five and twenty individuals, covers an area of about thirteen square kilometres. Lowland gorilla groups contain a greater number of animals, between fifteen and thirty, and range over an area of twenty-four to forty square kilometres. Gorillas move round over long-established pathways and each group is led by an adult male whose back is covered with silver hairs called "silver back".

In gorilla's group the males have dominance hierarchy and the most dominant is known as *alpha* followed by *beta* and *gamma*. But there is no dominance amongst females

Dominant male in gorilla society is not very aggressive and all other males have access to receptive females. Eisenberg (1978) called these groups as "age graded". This means that there is only one oldest male and other younger males are graded age wise. Bands of gorillas mix when they come into other's home range.

Lead males of individual gorilla groups hardly ever engage in fights. Whenever they met, two such dominant males will eye one another in silence with a threatening stare. In order to demonstrate its pacific intentions, a gorilla which encounters another will look towards it and not its head. If one of the two gorillas in such an encounter should adopt a threatening posture, the other will usually move on or adopt a submissive posture. The threat behaviour of the gorilla provides a good example of the ritualization of aggression. Never the less, these threats can be quite spectacular and it is perhaps undependable that they were misinterpreted by early explores and hunters. In the full threat sequence, a gorilla will rear up on its hindlegs, drum its cupped hands on its chest and then charge through the forest, uttering high-pitched screams and breaking branches or ripping up trees on its way. Given the size and strength of a gorilla, this exhibition is obviously quite terrifying. The sudden attacks inflicted on early travellers by gorillas were a result of complete misunderstanding of the natural behaviour of these greet apes, which only become dangerous when they are threatened.

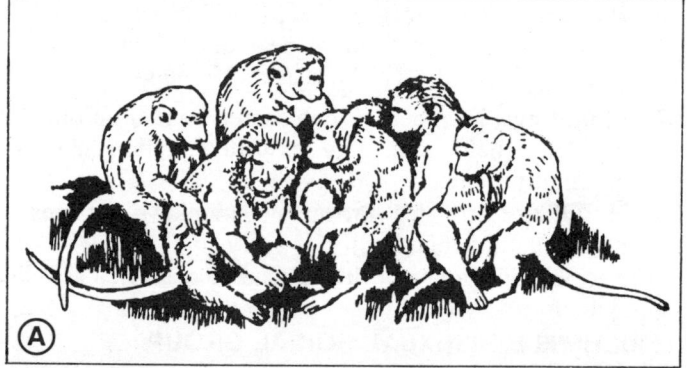

(B) Rhesus Monkey

Rhesus monkey (Macaca mullata) are inhabitant of India. They are mostly found in the religious places of India. They do not have families but the offspring of a particular rhesus mother stay close to her. As the troops move, the females and young males are always in the lead. The most dominant male is the leader of the group. The leader of the troop plans the day and area of foraging. The males have dominance hierarchy but an interesting case is that the bonded females acquire dominance form.

Suppose alpha is the most dominant male. Then his bonded females will enjoy high place in dominance hierarchy among females and rest of the group members. Even infants of

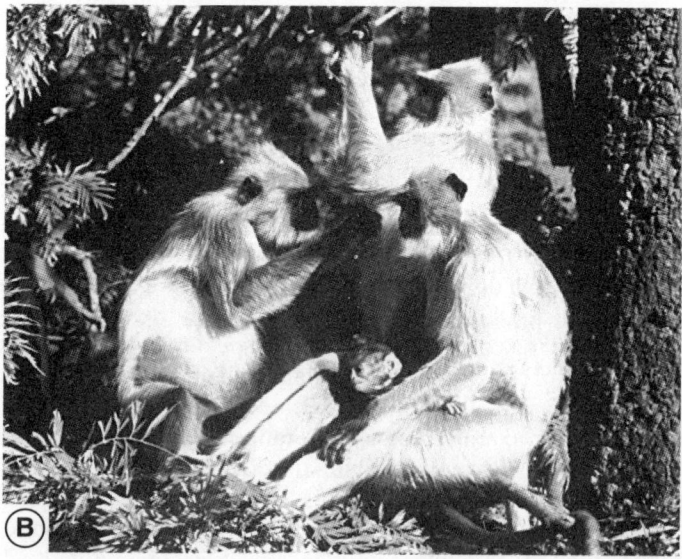

Fig. 5.25. (A) Rhesus Monkey society : Multimale bisexual social group of Rhesus monkey huddled together. (B) Hanuman langur huddled together at night.

bonded female acquire that dominance like the royal family of England. The dominant males can be identified by their majestic walk and by their long strides. They carry their tails up. A linear dominance hierarchy exists in a group of rheses monkey. Alpha male move with their tails up. A subordinate male tusk its tail between hind limbs.

A subdominant males walks carefully and tusk its tail between the hind limbs. If the *alpha* male goes away from group even for a short while the *beta* male will raise its tail and as soon as the alpha returns it will take the tail down. Social group of rhesus monkey may split into smaller feeding group temporarily for foraging but all family units remain in near vicinity and unite at the time of danger. Roosting behaviour is of common occurrence among rhesus monkey. Approximately 200 individuals of rhesus monkey roost together. In winter 6-10 members embrace each other and sleep together in night.

(C) Squirrel monkeys

Squirrel monkeys *(Samiri sciureus)* are found in northern part of South America. The group size vary from 30-100 individuals. Adult female and their young form the core of the group. During breeding seasons adult males intermingle in the groups of females for a few month. Groups turn into many male and many female type during breeding season.

(D) Baboon

Washburn and lrevene De Vore studied pattern and movement of cohesive band of baboons *(Papio)*.The band always move under the sway of a few dominant males. The group of baboons have 50 to 100 individuals which wander in an area of only 3 km in diameter.

Most dominant males live in the center of the group and the others (less dominant) spaced out around him. When the troop moves the females and infants remain in the center for the safety. At the edge of the group are the youngest males. At the time of attack of predators youngest male give alarm calls and

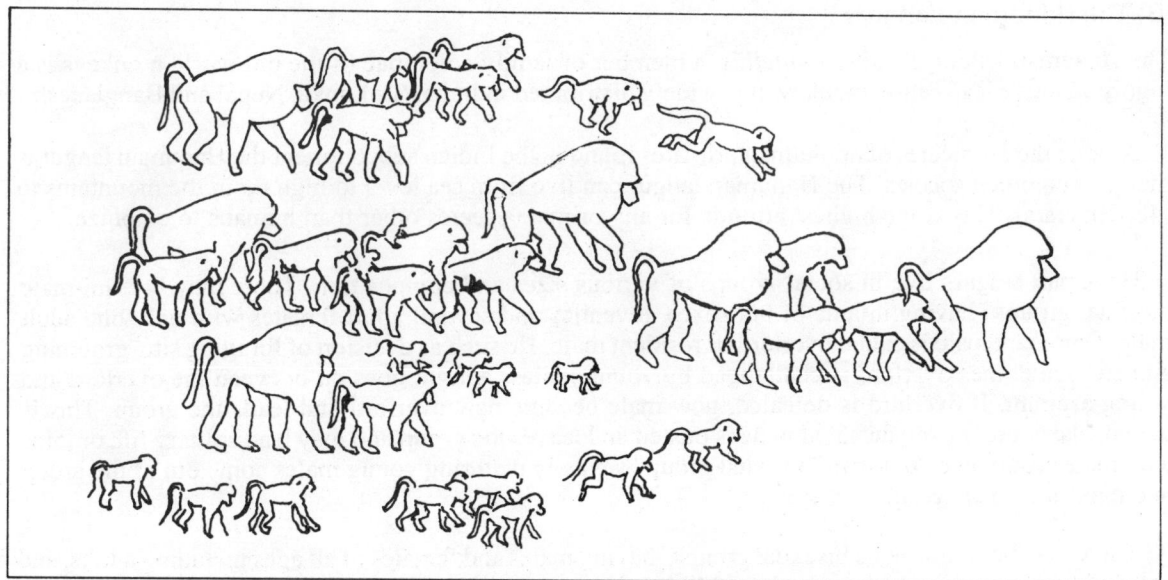

Fig. 5.26. Baboon Society : Troop of Baboon marching in home range.

males rush over and threaten the intruder. They spend night sleeping on certain trees. The male's position in the dominance order depends on his strength and ability for fighting. All the females subordinate to males.

The hamadryan baboon (*Papio hamadrys*) is a terrestrial primate inhabiting the plains of North East Africa and South West Arabia. The hamadryas baboon society has several levels of organization. The simplest level, the breeding unit is a harem of 1 to 10 females with a single male. At the next levels, several members of different harems may form larger bands while feeding, and these bands may act as a unit to defend a feeding site from a rival bands. The bands do confine their wandering to a larger area of about 25 square km. Still higher levels, several bands may join into larger groups for sleeping. As many as 700 hamadryas may sleep together. Gelada baboons (*Theropichacus gelada*) are large sized aggressive monkeys. The adult males are capable of chasing a leopard. These are found in northern Ethiopia. These monkeys sleep on cliff as one male family unit. In the morning, these units get together to from a large troop of many males and females which remain together all through the day while foraging. During night all get separated once again into smaller group of one male unit to sleep on a common cliff.

(2) SINGLE MALE BISEXUAL GROUP

Chacma baboons and Hanuman langur show single male bisexual social organization.

(A) Chacma Baboons (Papio ursinus)

Chacma Baboons are found in Angola and Zambia. They form one male family units of about 20 individuals. In day time many such units live close to each other and may appear as one group of many individuals. Their home ranges overlap considerably. Thus during the day time entire troop appears as a multimale bisexual group but in the evening they usually separate into one male many female & their young smaller group. The smaller groups occupy their own sleeping region.

(B) The Hanuman Langurs

The Hanuman langur, *Presbytis entellus,* a member of family coloninae of the old world monkeys is a highly adaptive leaf-eating monkey. It is widely distributed in India, Sri Lanka, Nepal and Bangladesh.

Among the 19 species of nonhuman primates found in the Indian subcontinent the Hanuman langur is the most common species. The Hanuman langur can live from sea level to high up in the mountains to (4267 meters). This is the highest attitude for any primate species other than humans to colonize.

Hanuman langurs live in social groups of various sizes and composition. There may be "uni-male bisexual groups" having infants of bot sexes, juveniles and several adult females with only one adult male. Dominant male is called overlord or resident male. He such as decision of foraging site, grooming site etc. sometimes overlord is challenged by young males. A fight goes on between the overlord and young aspirant. If overlord is defeated, new male become new overlord and leads the group. This is called take over. The old defeated male is ousted and leaves the group and may lead solitary life or joins a all male group. In a "uni-male bisexual group" sexually maturing young males come out of the group and make a all male group.

There may be "multi-male bisexual groups" having males and females of all ages including adults, and solely "male groups" which comprise of all ages except new borns.

Hanuman langurs are highly territorial and live in a fixed area, which is called their home-range. Home range often overlap to some extent, which may be quite extensive at times. In bisexual troops the home ranges have been known to very from 0.07 to 13 square km. In all-male groups, they are more extensive, 4.3 to 22 km. By and large, all groups use large trees as their sleeping sites. These sites constitute only a limited area of the total home range which is only about 100-150 sq. meters. It comprises either one large tree or 2-6 small trees or both.

The sleeping area is an important location as most of the groups' activities start and terminate here. In general the home range has been considered as the feeding, resting and sleeping sites of hanuman groups to which they restrict their daily activities.

Langurs in nature, have good association with other animals such as chinkara, chital, blue bull, sambhar, cattle etc. The langur's keen eyes and sharp sense of smell of these associates combine to make an extraordinary predator detection system.

(3) DIFFUSED SOCIAL GROUP OF CHIMPANZEES

Chimpanzee (*Pan troglodytes*) form diffused social group. They do not live in permanent troops. Unusually bands of males, group of females with or without offspring of large troops of males and females with young may be seen.

Chimpanzees form temporary groups which wander over ranges of several square kilometers and last for few hours or days. The group may have all males, all females and their infants or a combination of males and females.

Bonobo Society

A pigmy chimpanzee - bonobo *(Pan paniseus)* inhabiting Africa's most remote and dangerous tropical rain forest bounded by the Congo and Kasai rivers in the country once known as Zaire, now the Democratic Republic of the Congo, is our nearest evolutionary cousins. Bonobos look early human with their upright bipedal gait, long slim arms and legs, slender neck and narrow chests. Whole body covered with coarse black hair blessed with expressive faces, they look like smallish people. Bonobo walks upright with their straight backs. In fact the species shares more than 98 percent of human genetic material.

The first researcher to study the behaviour of this species named Tokayoshi kano, in 1973 entered jungle of Congo.

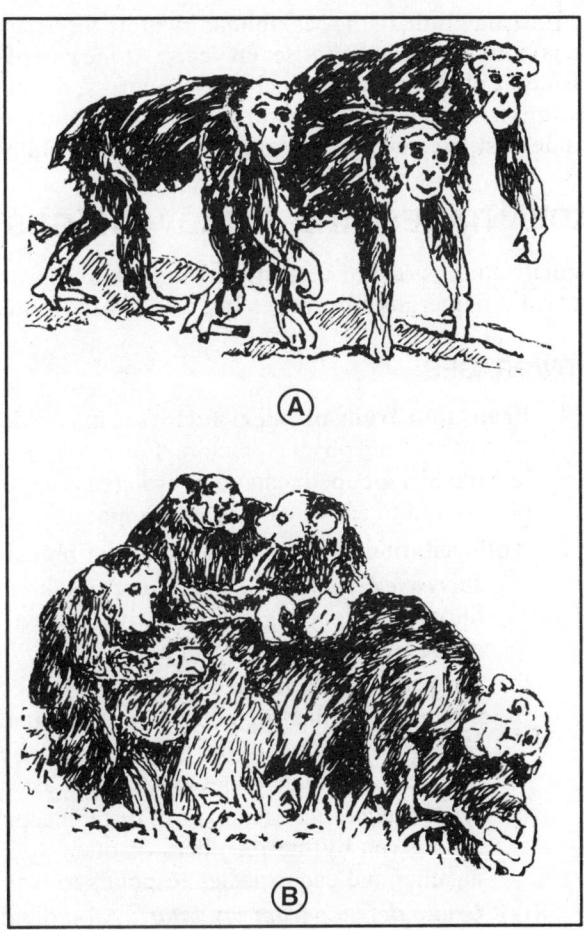

Fig. 5.27. (A) Chimpanzees form temporary groups having all females, adult females and their infants or a combination of males and females. (B) Social grooming in adult pan (Chimpanzees) provides a means of social cohesion within a group.

Kano was surprised to witness the bonobo females ruling the roost. They sat friendly together as they groomed each other, allowing favoured males to sit with them. If a male made a rare charge against females seated together, they either ignored his boorish display or chased him into jungle. Kano recognized 150 individual bonobos and noticed a close attachment between certain females and males. A highly ranked female he had named *Kame* was always accompanied by two males, *Ibo* and *Mon*. She groomed them, fed side by side, but never mated with them. They were mother and her two sons, bonded by familiar affection. Mothers are the core of bonobo society, holdings the group together. They even pushed their son's status by encouraging them to mate with other females in their social circle, because the more females a male can mate with the higher is his status. And if a male dared attack another male, his mother would marshal her female allies to defend him.

Chimpanzee males rarely have close contact with their mothers after they mature but male bonobos bonded with their mother for life.

Barbara Fruth, of the Max-plank-institute for behavioural physiology in Germany, has studied bonobo behaviour in the congo for seven years. At the end of each day, she noted each bonobo in a group would fashion a platform from branches high in tress, then weave 20-30 leafy side branches into a well-padded mattress. It was positively luxurious by comparison with Chimpanzee's rudimentary cradle, or a gorilla's crude nest, created by flattening grass with its bulky body.

ADVANTAGES AND DISADVANTAGES OF SOCIAL LIFE

Socialization is one of the ways to survive and get better opportunities to breed successfully. Society provides numerous advantages but a few disadvantages too.

ADVANTAGES

1. **Protection from physical factors :** In a colony numerous members live together and protect each other from physical factors. For example a bird bobwhite quail (*Colinus virginianus*) survive better when grouped than when isolated (Gerstell, 1939). *Lycus loripes* is distasteful beetle which birds avoid to eat when they are in mass.

2. **Antipredation :** Improved detection of predators depends on more than one factors.
   (i) *Increased chance of detection of predator :* Presence of numerous members means presence of more sensory organs and individuals will detect a predator quickly and be able to warn rest of the members of the group.
   (ii) *Members act as guard :* One or a few individuals assume the role of watching for the entire group while other members forage and remain busy in other activities. One Hanuman langur (*Presbytis entellus*) of the group occupy the highest canopy and remain vigilant for predators. Monkeys and male baboons often act as sentinels while other troop members forage.
   (iii) *Mutual vigilance :* Animals of different species living in the same habitat respond to the alarm calls given by the members of other species. Baboons, Zebras, Gazelles etc. often graze together and each species responds to warning calls of each other.
   (iv) *Group defence from predator :* All individuals of the group attack predator and kill or drive away the predator. Similar defensive formation occurs in elephants and ungulates to repulse lion, hyena, and wild dogs. Groups of baboons have also been seen chasing leopard, cheetah, and lions. Ground squirrel of California, Coatimundis Agoutis and various non-human primates have been observed mobing snakes. Many species of colonial or flocking birds (Gulls and Terns) also mob predators such as a fox.

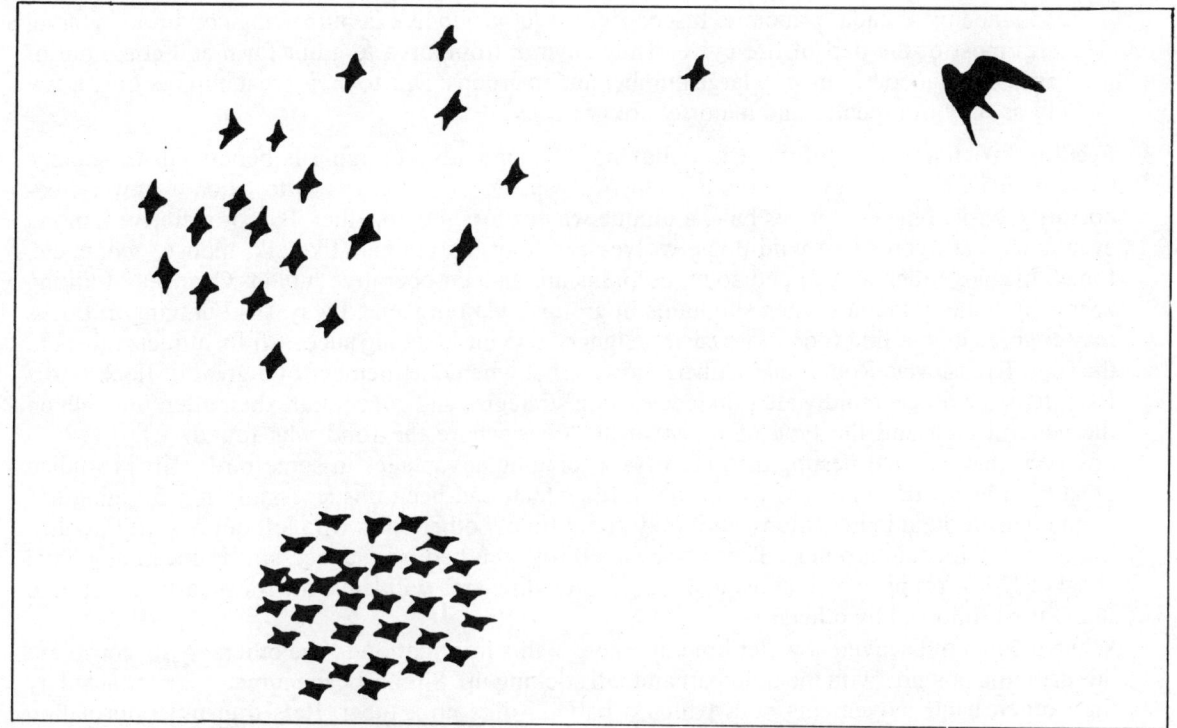

Fig. 5.28. The response of a flock of starlings to the approach of a bird of prey.

(v) ***Protection of young*** : Young of the group are helpless and need more protection. Musk ox form a defensive ring around their calves, while adult males form a ring around the herd. adult males collectively chase wolves in attempt to drive them off.

Predators avoid to attack group due to geometrical effects. Predatory bird hawk, prey upon wood pigeons. It was observed that attack success of hawk decreases as the flock size of the wood pigeons was increased. Predators attack individuals on the periphery of the group, prey animals in a group should therefore, gain protection by remaining or moving towards the center of a group. Sea gulls gather together in colonies during the breeding season. They form a united front to protect their nest and nestings against predator.

(vi) ***Confuse the predator*** : Members of a group act in such a fashion that predator becomes confused. Geese come near each other and flap their wings simultaneously and make water fountain when a hawk comes near them. This act of geese confuse and frighten the predator and they leave the prey.

The great ethologist Niko Tinbergen was mobbed by gulls on many occasions during his visits to their colonies. Question arised in his mind why the birds mobbed ? He imagined that mobbing helps gull parents confuse and distract predators intent on finding and eating their offspring. Zebra, deer and antelopes start running in all directions in a very confusing fashion when attacked by a lioness. Most of the time the lioness is unable to decide which one to follow, and in the meantime, all of them escape.

(vii) ***'Lost of group' principle*** : Individuals of a group try to hide himself in the group when attacked by a predator. This is based on *'lost in group'* principle. This principle is itself explained by 'cicada' principle. Insect of *'cicada'* group live in burrowing condition in larval form most of the part of life cycle. They emerge from larva to adult form and come out of earth simultaneously in very large number and in groups. Due to their great number only a few fall as prey of predator and majority are protected.

3. **Feeding efficiency and information sharing :** Co-operative foraging is beneficial for society. Co-opeative foraging may be divided into two aspects : (i) It is easier to catch a prey on co-operative basis. Nile crocodiles have a unique way of foraging together. By co-operative hunting even small carnivores like wild dogs, wolves can hunt big animals like elk, moose, zebras etc. Lions, hyenas, killer whales and some dolphins are also co-operative hunter. Chances of killing zebras by lioness doubles when she hunts in groups, in an organized way. (ii) Foraging in flocks may enable birds to find food more easily. Sight of one bird feeding successfully attracts others to the spot. Krebs, Mac Robert and Cullen showed that when one member of a great tit flock find a food item, the others rapidly alter their searching strategies and concentrate their attention both on the general area and the type of niche in the trees where the food was found. Ward (1965) observed that colonial nesting also conveys a foraging advantages in some birds. Krebs studied great blue heron colonies and found that birds which had been unsuccessful on a foraging trip would hang around in the colony until they could follow other birds who left quickly after returning from the feeding grounds. These were the birds who had been successful in locating a local shoal of fish. Groups, which know about a good feeding area will leave the roost early to return to it and then followed by others.

When a baboon discovers a water hole, it conveys this information to the others by its conspicuous drinking posture, with the hind part and tail sticking up. Similarly, the inmates are attracted by the excited hand movements with which a baboon digs up a tuber. Rats transmit information regarding poisonous bait to other member of the group living in a house. All rats leave the house simultaneously. If rats were living solitary they would be deprived off these informations.

In a group mutual vigilance for predators allow each individual to spend more time foraging, without increasing vulnerability to predators. In a group of hanuman langurs, the related adult females temporarily take away the infant from mother to enable her to forage. This behaviour is called *aunt behaviour*. The pups of wild dogs, wolves and lions are often attended by few adults while other pack member can go out hunting.

Social organization of carnivores help to protect caracasses from scavengers. A single lion usually cannot protect a pack hyenas or wild dogs, or crows or vultures from stealing a caracass, but two or more lions can.

4. **Stimulation and synchronization of breeding :** Group living facilitates reproductive success. In solitary animals like rhino and orangutan it is difficult for them to find a mate, they have to cover large areas in forest, spend much time and energy to find a suitable mate but it is easier to find receptive partner in a social group. Domesticated lions were unsuccessful in mating. Watching others courting and mating initiates, sexual behaviour in other members also. Experiments have showed that the hormonal cycles of some female bird and mammals are affected by the presence of males of species concerned (Chapter 3). Large number of sea-birds nest in dense colonies, even though they may vigorously defend their own small territory within the group. Fraser Darling was among all the first to point out that in such colonies a great deal of stimulation must result from the displays, which are a constant feature of a large group early in the breeding season. The effects of such stimulation, coming from neighbours as well as from a bird's own mate, will tend to accelerate and synchronize the reproductive cycle within the colony. Coulson has shown that birds breeding in the most densely packed central areas of a nesting colony are more successful than those in occupying more peripheral nest sites. They lay more eggs and lay

them earlier. There seems little doubt that heightened social stimulation in the central area is one of the factors contribution to these effects. Mating swarms are common in insects and among some vertebrates.

5. **Increases competitive ability :** Watson and his co-workers have shown that population size is effectively determined by territorial behaviour. In autum, the cock birds flight over the breeding areas and a proportion of them success in winning territories. The unsuccessful birds are driven away into the valley bottoms. Only the territory holders can breed and the next spring, the surplus birds are rendered effectively sterile and, in any case, have a far higher mortality in the unfavorable habitat into which they are forced.

6. **Division of labour and solution of Environmental problems :** Division of labour is useful and befitting in all aspects of life. Termitarium of termites is big and complex in which microclimate is even very regulated i.e. temperature, humidity, O_2–CO_2 quantity are maintained evenly hence, it is obvious that high social arrangement for successful mode of life is made possible due to division of labour.

7. **Energetic efficiency :** Role of energy in socialization of animals can be understood by two examples:

   (i) *Thermal and other forms of energy conservation :* Animals found in cold arctic regions such as vole, penguins, honeybee, etc. live in close groups. Thus, they reduce the relative surface area and make a common hot regions around the group which protect them from cold.

   (ii) *Efficiency in Movements :* According to principles of physics, a group swimming in fluid in a definite manner can swim more smoothly and spending very less energy than an individual. Application of this principle is applied while geese and ducks fly in group in air making a 'V' like shape.

8. **Transfer learning :** Socialization helps in transfer of learning from one generation to another. For example finding food source, food capturing technique, water source, avoiding danger and killing enemy etc.

DISADVANTAGE

The following are a few disadvantages associated with living in groups :

1. Competition is increased. Possibility of intense aggression as social organism crowd around a clumped resource.
2. Increased chance of spread of diseases and parasites.
3. Interference with reproduction, such as cheating in parental care or killing of progeny by nonparents.
4. Reduce fitness due to inbreeding.
5. Become distinct to predator.

EXERCISE

1. Define sociobiology. Write difference between aggregation and society. Mention properties of social groups.
2. Describe advantages and cause of social life. Mention disadvantage of social life if any.
3. What do you mean by social insects ? Describe various degrees of social development in them.
4. Give an account of social life in insects. (Civil services, 1997).

5. Write brief note about social organization in honeybee or ants. Explain nature and functions of different castes of honeybee and ants. (Civil services, 1981)

6. Write short notes on social behaviour of invertebrates besides insects. Compare insect and human society.

7. Describe school of fish, aggregation of amphibians and reptiles giving suitable examples.

8. Describe social organization of birds.

9. Describe interesting aspects of social behaviour of rhesus monkey and hanuman langur.

10. Describe social behaviour of Lion, Elephants, Vampire bat and members of order cetacea (Whale and Dolphins).

11. What factors are usually present in behaviour that is called 'social' ? What kinds of behaviour can be recognized in the schooling of fish ?

12. Describe the social signals given by spotted female hyenas by their pseudopenis. How it develops in female hyena.

13. Write short note on Bonobo society.

14. Give interesting points in social behaviour of Baboons.

15. Differentiate and describe 'lordship' and 'lordosis' in context of social behaviour and sexual reproduction in baboon and cat respectively.

16. What do you mean by altruism? Describe altruism in primates.

17. Describe communication in honeybees. How communication system help honeybees to maintain a society.

18. Describe wasp polities in forming an alliance. Mention how wasps choose their queen.

19. Write short notes on "Farmer ants" and "Honey collector ants".

20. How ant queen mutilate workers.

21. Write a short note on bossism in ants and honeybees.

22. Write short note on nepotism in social insects.

23. Write short note on "reciprocal altruism" in bats.

24. Write shorts on "allogrooming", "Roosting", "Mounting" and "Huddling" in primates.

25. Write short note on roosting of munia.

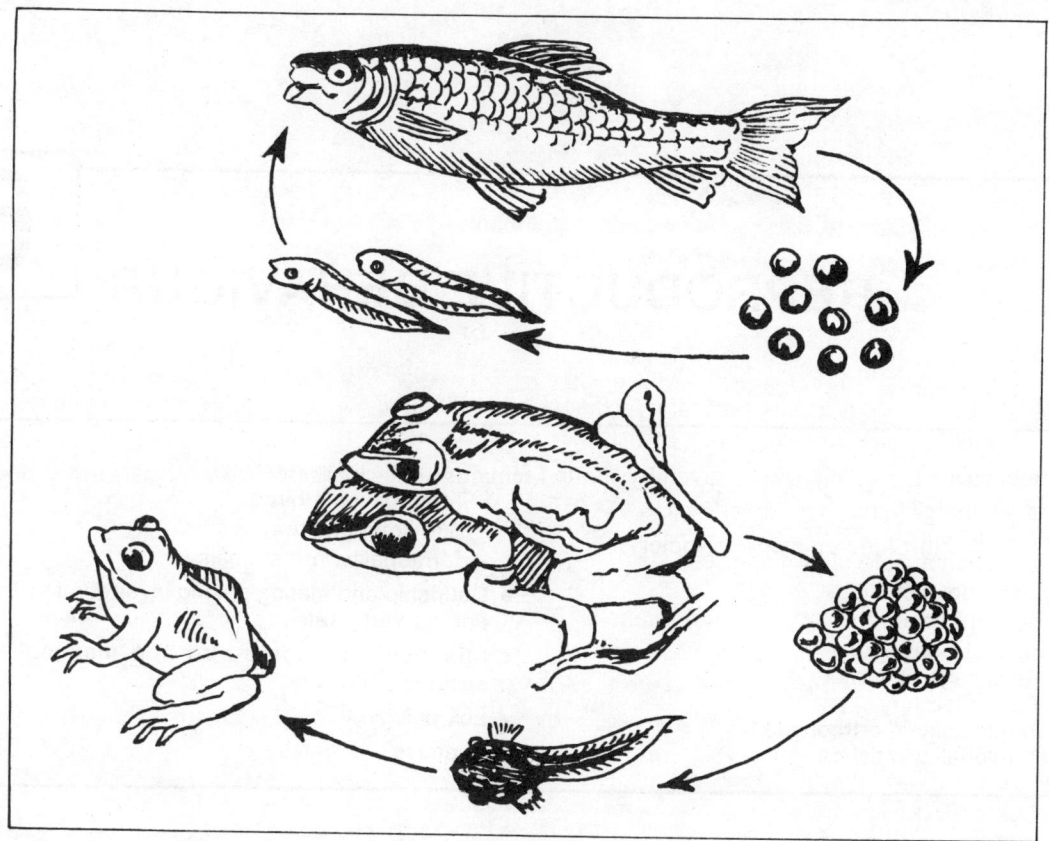

Reproduction, or multiplication of an organism to produce offspring of the same kind is a universal characteristic of all living beings. It results in the continuity of life from one generation to another. Reproduction is accomplished by two methods : asexual and sexual. Asexual reproduction concerns a single individual which produces new offspring exactly similar to the parent. It does not involve the production or fusion of sex cells (gametes). Barring blue green algae and some fungi; most plants and animals reproduce sexually.

The process of bisexual reproduction involves two partners of opposite sex to ensure fertilization (fusion) of two haploid gametes to give rise to a diploid zygote. The bisexual reproduction not only maintains the flow of life but also involves the transmission of genetic material from the parental generation to the offspring generation. Many synchronized activities between the opposite sexes are required in hierarchial patterns to ensure successful mating.

This chapter gives detailed account of some interesting aspects related to reproductive rituals in certain sexually reproducing species and also answers many intriguing and highly profitable questions regarding sexual behaviour of animals.

REPRODUCTIVE BEHAVIOUR $\boxed{6}$

INTRODUCTION

There are four major steps; *pre-courtship, courtship, mating* and *post-mating*; to complete the entire drama of sexual reproductive behaviour enacted by bisexual animals. Most of the episodes of reproductive behaviour are *pre-courtship* (sex dimorphism, sexual selection, sperm competition, territoriality) and this may appear to a lay man unimportant in comparison to *courtship* and *mating* part but these pre-courtship acts are equally important and interesting to an ethologist. However, it is true that pre-courtship is indirectly involved part of reproductive behaviour while courtship and mating is directly involved part of reproductive behaviour.

SEX DIMORPHISM

Male and female of many bisexual species differ morphologically and this condition is known as sex dimorphism. Differences among species in the degree of sexual dimorphism in body size were a possible measure of the investment of males made in fighting capacity. Although there are other factors besides sexual competition that might result in sexual dimorphism in body size.

FISHES

Very few species of fishes are sexually dimorphic. Male Sharks bear copulatory organs called claspers. The copulatory organs help in introducing the milt directly into the genital tract of the female. Among teleosts an intromittent copulatory organ is present only in those species in which the fertilization is internal. Tengra *(Mystus seenghala)* bear a conical genital papilla but fertilization is external. In Gambusia (mosquito larva eating fish) vas deferens is produced into a tube upto the end of the anterior rays of the anal fin which help in sperm transfer. Males of Poecilidae family bear a complicated intromittent organ, ending in curved hooks, spines and barbs. The male four-eyed fish *Anableps* bear a special tube for copulation. Male white sucker *(Catostomus commersoni)* bear enlarged anal fin which serves to transfer the milt. In clasping cyprinodont *(Xenodexia)* the pectoral fin is modified and used in mating by holding the gonopodium in position for insertion into the oviduct of female.

Male and female of many fish species can be distinguished only during spawning season. The body of male of many families – Cyprinodontidae, Cichlidae, Labrynthidae and Labridae – become brighter in colour during the breeding season. The male bow fin *(Amia)* bear a black spot at the base of the caudal fin. Male flat fish *(Bothus)* bear spines on snout. Male Sword fish *(Xiphophorus)* bear elongated caudal fin. The common dragonet *(Callionymus)* exhibit well marked sex dimorphism. The males are orange coloured with deep blue stripes on the sides and a row of blue or green spots. The female is dull yellow brown with green spots.

AMPHILBIA

A few species of Amphibia are sexually dimorphic. Male and female frogs *(Rana tigerina)* can be distinguished on the basis of certain external characters. Male frogs bear two *vocal organs* to produce crocking sound to attract females for *amplexus.* In male frogs, during breeding season, the first fingers of the fore hands swell and are provided with pads called *nuptial* or *copulatory* or *amplexusory pads.* *Articular* pads on the other fingers of the male frogs develops during breeding season only.

REPTILES

Some forms of copulatory organs are always present in reptiles except in a living fossil *Sphenodon*, but only a few species show distinct sexual dimorphism. Some marine ophididae males possess intromittent organs. In *Uromastix* sexual dimorphism is marked by the presence of one pair of protrusible copulatory organs called, *hemipenes.* In breeding season, colour changes is remarkable in reptiles. Male lizards bear the dark reticulation of the black against a general background of grey ; while females exhibit a pale, brownish tint.

BIRDS

Both sexes are alike in most of the bird species and it is hard to tell them apart. However, male and female of few species have slight difference in plumage colour, structure of beak, song and nesting behaviour. Budgerigar *(Melopsittacus undulatus)* is inhabitant of Australia. The male is distinguished by the blue colour round the nostrils, which area is brown in the female. Turquoisine grass parakeet *(Neophema pulchella)* a rare species of Australia exhibit minor sex dimorphism. The female differs from the male in that it lacks the red shoulder patch and the blue colouring is not so vivid. The Red-headed Lovebird *(Agapornis pullaria)* inhabits tropical Africa. The female's face mask is yellow, whereas the male's is vermilion, and her under-wing covers are green. Contrary to above examples there are a few species of birds which are morphologically so different that at times it is difficult to believe that the two sexes really belong to the same species. Male and female pigeon *(Columba)*, Peacock/hen *(Pavo cristatus)*, Electus parrot *(Lorius rotatus)* can easily be distinguished morphologically. The plumage of electus parrot bird is markedly different in the male and female, so much so that they were originally believed to be two distinct species. The cock is coloured a bright green whereas the hen is a magnificent red.

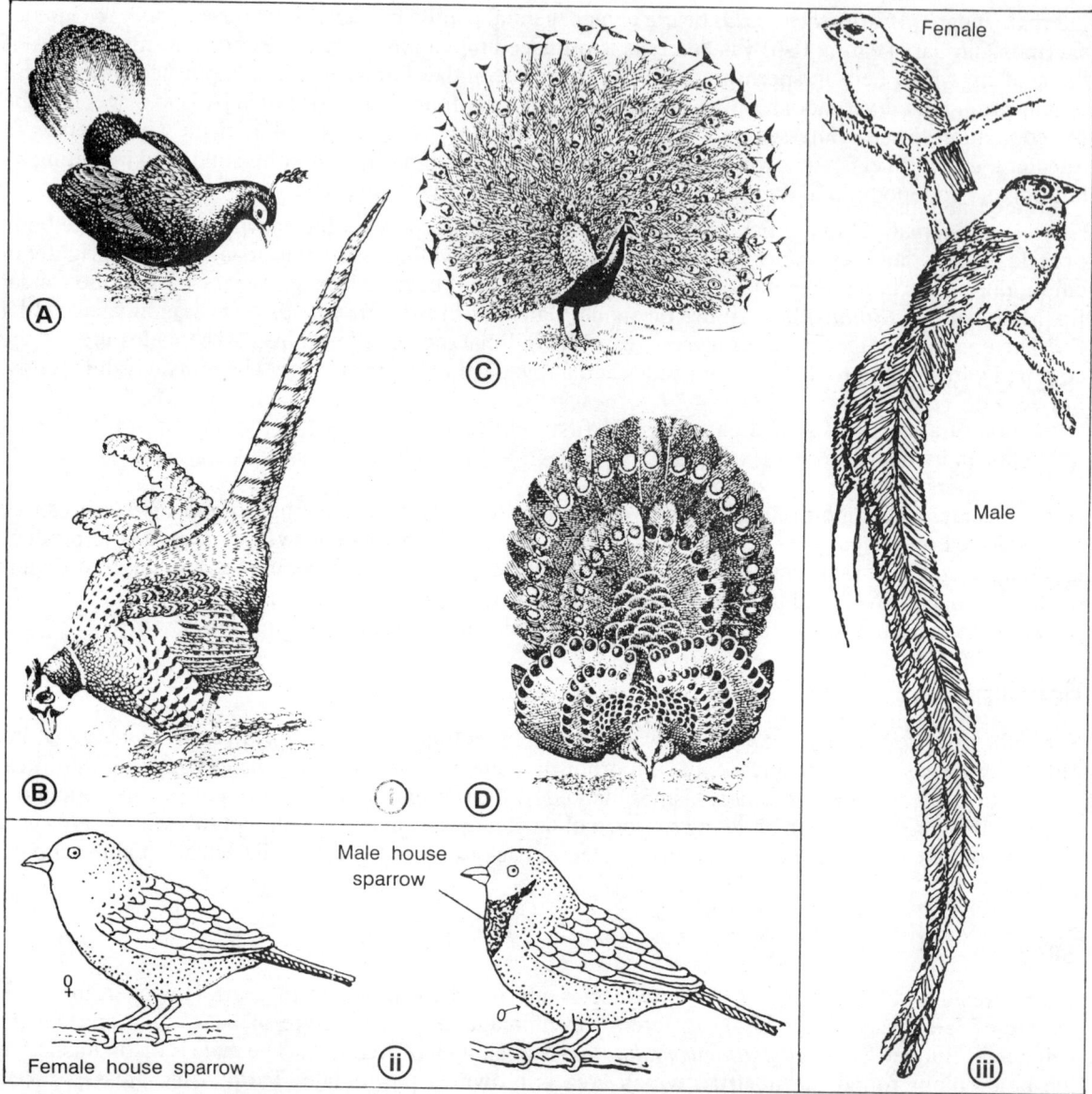

Fig. 6.1. Sexual dimorphism is clearly evident in some birds. (i) Male birds with well maintained plumage, dancing and nest building ability : (A) Himalayan monal, (B) Ring necked pheasand, (C) Indian peacock, (D) Myanmar peacock. (ii) Sexual dimorphism in house sparrow (*Passer domesticus*). (iii) Sexual dimorphism in African Paradise birds (*Vidus paradisea*) in breeding season.

MAMMALS

With a few exceptions mammals show distinct pattern of sexual dimorphism. Adult males are bigger than adult females. This is because males of most mammal species devote the bulk of their time and energy in attempts to introduce their sperms into as many females as possible. But there are few exceptions to this rule. Female hyenas are heavier and more aggressive than males. It is interesting to note that female hyena bear a pseudopenis.

The degree of sexual dimorphism is more evident in those species in which males can monopolize many mates, and less evident in those species whose males are limited to one or two mates per breeding season. Data on the ratio of body lengths of males to those of females, a standard measure of sexual dimorphism, in several mammalian groups supports this fact. Thus an elephant seal male may mate with as many as 100 females. Male seals are about 60 percent longer and about 5 times heavier than female seals.

Male Baboons and Hanuman langur are much larger than females and they compete for reproductive success. Dominant males indeed monopolize estrous females.

Sexual dimorphism is well marked among humans. The differences between the skeletons of male and female humans are primarily due to the greater muscularity of the man and to the fact that the female pelvis is designed to enable her to give birth to an infant with a large head.

SEXUAL SELECTION

Selection of a receptive sexual partner is the first link in the chain of events leading to fertilization of gametes. Individuals of one sex (usually the males) "advertise" that they are worthy of an investment, then members of opposite sex (females) choose among them. This is intersexual selection. Intrasexual selection involves competition within one sex (usually males) with the winner gaining access to the opposite sex.

The migration of Hilsa and Salmon fish from sea to river for breeding is a specialized kind of sexual selection. It serves as a means of selecting the healthiest male for breeding. Weak males reach late at breeding site and are eliminated automatically.

Peahen pheasand show preferences for peacock pheasand with well maintained plumage and spectacular dancing ability. Female Baya (a weaver bird - *Ploceus phillipinus*) choose a male whose nest catches her fancy. In some cases females may incite competition among males and thus may gain some control over the choice of mate. For example, female elephant seals (*Mirounga angustirostris*) vocalize loudly whenever male attempts to copulate. The vocalization of female elephant seal attracts other males and tests the dominance of the male attempting to mate. Dominant harem master will drive off low ranking potentially inferior mating partners.

There are numerous differences in sexual selection among the various human races. Darwin was of the opinion that of all the causes which have led to the differences in external appearance between the races of man, sexual selection has played for the most efficient.

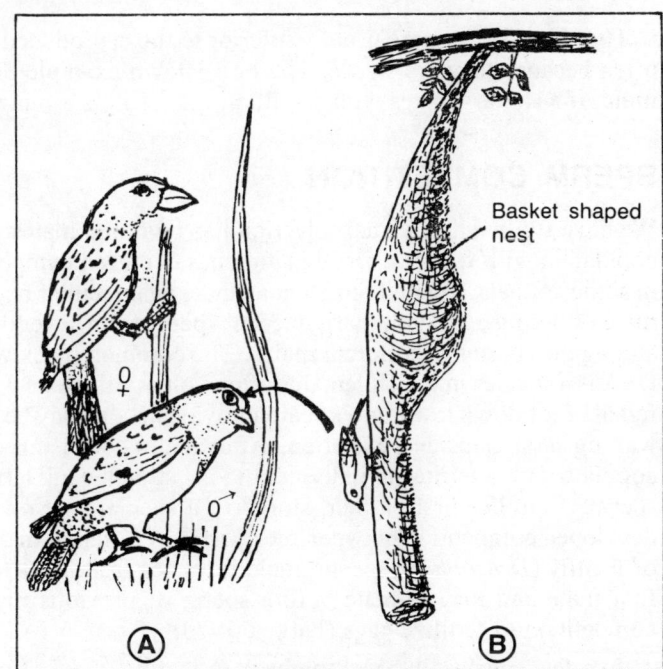

Fig. 6.2. (A) Male and female Baya weaver birds (*Ploceus philippinus*). (B) A Baya male weaving nest and female baya watching the process. The best woven nest is selected for mating sites and its builder gets an opportunity to mate with female baya.

Smith (1958) put forward a theoretical analysis to explain the role of sexual selection in the evolution of mankind. Imagine a society in which man prefer white complexioned wife and in which this preference is determined genetically. White complexioned women will have a choice in the selection of mates and are likely to mary early and to produce more offsprings. Smith's analysis suggests that degree of polygamy is an important factor in determining the effectiveness of sexual selection in human society. Among the Xavantes and Yanomamas, two of the surviving primitive tribes of South American Indians, the man vary considerably in their reproductive performance. In one of the villages studied, a quarter of the total population were the offsprings of two head man. Statistical studies of urban man show evidence that active mating preferences (assertive mating) occur for physical traits like stature and for psychological traits such as intelligence and academic achievements. Although it may be true that female hips are sexually attractive to men and strong man may be attractive to women, this does not necessarily mean that sexual selection is responsible for these features only.

CHOOSING A MATE OF OWN SPECIES

Mating between members of different species is very very rare in nature. Numerous factors keeps a species isolated. Important isolating factors are :

(i) Lock and key system of genitalia.
(ii) Physical isolation
(iii) Psychological Isolation
(iv) Gamete Isolation.

Hybrid offsprings are usually inferior to those produced by matings of members of the same species, often because they are sterile. The best known example of a sterile hybrid (produced in nature) is the mule; if a she-ass mates with a stallion the result is a mule, which is sterile.

SPERM COMPETITION

We have studied that sexual selection has favoured males with the ability to cope with competition for copulation with females. Once mating has occurred competition for fitness should essentially stop. But in some animals, a mated female may mate again, either because she is compelled to do so by a coercive male or because she voluntarily accept sperm from several males. This is the microscopic battle fought among the sperms of different males. The common black winged damselflies (*Calopteryx maculata*) of USA is a species in which females often voluntarily mate with more than one male. When an egg-ladden female flies down towards a stream to oviposit, she may be intercepted by a non-territorial satellite male waiting in streamside vegetation. After mating with this male, she may subsequently encounter and copulate with a territorial individual in his stream bank territory, even though she already has plenty of sperms from her first partner, stored in a special sperm storage sac in her body. Thus damselfly has developed competition between the sperms of different males to fertilize the same female's eggs. In case of fruitfly (*Drosophila*) second male fertilizes from 83% to 99% eggs. Female spiders store sperms of first mate and may re-mate before sperm of previous mate are used up. Thus she create the sperm competition to fertilize eggs (Farker, 1970).

In a few species, in order to check re-mating, the first male of some species has developed interesting methods. Members of order Lepidoptera (Moths and Butterflies) produce two kinds of sperms. One kind is the usual type (*eupyrene*) that fertilizes the eggs. The second type (*apyrene*) contains no nuclear material but may comprise more than half the sperm complement. The question arises why should ␣les waste energy on these dead sperms? Silberglied, Sphepherd, and Dickinson (1984) suggest that ␣ the result of sperm competition, possibly displacing *eupyrene* sperm from first male or delaying re-mating by female. First male fruitfly (*Drosophila melanogaster*) copulating with the female may transfer "anti-aph-rodisiac" substances that inhibit court-ship behaviour of other males. The male Acanthocephalan worm (*Moniliformis moniliformis*) sticks a '*chastity belt*' on a female after mating, probably to pre-vent other males from copulating with her.

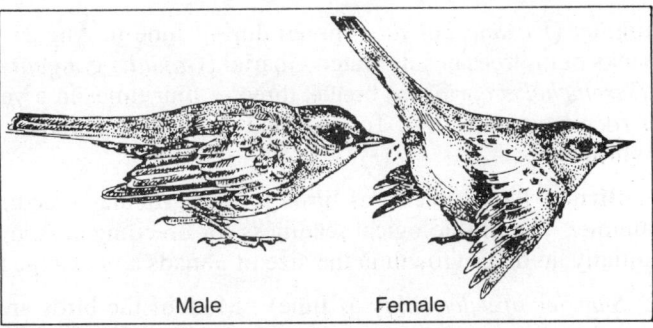

Fig. 6.3. A male Dunnock pecks at the cloaca of his partner after finding another mate near her ; in response she will eject a droplet of sperm-containing fluid.

Some male damselflies use their pe-nis to remove other male's sperms from female's storage organ before transfer-ring his own sperms. The males are also known to '*rape*' other males, cement-ing up the victim's genital opening to render them incapable of copulation. An interesting kind of sperm competition has been found in the hemipteran insect *Xylocoris maculipennis* by J. Caryon. Copulation in this insect is performed not by common method of mating but by injecting sperms. The male punctures the side of the female with his genitalia and squirts his sperms in. A totally different type of sperm transfer method has also been observed in this insect. A male *Xylocoris* sometimes copulates with another male. His sperms then migrate to the victim's testes, and when the second male happens to copulate with a female, the first male's sperms are also injected into her.

Male dunnock (a small European songbird species) may induce his partner to void sperm after finding her in close company with a rival male. Similarly, some male Sharks give their mates a contra-ceptive drouche prior to passing his own sperm. A Shark clasper has two tubes. Through one tube, a male can spray sea-water at great force, perhaps washing out the female's reproductive duct before passing his own sperm into his partner through the other tube.

After a new stallion has taken a band of wild mares from another male, any pregnant mare may abort after having been forced to copulate by the new harem owner. After a similar take over in certain mice, exposure to the odour of the new male's urine causes pregnant females to reabsorb their embryonic offsprings.

BREEDING SEASON

Most of the animals breed in particular time of their life or season, that is why they are called seasonal breeders. In lower animals the timing or seasonality is less understood. However, few examples are notable. Paloloworm (*Eunice*) of the Pacific ocean spawn when the moon is full, during October/November but the Atlantic Paloloworm spawn about the last quarter of the moon in July. Timing of breeding in the higher animal is a more complicated affair. Migration of some species of fishes, birds and mammals is also related with breeding season.

Fish : Grunion fish exhibits lunar rhythm and breeds on full moon nights during March to July.

Amphibians : Frogs and toads e.g. Malabar tree toad (*Nectophryne tuberulosa*), Goro hills tree toad (*N. kempi*) breed in rainy season (June-July). Himalayan Newt (*Tylototriton verrucosa*) congregate in pools after one or two pre-monsoon showers (April-May) and breed in monsoon months.

Reptiles : Indian moniter (*Varanus bengalensis*) breed during July to September. They lay 19-30 eggs in clutch. These eggs are deposited in holes and are covered with leaves, garbage and sand. Water moniter (*Varanus salvator*) breed during June to August. 15 to 30 eggs are laid in holes on the river banks or on trees beside water. Gharial (*Gavialis gangeticus*) breed in March/April. Leather back turtle (*Dermochelys coriacea*) breeds three to four times in a year but the peak period is May-June. Mugger (*Crocodylus palustris*), Tortoise and shell turtle (*Eretmochelys imbricata*) breed during November to February.

Birds : Each species of birds has a particular breeding period usually a few weeks in spring or summer. The physiological readiness for breeding season appears to be geared to the right season and initially involves growth in the size of gonads and change in behaviour.

Summer breeder (May to June) : Most of the birds are summer breeder, when day length become longer and temperature rises. Kea (*Nestor notabilis*), Lyre birds (*Memura*), Emus (*Dromiceius*), Tragopan, Ducks, Black necked Crane (*Grus nigricolis*) breed in summer.

Rainy Season (July, August, September) : Australian birds (Tree Swallow, Wood Swallow, the Budgerigar and Zebra finch) breed in rainy season. Flammingo breed in the Runn of Kutch after the monsoon. It is very particular about waiting for the right condition. In some years when the rainfall has been too heavy or too slight, it refuses to nest at all.

March–June : Malabar Pied Hornbill (*Anthracoceros coronatus coronatus*) is found in Peninsular India. Indian Pied Hornbill (*A. malabarieus malabarieus*) is found in Malabar region of India. Assam wreathed Hornbill (*Rhyticeros undulatus ticehursti*) is found in Assam. Koklass Pheasant (*Pucrasia macrolopha*) and Cheer pheasant (*Catreus uvallichi*) all breed in between March and June.

March–September : Great Indian bustard (*Ardeotis nigriceps*) is endangered species and the male is polygamous. Peacock-Pheasant (*Polyplectron bicalcaratum*) male show a spectacular courtship display and breed between March to September.

January–April : Pigeons and Himalayan Golden eagle (*Aquila chrysaetos daphanea*) breed in between January to April.

December–March : Himalayan bearded Vulture (*Gypaetus barbatus aureus*) has an elaborate courtship display and both the sexes take part in incubation and bringing up of the young ones.

Several sea birds such as Brown booby (*Sula leucoaster*), the sooty tern (*Sterna fuscata*), Lesser noddy tern (*Anaus tenuirostris*) breed at intervals of 8-10 month.

Mammals : All mammals are seasonal breeder. Exceptions are man (*Homo sapiens*), Leopard or Panther (*Panthera pardus*), Sea cow, Jackal (*Canis aureus*), and Lion (*Felis leo*). These breed throughout the year.

Summer Breeder : Himalayan brown bear (*Ursus arctos isabelinus*), Mouse-deer (*Traqulus meminna*), Sloth bear, etc. breed in summer.

Winter breeder : Gaur (*Bos gaurus*), Blackbuck (*Antilope cervicapra*), Striped hyena (*Hyena hyena*), Leopard cat (*Felis bengalensis*), Musk deer (*Moschus moschiferous*), Swamp deer (*Cervus duvauceli*), Clapped langur (*Presbytis pileatus*), Golden langur (*Presbytis geei*), Phayre's leaf monkey (*Presbytis phayrei*), etc. breed in winter. Rhinoceros mate during February, March and April. Gestation period is 12 to 19 months. The calf usually a single is born around October. Asiatic lion (*Panthera leo persica*) mates between October/November Gestation period is about 4 months. Indian Fox (*Vulpes bengalensis*) breeds between Nov. and January. Indian wild dog (*Cuon alpinus*), Blue Whale (*Balenoptera musculus*) migrates to temperate region in winter for breeding.

Rainy Season : Tiger (*Panthera tigris*) mates after rains, and the young ones, usually two to six are born between February and May. The cubs are looked after the mother. Male Hoolock Gibbon (*Hylobates hoolock*) is monogamous and remains contented with a particular female. The mating period is early in the rainy season and young is born in winter. Wolf (*Canis lupus*) breeds mostly at the end of the rains and young once, usually 3 to 8, are born about December. Four horned antelope (*Tetracerus quadricornis*) ruts during the rains.

September-October : Hangul (*Cervus elaphus hanglu*) rut in the month of September and ends by the end of October. The stag establishes a harem. The young is born in April - May.

BREEDING TWICE IN A YEAR

Some birds and few mammals breed twice in a year. Shahin Falcon (*Falco peregrinus*) breeds during March/May in the Himalaya and from January to April in the penisnsular Indian Hills. Great Pied Hornbill (*Bucerus bicornis homrai*) breeds once in March/April in the northern area of its distribution and twice in February/April in southwestern India. Towhee (*Papilo alberti*) of Arizona nest twice in a year, once in March/April and again in July of the same calender year. The sooty terns of Christmas island in the Pacific Ocean have two breeding seasons at six months interval.

Pig tailed Macaque (*Macaca nemestrima leonina*) breeds twice in a year. Once in June and twice in December. Jungle Cat (*Felis Chaus*) breed twice in a year.

TERRITORIAL BEHAVIOUR

A territory is an area held and defended by an individual or group of animals against animals of the same or different species. Why males of a species living together peacefully become aggressive to other males of its own species in breeding season ? Aggressiveness among males increases during breeding season for breeding territory. The increase of aggressiveness is due to the increased level of male hormone. For many animal species the territory must be extremely important for survival, since a great deal of time and energy is spent in defending it. Territorial defence behaviour is particularly common among mammals, birds, reptiles and fishes.

A wide variety of natural weapons may be used by males involved in territorial fighting. In fishes and reptiles teeth play an important weapon and the tail is used to batter the opponent. A hook develops on the lower Jaw of the male Salmon during the breeding season that acts as offensive organ. Some fish species beat the water with its tail, producing turbulence which drive away the opponent. Birds mainly use their beak and claws as weapon to defend their territory. Among mammals, big herbivores have horns or antler + heavy hooves while carnivores have powerful canine teeth and claws used to defend territory. Two male giraffe fighting for breeding territory tries to cut the neck and head of opponent. They also try to injure genitalia of the opponent male.

ADVANTAGE OF TERRITORY

Territorial behaviour forms an important part of social behaviour. Owing a territory advances the owner's reproductive success has been found in many species. Territory provides a base which the male can advertise himself to female. It provides a protected place where courtship, mating, parental care to young can occur freely and without any interference.

SIZE OF TERRITORY

Territory size varies enormously among species. Poplar aphid defends a territory of a few sq. mm area only, whereas Wagtail defends an area of 600 meters of river bank. Robins and Wablers have territories smaller than 200 sq. meters. Eagle may dominate an area of 70 sq. km. An African antelope (Male Gerenuk) occupy small territory, a termite mound only, smaller than his body size. The winter feeding territories of a hawk called the northern harrier varies from 4 to 125 hectares in size, a remarkably large range.

Tiny siphonoectine amphipods live in great numbers in the fine gravel of shallow marine bays. They may create and control clusters of mates by herding them together. Male siphonoectine amphipod construct elaborate cases composed of bits of pebble, fragments of mollusk shells. Males move about in their "houses" searching for females in their abodes. Single female is "captured" and their house glued to that of the male. A male may construct an apartment complex containing his case cemented to the abodes of three females (Fig. 6.5).

Territoriality in Arthropoda

By passing the tissue of a tree through her digestive tract, a female bark generates some volatile metabolic-by-products that carry information about her existence and location. This information helps male beetle to locate his partner. Male bark beetle traces the female through this volatile chemical and copulate with her.

Some insects (crickets and dragonflies), fiddler crabs, poplar aphid etc. are highly territorial. Generally males make a territory but contrary to general rule female poplar aphid chooses a young poplar leaf as territory. She continuously probes and feeds on tissue at the base of the expanding leaf, creating a depression that will eventually grow into the gall in which she will raise her offsprings. But if a second female tries to occupy the leaf the initial owner and the

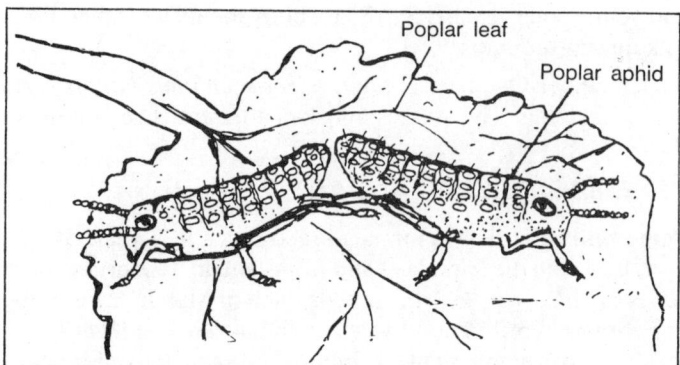

Fig. 6.4. (i) Territorial Dispute between two Poplar aphids. Female may spend hour kicking one another to determine who gets to occupy a preferred leaf or the superior location on the leaf.

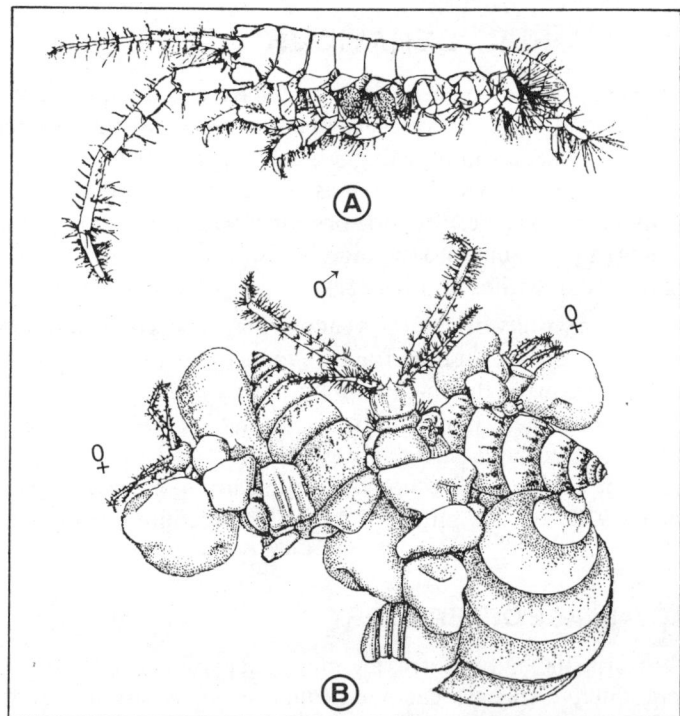

Fig. 6.5. Female defense polygyny in a marine amphipod (A) One individual is shown without his house. (B) A male has glued the houses of several females to his case.

newcomer may begin a kicking and shoving dual that may last two days. Long territorial fight causes delayed gall formation and the size of the gall reduces.

Black winged damselflies defend mating territory vigorously. Male black winged damselflies wait for mates to come to them at their resource rich territories. Female damselflies mate at these territories and then lay their eggs in the aquatic vegetation that the male controls. Two male antlered flies lung at each other and show their strength by using antler (Fig. 1.6A).

TERRITORIALITY IN FISHES

Few fish species become territorial during breeding season. The male three-spined stickleback selects an area and defend it vigorously. They make nest in their territory and attract females for breeding. The red colour spot on belly of male stickleback acts as a prenuptial signal for the female and intimidatory signal for rival males. The male fish regains its original dull colour after breeding. Their aggressiveness also diffuses after mating.

TERRITORIALITY IN REPTILES

Male Yarrow's spiny lizards are found in South Arizona and are highly territorial. Marler and Moore have studied the costs of territoriality the species has to pay. They inserted small capsules containing testosterone beneath the skin of some male lizards captured in June-July – a time of the year when the males are not territorial. The experimental animals were then released back into their habitat. Marler monitored the territorial behaviour of the experimental lizards as well as sham treated control group. The testosterone - implanted male Yarrow's spiny lizard patrolled more and performed more push-up threat display than the control group did. As a result, testosterone implanted males had less time to feed than the control group. As a result death rate was higher in experimental group. If the expense of territorial defence is worth paying then why territoriality is found in many species ? The answer is for reproductive compensation from the defended resource. In nature male Yarrow's spiny lizards become highly territorial during breeding season (Sep/Oct) when receptive females are available.

Female tree lizards of the Sonoran desert do not form tight-knit herds or

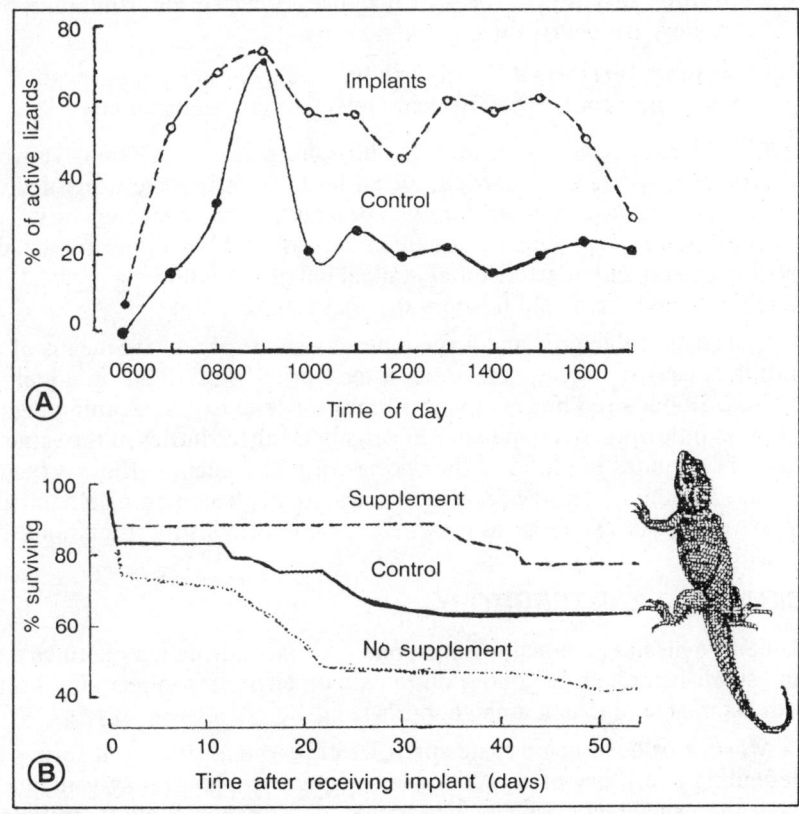

Fig. 6.6. Males of Yarrow's spiny lizards are not normally territorial during the summer (June/July) but will become highly territorial at this time when they received a testosterone implant. (A) The experimental males spent much more time moving about than did control males. (B) Testosterone - implanted males that received a food supplement survived but high mortality rate was there in comparison to unfed testosterone-implanted males.

bands but 3 or 4 commonly coexist in a single mesquite tree. A male that succeeds in keeping other males out of one or two mesquites will have access to three or more mates.

In turtle and tortoise reproduction is initiated by fighting between males for territory. Males of Harmann's tortoise injure other males quite seriously during such encounters..

TERRITORIALITY IN BIRDS

Nice (1941) and May (1953) recognized four main types of territory for different species of birds.

1. **Mating, Nesting and Feeding Territory :** All acts of reproductive behaviour i.e. the courtship, mating and nest building take place here. Song sparrow, Wood peckers, Warblers, Shrikes etc. make this kind of territory.

2. **Mating and Nesting Territory :** Only mating and nest building is done in this territory. Common examples are Grebs, Finches, Swan, Willet etc.

3. **Mating Territory :** Birds of paradise, Bower birds, Humming birds, Mannakins etc. establish territory for courtship and mating only.

4. **Nesting Territory :** Small territory meant for nesting purpose. Examples are colonial birds like Penguin, Acord, Wood pecker, Gulls, Herons, Pellican etc.

Many bird species are territorial in breeding season. An extensive work into the nature and function of territoriality has been carried out on birds. Mostly male birds make breeding territory but female Chinese Jacana establish territory and defend her territory efficiently. The female Humming bird has a separate nesting site which she defend herself. Old territories are usually deserted at the close of the nesting season and new territories stalked out of the following season. Song sparrow are exceptional as they retain their same old territory the year round.

The song of the birds and some times a visuals display are means of asserting territorial claims, and intruders usually retreat, sometimes after a brief 'ritual fight' in which neither competitor is seriously injured. Robin's red breast is sign stimuti for females but warning sign for males of same of species. There is little or no overlap between neighbouring territories of the same species and, in areas where the territory includes the food of the species, it will contain sufficient food to support the birds and their young. As population size grow, territories usually become smaller and able to support fewer new birds. In extreme cases, some birds may be unable to establish territory and therefore, fail to breed.

BIRD SONG AND TERRITORY

Robert Payne has demonstrated that one year old male indigo buntings that are able to mimic the song of an established older neighbour do remain on territories longer and produce more fledglings than individuals unable to match a neighbour's song.

Most of us have heard male sparrows or warblers singing in spring, which they generally do while defending a territory of an acre or less. A male songbird may generate several thousand full-throated songs in a single day. Singers also provide information about their location to individuals of their own species.

European songbird defend feeding territories during the non-breeding season. In Southern Britain, wagtail winter territories are 600 meter stretches of river bank. Territory owners consume the aquatic insects that are constantly being washed up by the river. Wagtails, like sunbirds and bee-eaters, have the ability to switch back and forth between territoriality and non-territorial behaviour. When insect renewal rates drop within an area, the territory owner often temporarily joins flocks of non-territorial birds that forage widely over the country-side. When the river edge is full of aquatic insects, a territorial bird will remain at its site and vigorously defend it against outsiders.

But how can we account for the territorial birds's persistent return to areas that yield less prey than non defend regions visited by flocking birds? Why bother to be terrestrial when the hunting is better elsewhere? Davies is of the opinion that when snow

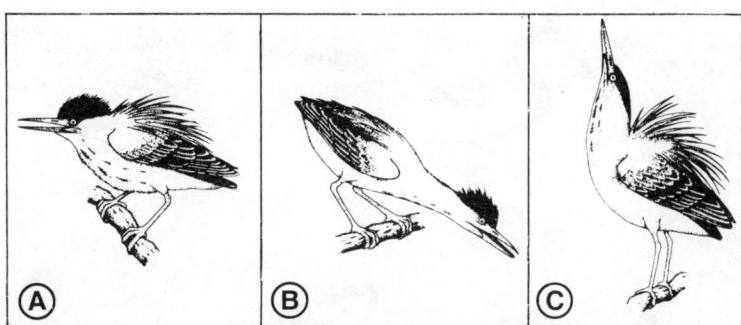

Fig. 6.7. Displays of the green heron *Butorides virescens* (A) Forward threat (B) Snap display (C) Stretch display.

covers the meadows, the river edge may be the only place with a predictable and constant supply of food. To maintain its weight, a wagtail must feed 90 percent of the time and collect about 7,500 food items per day. A single day of starvation can kill it. Thus, territorial ownership may provide an element of insurance against exceptionally bad weather.

American Green herons (*Butorides virescens*) nest in dead trees in salt marshes. The male arrive in spring and defend a nest tree against rival males. Intruders belonging to the same or other species are challenged by a forward threat display. The male adopts a horizontal posture, points its beak towards the opponent, erects its feathers, and vibrates the tail. Females are attracted by the male's advertising call but initially are threatened by the male. As female persist, the behaviour of the male modifies and his readiness to accept the female is signaled by the snap display. The beak is pointed diagonally downward and the mandibles are snapped together. After accepting the female, the male performs the stretch display, which is a ritualized form of flight intention. It is the antithesis of the forward display in many respects. Whereas the forward display is accompanied by a harsh call and ruffled feathers that increase the bird's apparent size, the stretch display is accompanied by a soft call and sleeked feathers. In the forward display the beak, and bird's main weapon, is directed toward the opponent, thus exhibiting the bright red lining of the mouth. In the stretch display the beak is directed away from the female. Whereas the forward display signifies threat, the stretch display symbolizes appeasement and is followed by mutual displays on the part of male and female.

Various threat postures exhibited by great tit (*Paras major* – in territorial boundary disputes) are summarised in Fig. 6.8.(a) is the normal relaxed posture, which grades into a head-up threat display, (b–d) into a head-up threat display, (e–g) the horizontal display, (h–i) is sometimes accompanied by a wings-out display (j–k). The male sage-grouse (a North American bird) fluff up their plumage and thus increase their apparent size while defending his territory.

Male satin bower birds protect a site at which they build their bowers and await the arrival of females, to whom they offer only elaborated display and the chances to mate, an opportunity often ignored.

TERRITORIALITY IN MAMMALS

Most of the mammals select and defend an area for breeding purpose. Competition for territory among males of conspecific goes on prior to mating. Bull elephants become very aggressive during the breeding season. Spotted hyenas actively mark the boundaries of their territories with their dung and urine, which clearly announces the presence of particular hyena. This warns intruders to stay away or take risk to fight with the owner of the area.

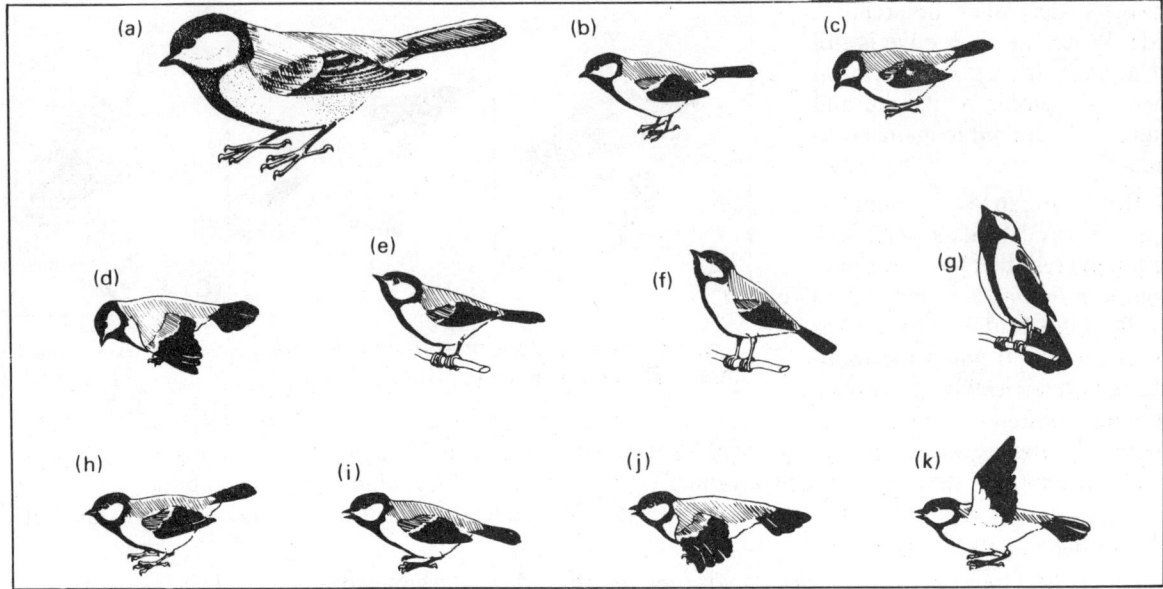

Fig. 6.8. Postures of the great tit *Paras major* seen in territorial dispute.

Females of a tropical bat form groups that forage together at night, always returning to the same spot in their home cave to roost during the day. The existence of these roosting groups is tailor-made for female defense polygyny because one male can readily guard the clusture. (Fig. 6.9) Successful territory holders father 60 to 90 per cent of the offspring of the female in their roost and that one male may sire as many as 50 pups during his territorial tenure.

Males of bighorn sheep defends their breeding territory vigorously. Bighorn rams visit the place where potential males are fighting with other males to monopolize the females. Males of family Ervidae (deer) and Bovidae (antelope and gazelles) of order Artiodactyla live most of the year in all-male herds. As the breeding season approaches, males engage in battle using their ant-

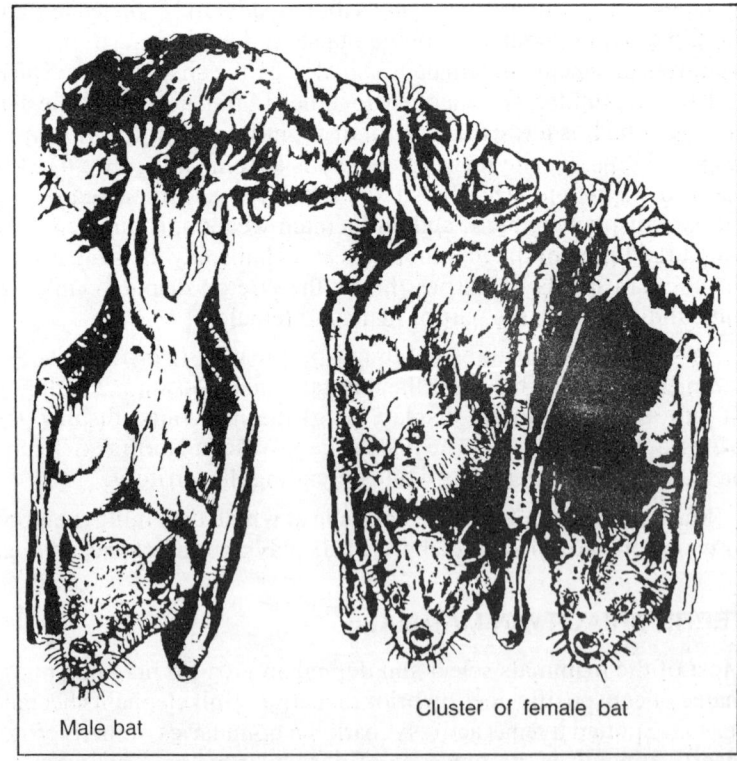

Male bat

Cluster of female bat

Fig. 6.9. Female Defense Polygyny Vampire bat. The male at the top (left) guards a roosting cluster of females.

lers. The winners of the battle gains dominance and it do most of the mating. Antlers are better developed in those cervidae species where males compete strongly for large groups of females.

During breeding season male red deer have aggressive displays in which opponents lock antlers, permitting them to accurately judge each other's relative size and strength.

Male cats spray urine to mark territory. To defend this area it fight vigorously with other males. They cease to mark territory by spraying urine when their testes are removed surgically. Every year after monsoon lions and tigers mark their territory by urinating on trees of jungle. Rain wash out the previous territorial marking.

Male Mongolian gerbil mark its territory with an oily secretion from a gland present on ventral surface. Castration of testis leads to regression of the gland and disappearance of marking behaviour. Testosterone injection causes castrated male gerbil to go through the full pattern of marking behaviour.

Male elephant seals are the first to move on to dry land to establish territories which they fiercely defend. Females join male in a territory after one month. Only those males which have been able to maintain a territory will be able to receive and mate with a group of females.

Aggression of males of deer and giraffe is controlled type and considerably less deadly than one might imagine. In fact, it is quite rare that costing between two stags during the rut leads to the death of one of the combatants, or even to serious wounds. Everything takes place as if the aggression were being kept under tight rules. It is significant that such "control" of animal aggression is most noticeable among animals living in families, groups or colonies which would be rapidly disrupted by persistent aggressiveness among their members. So such aggression, while it continues to exist, has generally been transformed into a kind of ceremony – it has become ritualized.

COURTSHIP AND MATING RITUALS OF ANIMALS

The urge to mate is one of the greatest driving natural instincts of animals. Before mating opposite sex attract her/his partner by various activities so that they may come close to each other and mating occurs. Courtship refers to *"the activities of two individuals of opposite sex which follows the mating"*. *Mating refers to "the aspects of a species organization which determine ways in which the opposite sexes come together so that insemination and fertilization of the female by the male takes place"*.

Charles Darwin pointed out that the winning of a mate is an exceptionally complicated process in which display gives one mate an advantage over other. It may help to break down barriers which prevent the mates from coming together. It helps male and female to find one other, to indicate suitable breeding sites and to synchronize physiological processes for fertilization.

A female's reproductive success is not often increased by having many mates. Instead, a female's fitness is primarily a function of how many eggs she can produce and by what happens to the eggs after they have been fertilized. If males vary in their effects on offspring quality and survival, then females should discriminate in favour of those individuals that will contribute the most, creating mate choice selection via their preferences. During courtship male actions are of two types : those involved in male-to-male encounter and those of male-to-female encounter. In most of the cases, the forelegs, wings, mouth, vocalization of the male serve as signalling structures. Female signalling is limited mostly through pheromones.

FUNCTIONS OF COURTSHIP

Generally, the animals tend to avoid contact with one another, as a behavioural adaptation to reduce the transmission of parasites and diseases. The function of courtship is to break this barrier and bring opposite partner together to facilitate mating.

Tinbergen (1954) mentioned four main functions of courtship :

1. One of the functions of courtship is to break down the natural inhibition towards contact between two opposite partners. Male attracts female by different acts. Female are attracted by such displays and come to the male's territory.
2. Courtship displays serve to supperess non-sexual responses in the female.
3. Courtship displays serve to facilitate the sex and species to synchronize the copulation.
4. Courtship displays and song pattern are species specific. They ensure that pair bonds and copulation take place between individuals of the same species.

In some animals courtship is brief and done merely for the sake of getting through the act of mating. But in others it lasts for a long time and involves vigorous and elaborate displays. However courtship may be brief or elaborate it fulfills four major functions :

1. Mate finding,
2. Persuation,
3. Synchronization, and
4. Species specific courtship.

MATE FINDING

In higher animals, search of a suitable mate is a highly organised process which involves many senses such as sense of sight, smell, sound, touch, surface vibrations, electrical stimulation and even taste.

For a large number of diurnal and some nocturnal animals vision is the primary factor which plays an important role in recognising a mate. Owls (bird) and certain insects have special lenses which enable them to find a mate by straight site. Fire flies, glow worms and many of the inhabitants of the deep sea have luminescent organs which help in mate finding. Many species of insects, moths, sea cows etc. rely upon chemical trails (Pheromones) for mate finding. The chemical secretions produced in urine by a bitch attract all the male dogs in the neighbourhood. Dogs show no interest at all if her (bitch) odour is somehow suppressed. Same is the case in horses, Zebra, Giraffe etc. Mare in heat attract stallions by chemical substances contained in urine. White whales (Beluga) emit a series of high-pitched mating calls which can be heard 300 meters away. Male cichlids (a family of tropical fish) raise their dorsal fins and beat the water with tail. Such behaviour enables breeding partner to locate each other. Croacking sound produced by male frogs attract female frogs for amplexus.

In predatory species including cannibals, courtship inhibits the aggressive response evoked by the presence of other individuals within a certain territory. Scorpions and spiders are cannibalistic. Male scorpions and spiders not only stimulates the female sexually but he has to suppress the non-sexual behaviour of the females so that she may not eat him. In ethological terminology courtship provide releaser stimuli which inhibits hunger drive. A young polar bear attacks all other polar bears, male or female, that try to invade the hunting territory it has stalked to itself during the non-breeding season. However, male polar bear suppresses his ferrosus nature toward female polar bear during breeding season. The female polar bear approaches to male polar bear for breeding only after assurance that it is safe to approach the male.

PERSUASION

In most of the species the male plays active role in mate finding, persuading and mating, than females. After mate finding and recognising a potential female the next duty for the male is to bring the female into close proximity. Male performs certain behaviour patterns whose function is to stimulate the female until she is sexually receptive. Lions persuade lioness many kilometers and invest lot of time in alluring her.

Male baya allure female baya by melodious song and well woven nest. Peacock pheasand attract Peahen by magnificent dance. In human beings feminine coyness probably stimulate the male, a show of resistance often serves to encourage the male and lead him on.

SYNCHRONIZATION

Two individuals of opposite sex ready to copulate, co-operate, move and turn at the same time and speed to facilitate mating is called synchronization. Cats, rats, lions etc. assume a posture called *lordosis* to facilitate smooth mating.

Precise synchronization of male and female courtship activities is especially important for species in which there is external fertilization. It occurs because both respond to external cues such as day length, lunar cycle, tidal rhythm etc. Grunion fish, palolo worm etc. show synchronization with physical factors of environment for successful breeding.

SPECIES SPECIFIC COURTSHIP

Courtship displays are species specific i.e. the signals used for mate finding, persuasion, appeasement, synchronization etc. vary in different species. The partner that received such signals is usually responsive only to the displays of its own species.

Song produced by male cricket and croaking sound produced by bull frogs are species specific in terms of their pitch and timing. Female respond only to the calls of their own species. The antennae of many male moths e.g. silkworm moth are selectively responsive to the pheromone emitted by females of its own species. Songs of male song sparrow, swamp sparrow and white crowned sparrow attract females of their own species only.

Reproductive isolation by breeding habit in tree frog (*Hyla*) is interesting to note. *Hyla versicolor* (gray tree frog) and *Hyla femoralis* (Pine wood tree frog) are found in the same pond near new Orleans. They breed at the same time. Both species are very similar in their external features but their male's breeding calls are extremely different which are well recognised by their females, and hence no mixed mating occures.

DIVERSITY IN MATING SYSTEM

There are two principal types of mating systems which occur in animal world.

1. MONOGAMY

A male pairs with a single female of same species. This is rare in insects. However a queen and a king form a pair for life in termites. In birds a male pairs with a single female during one full breeding season. House sparrow, Parakeet, Blue rock pigeon, Black drongo, Wrens (*Troglodytes troglodytes*), Robin etc. are monogamous. Many migrant birds e.g. crane are monogamous during the breeding season but live separately for the rest of the year. Many gulls have a strong tendency to return to their exact nesting locality where they join up with their partner each year. The pair remains together for life, unless a divorce takes place as a result of the failure of one partner to fulfil its duties. Crool (1964) observed that the primarily insectivorous species which inhabit forests are monogamous whereas Savannah-dwelling seed eaters are colonial and polygynous.

There are certain exceptions to seasonal monogamy. Gees and swans (*Cygnus*) live in permanent lifelong pairs.

2. POLYGAMY

The adult males with two or more partners and none of them mates with other individuals. The polygamy is of two types :

(a) *Polygyny* : A male mates with more than one female during a single breeding season. In all cases polygynous system benefit the male by increasing his access to fertilizable eggs. Polygyny occurs more frequently in insects, birds and mammals. Among birds polygyny occurs among pheasants. During rainy season male peacock pheasant forms a flock or harem of 4 or 5 peahen.

(b) *Polyandry* : A single female mates with several males during one breeding season. It is relatively rare in insects. Example : queen honeybee mates with several drones in succession during nuptial flight. Polyandry is also found in birds. Examples are painted snip (*Rostratula benghalensis*), Bronze winged Jacana (*Metopodius indicus*), American Jacana (*Jacana spinosa*), Tasmanian Hens etc. The female is more conspicuous, territorial and dominant than male. After courtship female lay a clutch of eggs for each of her male and it is the male who incubate the egg and rear the young, unaided by the female.

An intermediate between Polygyny and Polyandry, in which females lay a second batch of eggs which the male incubates or guards but where the male may also mate with other females was called multiple clutch polygamy by Emlen and Oring. This is common in fish and occurs occasionally in birds. Polyandry has not been reported for mammals. (Eisenberg. 1966). Jenni (1974) describes Polyandry in several species of birds. Most are in order chondriiformes. The females of the American Jacana (*Jacana spinosa*) defend large territories in marsh areas which include the smaller territories of several males. The males perform all duties of incubation and parental care they also defend their territories against other males.

COURTSHIP AND MATING RITUALS IN INVERTEBRATES

Ethologists have shown less interest in studying courtship and mating behaviour among invertebrates in comparison to vertebrates. However, interesting cases of courtship and mating among annelids and arthropods is described here.

ANNELIDS

A pacific palolo worm (*Eunice viridis*) is a deep sea annelid. The courtship and reproduction of this worm is very peculiar and interesting to watch. On the first day of the first quarter of the moon in November, which is its breeding season, the hinder part of its body becomes packed with reproductive cells. During this period the palolo worm swim to the ocean surface in large numbers. During swarming spawning takes place. On the surface of seashore gametes are discharged and external fertilization takes place. The Atlantic palolo worm (*Eunice schemacephala*) swarms in July during the first and third quarters of a lunar cycle. In the early morning, worms emerge from their burrows and make spiral swimming movement, breaking their hinder part of body bearing reproductive organs called *eptitokal part*. Sperms and ova are released on floating water where external fertilization takes place.

West Indian worm (*Odontosyllis enopla*) swarms during the night at the third quarter of the moon and the shining light from the females attracts the males. The luminescent glow at the surface of the sea that lasts only for 5 to 10 minutes. The females appear first at the water surface and emit a stream of brilliantly luminous secretion with the eggs. Males rush in with short intermediate flashes and release sperms for external fertilization.

Some species of Nereis (*Platynereis dumerii*) assumes a sexual form called *heteronereis* which swims actively at seashores during the full moon. This form i.e. heteronereis perform nuptial dance, in which males and females swim rapidly in a circle. The females produce a substance *fertillium* which attracts the males and stimulates them to shed sperms. Shedding of sperms excites the female and she shed eggs for fertilization.

ARTHOPODA

Male ghost crabs modify its environment to make himself conspicuous to potential females. It dig a deep burrow and make the excavated sand into a pyramid that enables females to find them. Male fiddler crabs (Fig. 10.4) have evolved 'signals' - special conspicuous behaviour patterns often combined with special structures whose chief function is to send stimuli to opposite sex. The single large claw of the male fiddler crab is for giving signal to female. One claw is enlarged way beyond its need for any other function. It is often brightly coloured and is waved rhythmically in the air during courtship displays to attract females and in defence of the burrow against other males.

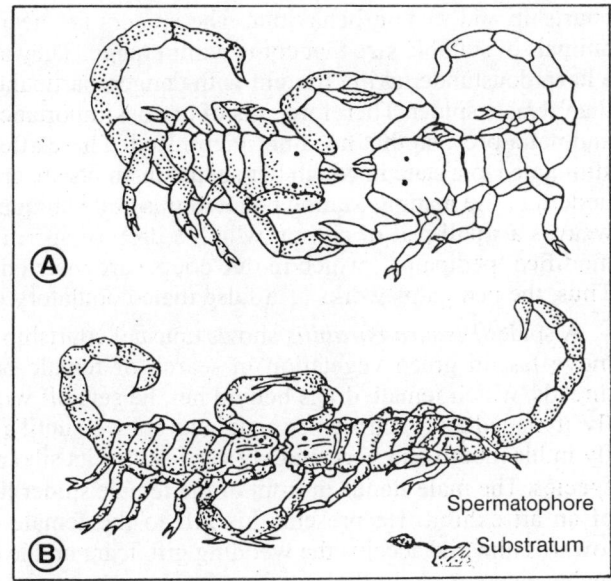

Fig. 6.10. (A) Courtship dance by a pair of scorpion. (B) Male scorpion pulling the female over the spermatophore.

Fabre described the courtship and mating behaviour of scorpions. In scorpions courtship takes the form of a dance called "*Promenada a deus*". On finding a suitable mate, male and female scorpion face each other, extend abdomen high into the air, and move about in circle. The male then seizes the female with his pedipalps, and together they walk backward and forward. This act may last hours or even days. In scorpions, Mites, and millipedes, sperms are "packaged" in a bag called spermatophore. The male deposits a spermatophore on the substratum and the female is dragged over spermatophore to pick it up. A wind like lever extends from the spermatophore. The male then manoeuvers the female so that her genital area is over the spermatophore. Pressure over the spermatophore lever releases the sperm mass, which is then taken up into female orifice (Fig. 6.10).

SPIDERS

Web builders viz. spiders exhibit a very unique way of courtship and mating. The very strange aspect of their mating is that as soon as the mating is completed, male is devoured by the female; though sometimes the male escapes by adopting some tricks.

For successful mating male spider perform various activities meant to calm down their prospective brides or to appease her and to make her busy during the course of mating. The prime function of courtship in predatory species is appeasement and inhibition of the normal predatory behaviour of the females.

In spiders, the male appeases his prospective partner so that she does not eat him. There is an indirect method of sperm transfer, which is highly unusual. Moreover, Spiders also show different patterns of courtship and mating behaviour. The spiders are nearly offensive and are ready to kill and eat most animals of suitable size that come within range. They are cannibals. The mating in spiders is, therefore, a hazardous undertaking fraught with danger, particularly to the male spider that is smaller and weaker than female spider. Therefore, it is of utmost importance to the male to indicate that he is potential mate and not a prey, so that he is not victimised. There after the courtship must proceed until the female is stimulated to a state in which her sexual instincts are aroused to the extent that she permits male mate to undertake the mating. Mating behaviour is quite unique in most of the spiders. The matured male spider, weaves a small pad of silk on which a drop of sperm is deposited and this is sucked up by specially modified 'pedipalps', which in due course are inserted into the genitalia of the female for fertilization. Thus, the pedipalps works as a false male copulatory organ.

A spider *Pisaura mirabilis* shows unusual courtship behaviour. In the month of may, the male spider move fast in green vegetation in search of female partner. As soon as he comes across her signal threads, which female drags behind her, he sets off with new energy to hunt for flies. After catching a fly, it immediately starts twisting it in its cobweb until a white ball is formed. Then he carefully holds the fly in his mouth and very quickly carries it in its silken packet to offer to the female spider of his own species. The male stands in front of the female spider like an enigmatic and incomprehensible sculpture of an art exhibit. He presents his gift to the female counter part. The female spider slowly moves towards him and accepts the wedding gift, tears up the packet and starts sucking on the gifted fly. Some male spiders pack up the remains of a fly caracass for their next dating while some male spiders cheat their female partners by providing false gifts.

Another species of spider *Pidippus johnsoni,* male court adult females that are outside the nest by using visual signals. Inside the nest, females are courted nonvisually by a series of movements that create specific vibrations on the silk thread of the female web indicating that the caller is a mate not a prey. Females are subjected to this vibratory courtship until a cohabitation situation is established.

Salticid spiders belonging to family salticidae are called jumping spiders. Here communication occurs *via* visual displays and colour pattern. The zig-zag and other dances of salticid males have all the characteristics of approach - withdrawal conflicts, to which the courtship have been ascribed. Almost all salticid spiders are well trained dancers. In the spring, they occasionally dance for up to half an hour. They raise their legs up and spread them apart, stretch them forward, flap them as if they were wings or sway them in time. They execute stunts in front of the mate.

The tiny spider, Attulus, exhibits movements and postures reminiscent of classical ballet when he dances to attract his mate. Male spider of *Hasarius adansoni,* species attracts the female by moving slowly in zig-zag fashion, waving his palps up and down. Soon as female turns towards him, he stops and remains motionless with his large forelegs held horizontally. He jumps and comes near the female. The display continues time and again until he is permitted to insert his pedipalps.

Members of family Lycosidae are known as wolf spiders. They have visual capacity. Courtship signalling involves the substrate vibration, airborne sound, pheromones and visual signals. The palpal drumming of male *Lycosa rabida* has communicator function in courtship. Many other species of lycosids produce audible sounds that are mainly substrate coupled. The visual signal is derived from movements of pedipalps, fore legs and abdomen and with additional dorsoventral movement of the entire body. In juvenile lycosids, the courtship occurs in the form of leg waving behaviour.

In web spinning spiders, the female in a web is continuously approached by a male who rhythmically taps on the suspension cord of the web. This tapping differs from the thread signals produced by a struggling prey. When female moves, the male usually retracts to resorts, but soon the tapping is repeated. When the pair comes together, the female is stroked by the palps or legs of the male. Now then she turns back and allows the male to deposit the spermatophore. The male taps the web characteristically to announce his arrival and not to be mistaken for the prey. To overcome the depression and fear, the male provides some food or a drop of saliva or an empty web to the female for keeping her quiet during the course of mating as a part of appeasement.

Male crab spider, *Xysticus cristatus* fear that he may be devoured by the female spider because of her carnivorous and cannibal nature. The male spider strategically binds his mate with strands of silk attached to the substrate prior to attempting his sperm containing pedipalp into her genital aperture.

Most members of family Arenidae build cobwebs. One species of this family *Meta segmentata*, is a linkage between the sexual and predatory behaviour. Male, being agile, either approaches the female across her web or the female off her web. He attaches the single line mating thread or silk line to the female web and starts giving signals by vibrating the thread. In response to the signals, female leaves her web and moves onto the thread line. She may do so by varying the speed more or less vigorously. Male frequently spots signalling and may jump off if he finds the female is approaching him rapidly and vigorously. He may cut the end and attach the end leading towards the female to his spinnerets. Thus, he provides a virtually endless thread on which female is running and finally she gets exhausted. This is a good time for male to mount on female and insert his pedipalp.

Courtship in female web is possible when the female is immature or she ecdysing. At this juncture the female is too soft and weak to attack. Courtship may also be facilitated in female's web when she commences feeding on prey; the feeding suppresses her cannibal nature.

At the moment of separation, the life of male spider is always in danger, if the female predatory drive is disinhibited. In some *lycosids*, the male pinches the female with his chelicerae trying to temporarily inactivate her as he dismounts.

In araneids, the male leaps off the female, be laid on his thread silk line, and uses gravity to escape. Male also gathers up the elastic mating threat and then uses it like a tension spring to pull himself away from the female at the moment of separation. Males, if seized sometimes, may also escape by autotomizing their legs. Despite all these escape mechanisms, the males may be caught and eaten away by the females.

Horse shoe crab (*Limulus a living fossile found in the bed of sea*) hooks himself on behind the female and remains there until eggs are released.

INSECTS

The courtship and mating behaviour have been studied extensively, spread over the different insect orders. In adult insects, mating is a frequent and easily observable process. It is also interesting to know that male insects show sexual selection. The behaviour of insect which leads to the insemination and the fertilization of the female by the male is termed as mating behaviour.

COURTSHIP AND MATING IN APTERYGOTE INSECTS

The male silverfish, *Lepisma saccharina* deposits the sperms in droplets without any protective capsule covering. Male *Lepisma guides* the female towards the externally deposited spermatophore by spinning a series of threads which restricts her movement and brings her closer and closer to the spermatophore to make contact and pick it up. During courtship male silverfish approaches towards wall and affixes thread to wall and floor. One main and several secondary threads are produced by the male. This excite female silverfish to accept the spermatophores.

COURTSHIP AND MATING IN PTERYGOTE INSECTS

Interesting methods of courtship and mating are evident in higher order of class Insecta. Copulation involves linking of the male and female genitalia to form a firm connection between the opposite sex and male transfers the sperm to female while they are joined in this fashion.

ODONATA

The courtship pattern is some what complex in dragon-flies. The female flies over the pond and male dashes her and follows her while swaying from side to side. He then turns and flies after her again. Male flutters his wings and occasionally bends his abdomen towards the female. After first courtship or after a few such courtships, the wings of the female beats more slowly. Finally wing beating stops when she perches on the site. The male catches her as she flies slowly and fastens his abdominal claspers to her head. In initiating copulation the male fly embrace the female whose wings are at rest. He then perches and the copulation continues (Fig. 6.11).

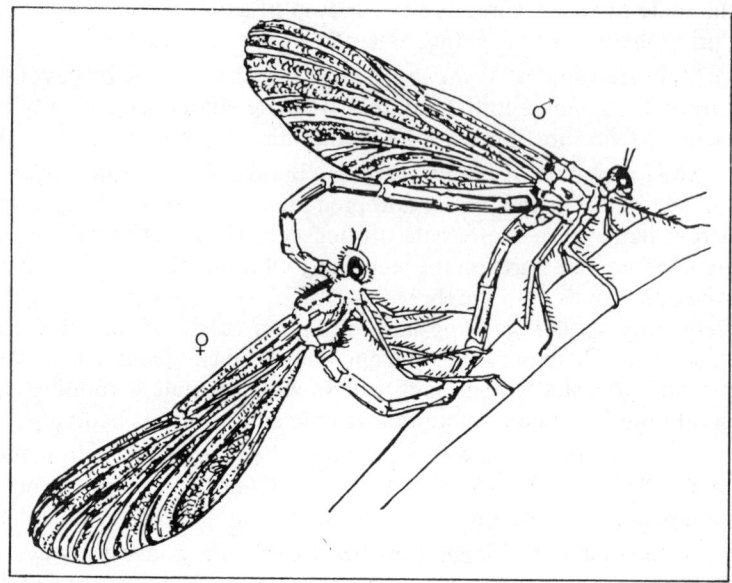

Fig. 6.11. Copulatory encounters of dragonflies. The male seizes the female with terminal pincers on his abdomen. She in turn covers her abdomen towards to contact the appropriate spot on the Ventral surface of the male's abdomen.

LEPIDOPTERA

Nuptial dance in diurnal butterfly of Europe was observed by Tinbergen. During the breeding season, as soon as male butterfly spots a female, he sets off on a whirling flight in which he circles round the female, coming closer and closer until she is forced to land. As soon as the female has landed, the male lands beside her and begins to walk around her, spreading his wings every time he passes in front of her. His wings in fact bear special scent producing areas which evoke the female's interest. Now female approaches the male and passes her antennae (feelers) between the male's wings as if to "sniff" at them. After being "seduced" the female allows the male to mate with her.

Gypsy moth (*Porthetria dispar*) shows a characteristic courtship. The virgin female moth releases sex attractant and begins a rhythmic protraction and partial retraction of the last abdominal segments. In calling position virgin female rests head upward on an upright surface. If she is not disturbed, she spreads the wings, slightly lowers the abdomen and begins a new rhythmic protraction and partial retraction of last segment of the abdomen. Female Gypsy moth exhibits a marked change in behaviour soon after mating ends. In satiated condition she does not call and avoids the attempts of male to copulate.

The courtship in different races of mulberry silkmoth, *Bombyx mori* starts within 5-10 minutes of their emergence. Female moth moves a little after emergence and sits quietly until the male approaches her. The male moth just after 5-10 minutes of emergence, raises antennae and starts fluttering of his wings. When male moth reaches near female, wing fluttering becomes more swiftly and turns his abdomen towards her. He touches the abdominal end of female with his antennae, wings and legs. Now he rubs his abdomen with the abdomen of female from end to end. At this time wing fluttering of the male reaches at the peak. The abdominal rubbing between two partners continues until they succeed in making genital contact. During mating the female co-operates by slightly up turning her abdominal end and maintains this posture. The mating duration varies from 30 minutes to 20 hours in different races of *Bombyx mori*.

Female erisilkmoth, *Samia cynthia ricini* releases the pheromone *"bombykol"* to attract the male moth. In response, the male moth flutters his wings and vibrates his antennae to recognise his partner. When a male moth finds a suitable mate he tries to mount the female. During mounting the male moth tries to hold the female with his legs, moves towards her head and starts rubbing the antennal and head of female. Non receptive female moves off with raised antennae to avoid the mounting. Receptive female remains passive and exhibits sexual recognition by keeping antennae just parallel to the forewings. The male moth moves downwards ventro-laterally and the female turns her abdomen exposing her genitalia to the male and then gential contact takes place.

In polyphemus moth, *Anthaerea polyphemus* female calling behaviour is initiated after exposure to a volatile substance present in the leaves of the host plants only at a specific time of the photoperiodic cycle and the mating occurs on or near the larval food.

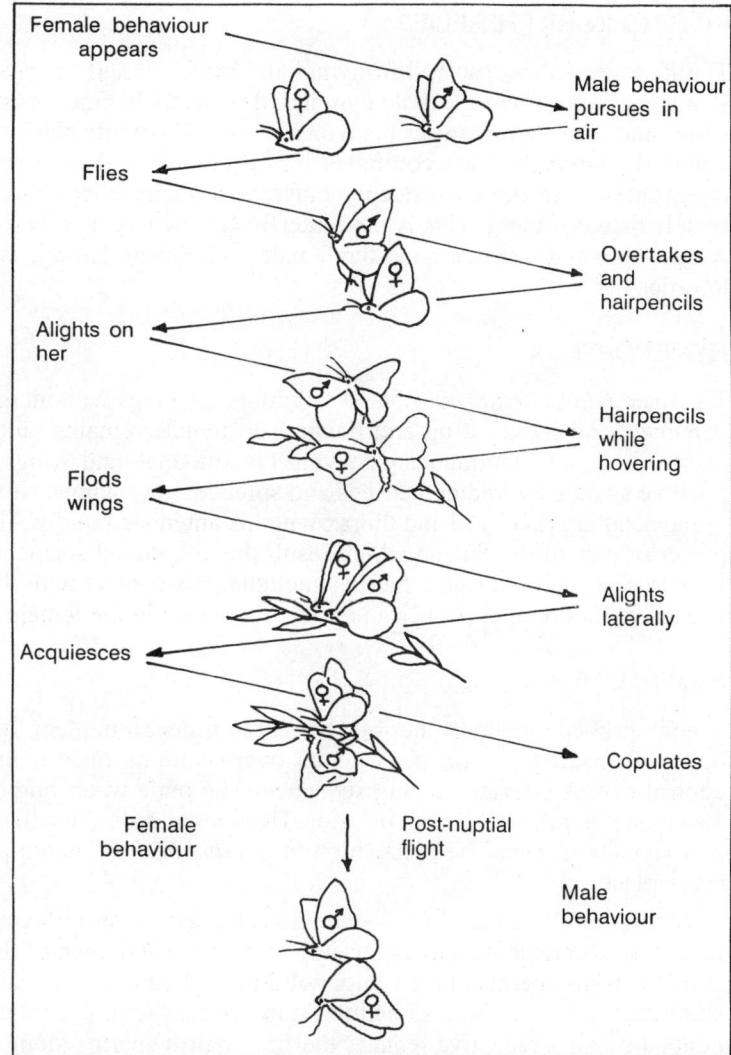

Fig. 6.12. Courtship and Copulation in the queen butterfly. (The arrows indicate the stimuli and responses involved in the courtship behavioural activities).

Male argynnis butterfly performs a zig-zag flight. He flies around the female. Unreceptive female fly away but the virgin butterflies flutting at the same spot and make a continuous low sound by the wings. Female darts out in a special pattern of flight and the male follows her. When the male comes closer to her, he overtakes her from below and raises swiftly above her head. This up and down movement forms a dance ritual. The male flies in a circle above and the fluttering female lifts her scent brush up and moves the abdominal tip up. The male argynnis butterfly settles down in a stand on one side of female and the quiet female gently moves the wings apart. The male butterfly clasps the female between the wings. He bows her body standing on a side of the female and contact her on his own. At the same time, one of the feelers moves gently over and lies on the head of the female. Mating is attempted and the female co-operate and mating is achieved. A chain of copulation takes place in argynnis butterfly.

KISSING IN BUTTERFLIES

The kissing is also observed in nymphalid butterflies. If the male approaches a receptive female she stands motionless and the male nymphalid butterfly begins his courtship activities. First, he flutters his wings and then slightly raises his wings to show the white black-rimmed spots. He opens and closes his wings rhythmically. This continues for several seconds to minutes. The male raises his forewings, opens them wide and bows deeply. Later, he folds his wings back tenderly pressing the antennae of the female between them. This is the butterfly *kiss*, where he presses her scent glands and then opens his wings again and moves around the female with the air. Kissing is also observed in craneflies belonging to order Diptera.

HYMENOPTERA

The male *Diaeretiella rapae* starts vibrating his wings without touching the female. He raises his right antennae, and moves it up and down. The female remains quiet. Gradually the male becomes more excited and runs continuously moving his antennae and wings fastly. Sexually excited female gives positive signals by folding her legs and spreading her wings. Now male quickly mounts on the back of female and taps her head and thorax with his antennae rapidly. The male places his hindlegs against the posterior pair of the female which result the abdominal segment of the male to bend downwards and forwards in such a fashion that his genitalia gets contact with the female genitalia. During copulation male gives abdominal strokes and inject the sperm in the female genital pouch.

HEMIPTERA

True bugs, bed bug and water bug belong to order Hemiptera. In water bug (belostomid bug – *Abedus herberti*), courtship takes place under overwhelming male domination. The male maintains absolute control over the female mating sequence. The male water bug commands the female to copulate and also guides her the copulatory position. He gives signals about his willingness to mate and determines the preoviposition time. The oviposition in *Abedus herberti* is not permitted by the male until the mating takes place.

Mating in *Sylocoris maculipennis* is achieved by an indirect method of transfer of sperms i.e. by injection. The male punctures the side wall of the abdomen of the female with the help of his genitalia and injects his sperms in the coelom of female. Sometimes a male *Xylocoris maculipennis* adopts more short cut method. A male sometimes transfer his sperm to another male's testes. When the victim male copulate with a receptive female, the first male's sperms along with the mating male transferred into female.

ORTHOPTERA

We have studied in chapter 3 that different species of crickets and grasshoppers make mating calls different from one another. In *Corthippus brunneus* and *C. biggutuliasis*, the male sings differently and the female replies the male song of her species with a closely similar song. The male distinguishes the female song of his species. This helps in finding the partner of its own species which ultimately help in copulation.

Some times cheating in mate finding is also found among the insects of desert Orthoptera. Silent satellite males become courtship parasites on calling by intercepting females. The males are attracted to the acoustic signalling of the latter.

The female praying mantis sometimes devours the head and part of the thorax of a male mantis attempting to copulate. One may be surprised to know that this is not as tragic as it seems, because removal of the head, especially the sub-oesophageal ganglion, increases the vigour of the male's copulatory movements. How a headless male mantis may still be able to copulate under this difficult circumstances is a matter of great research (Fig. 6.13).

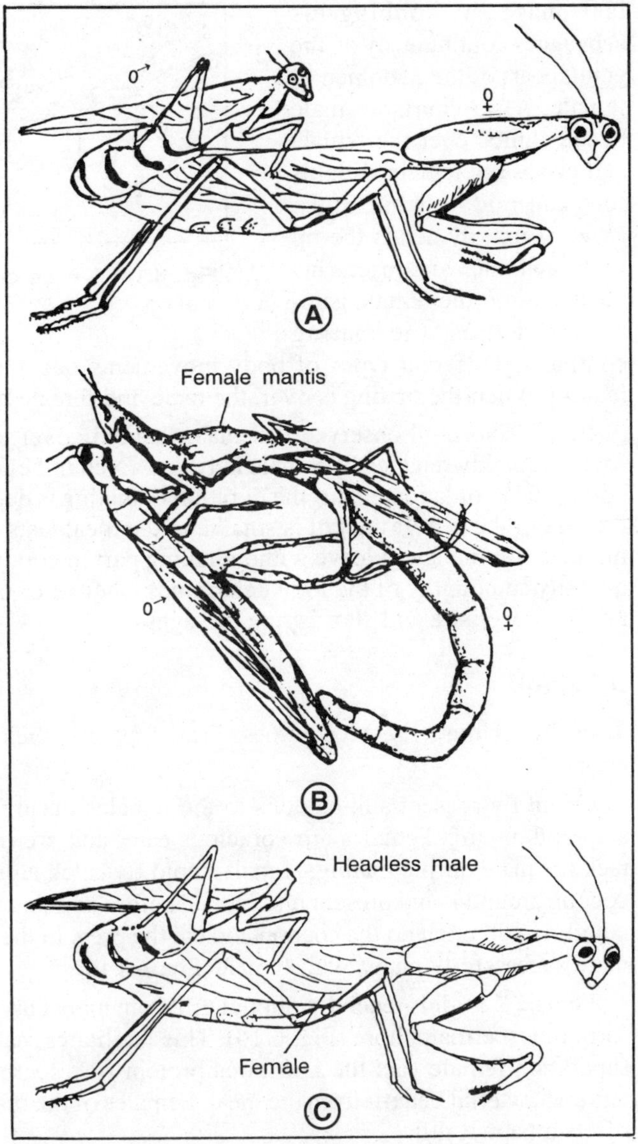

COLEOPTERA

Non-predatory male beetle (*Stilbocoris natalensis*) also give nuptial gift to his prospective wife. Male offers the female *fig seed*. She then feeds upon his gift and accepts his sperms which she presumably uses to fertilize the eggs she lays during her non-receptive phase. Females exercise active mate choice, creating sexual selection favouring males that provide large nutritious nuptial gift.

The courtship in *Arrhenodes* (Brentidae) beetle is interesting. When the male encounters the female, he taps her gently with his antennae. He gradually shifts his position until reaches up to her antennae and then the drumming begins faster and softer. Female comes into contact with his antennae. The male pours his saliva on to the seed (collected as nuptial gift) to make it more palatable and acceptable to female beetle. Female inserts her proboscis into the gifted seed to take as food, in the mean time the male approaches her and copulates.

Male and female fireflies (*Photimus pyralis*) emerge out separately from the grass. The male flies about two feet above the ground and emits a single short flash at regular intervals. The female climbs over a blade of grass, and waits there. If a male flashes with a decorous interval then female flashes spontaneously. If a male flashes within 3 or 4 meters of her

Fig. 6.13. Sexual cannibalism by a female praying mantis. (A) Male mantis take a jump and quickly copulate. (B) The female mantis has reached back to consume the head of her partner during mating. (C) A headless male mantis continues copulating the female.

location and glows again, the female responds once more with a flash and the exchange of signals is repeated usually not more than 5 or 10 times until the male reaches the female waiting in grass and then they mate.

Coecinellids, the male ladybird beetle initially gets excited by pheromone of the female and later he stimulates the female by a few antennal drummings, rubbing her elytra with his mouthparts and in the last phase, by rubbing his aedeagues continuously on the genital part of the abdomen of female. After courtship male beetle climbs over the female and clasps the female with his fore and middle legs firmly. Now he rapidly bends the tip of his abdomen and inserts his genitalia into the female genitalia and thus, the mating

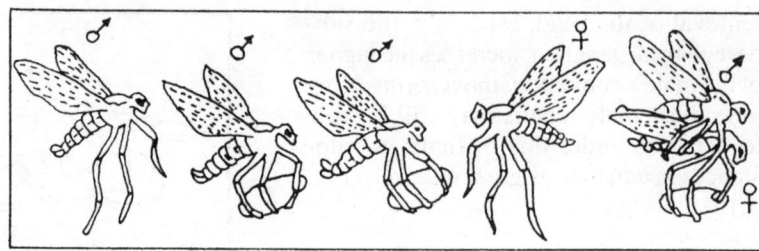

Fig. 6.14. A male cupid fly presenting gift to a female for successful mating.

continues. Different types of body movements occur in different species of ladybird beetles during mating. When the mating is over, the male and female move in a random fashion.

Randy Thornhill observed that males handing over unpalatable food, is quickly rejected by female ladybird. Even if the food item is edible and copulation begins the duration of mating is dependent on the size of the gift. If the gift is small and the meal lasts less than 5 minutes, a female will leave without taking part in copulation. The quantity and quality of the food determines whether or not she will become receptive and start laying her eggs.

DIPTERA

True flies, House fly, Mosquitoes, Fruit flies etc., belong to this order.

Cupid fly present silk baloons to the females during the courtship and mating. Females are voracious eater and are likely to attack the male during mating. A male cupid fly catch a prey, form a cocoon around it and present it to female before copulation. Female cupid fly will open up the cocoon and eat the prey. In the meantime male successfully mates with female (Fig. 6.14).

Female Katydids receive a nuptial gift from male katydids in the form of a spermatophore (Fig. 6.16). This facilitates mating, After separation female eats the nutritious protein rich spermatophore,

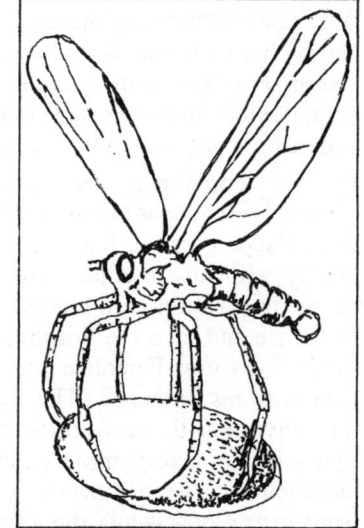

Fig. 6.15. A male baloon fly gift a baloon like prey to female.

gaining material benefit from the meal. Females of the black-tipped hangingfly choose among males that offers a nuptial gift.

Courtship and copulation of lovebugs during swarming is an unforgettable experience to the natives or tourists of north Florida. Lovebugs are not true bugs but a fly. They are called as lovebugs because of their prolonged aerial copulation. These lovebugs remain in air for several hours in copulatory position. Such pairs can copulate for an average of 56 hours.

Trycholyga bombycis, flies start vibrating the antennae, lifting of the abdomen and rubbing off the legs against the wings as well as the posterior part of the abdomen. After a brief courtship, the male mount on the dorsal side of female by clasping her head with his forelegs, thorax with his middle legs and with his third pair of legs resting on the floor and mates with her. It is ashtonishing to note that the female flies mate only once in their life time.

The female craneflies often starts the courtship by touching the male's long thread like legs. The male plays the most active role in courtship as a whole. When opposite sex happens to contact, the male grabs her legs with his own. The male then tries to pin down the female legs. After pinning, the female becomes motionless and male begins to search for head, by licking her with his mouthparts and moves progessively forward over her body. Later, he moves towards her back and *kisses* the back of female fly. The male fly stops at the posterior end of female fly and the mating occurs. If the courtship of craneflies is interrupted by removing the female, reintroducing the same female never allow the pattern to resume. Each time the male begins courtship with a new female cranefly. The first

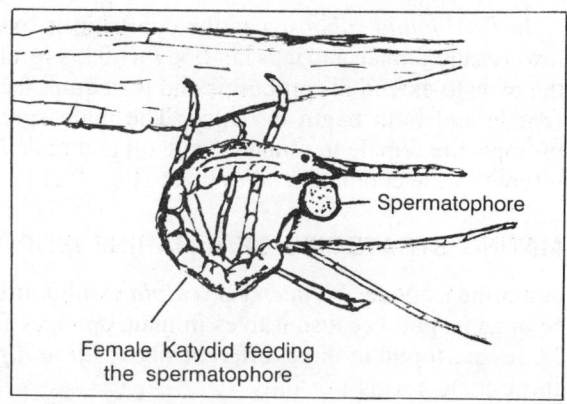

Fig. 6.16. Female katydid feeding the Spermatophore. Female has bent her head down to feed on the spermatophore.

detectable step of cranefly courtship occurs when two individuals happen to contact the legs of each other. Receptive female responds to the male grasps by raising one or more of her legs upwards where upon the male assumes a mounting position above the body of the female. Sexually unreceptive female keeps one leg continuously raised, eventually causing the male to leave.

Female *Drosophila melanogaster* is stimulated by male's courtship acts. The male touches any part of the female with his forelegs. This enables him to recognize whether the female is receptive or not. Male approaches the receptive female, opens and vibrates the wings near the female, circles the female and repeats wing vibration several times until the male mounts the female and copulate by curling the tip of the abdomen under and forward, simultaneously lunging upwards and forward thrusting his head under or between her wings. If she has spread wings then male grasp her body with his fore and mid legs and then achieving intromission.

During copulation the female may walk about and even feed while male is inert except that they periodically stroke the

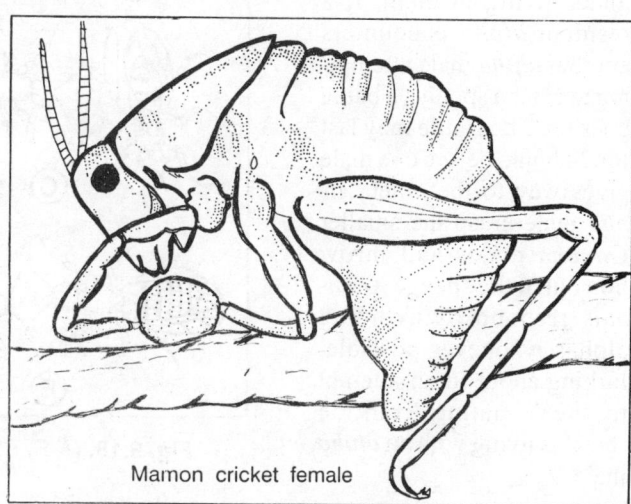

Fig. 6.17. Mamon cricket female eating the spermatophore gifted by male partner.

area of genitalic contact with their hind tarsi. At the end of copulatory period, the female typically kicks vigorously rearward with her hind legs against the face and thorax of the male. These actions may influence the male's behaviour but the physical force is never effective in breaking the genitalic union. Here the male determines the termination of copulation. When the male withdraws and separates from the female, he falls inertly to the substratum and remains quiescent for a short period before jumping to a standing position. The duration of the copulation is species specific. The shortest time is recorded 5 seconds in *D. enigma* and longest time is taken by *D. acanthoptera* with 1 hour.

In *Drosophila subobscura*, the courtship is exhibited by a series of responses. The male orientates towards the female and taps her body with his forelegs. The visual and tactile stimuli of the female cause the male to extend his proboscis and to acquire face to face position. The male then taps the head of the female and both begin to dance. The male spreads his wings when the dance stops. This posture prompts the female to remain standstill and male finally jumps over her body, attempts to copulate and ultimately the copulation takes place (Fig. 6.18)

MATING STRATEGIES OF A MARINE ISOPODE

A marine isopode, *Paracerceis sculpta* exhibit three different sexual strategies. This isopod is called the Sponge isopod because it lives in main sponges found in the intertidal zone of the Gulf of California. Males are found in three different sizes : *large Alpha, medium Beta* and *small Gamma* (Fig. 6.18). The three male forms not only look different, they also exhibit three different behavioural patterns for acquiring mates. The big forms, or *alpha* males, attempt to exclude other males from the interior cavities of sponges that have one or more females living in them. If a resident *alpha* encounters another *alpha* male attempting to enter a sponge, a battle goes on. The Battle may last for 24 hours before one male gives way to the other. *Alpha* male grasp the smaller *Gamma* males and throw him out of the sponge. *Gammas* respond by avoiding alphas whenever possible, lurking about in an attempt to sneak mating from the females living with an *alpha* male.

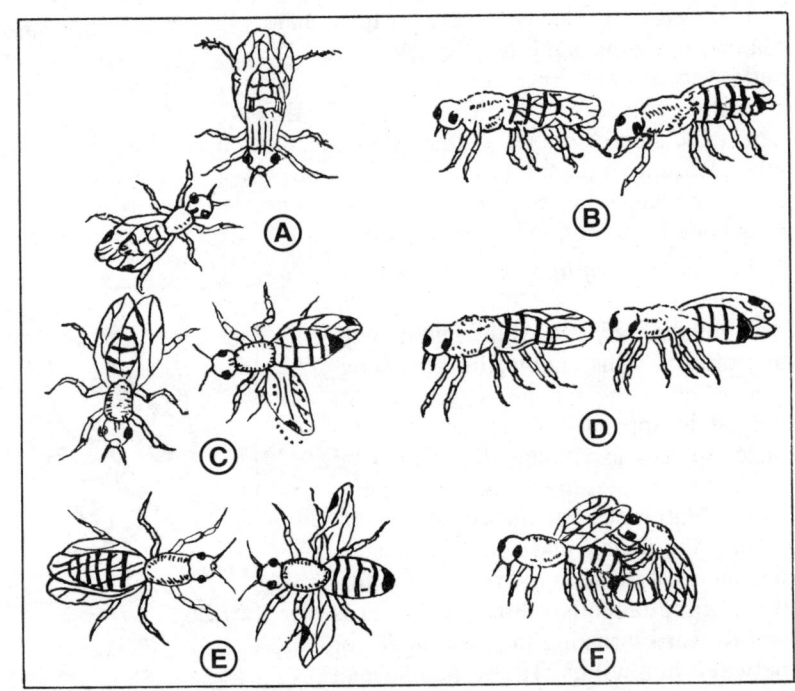

Fig. 6.18. (A-F) Stages in Courtship and Mating in *Drosophila*.

Whenever a *beta* male gets a chance to meet *alpha* male inside a sponge cavity, it behaves like a female, soliciting courtship, which the *alpha* is likely to provide – but to no good effect from the *Alpha's* perspective. Through female mimicry, female-sized *beta* males can coexist with much larger and stronger rivals and gain access to the females that the *alpha* male attempts to monopolize.

Male Panorpa scorpionflies are similar to sponge isopod in exhibiting three different ways of acquiring mates :

1. Some males defend dead insects that attract receptive females which feed upon the carrion;

2. Others secrete saliva on leaves and wait for female to come to consume this nutritional gift ; and

3. Still other offer their mates nothing but instead force them to copulate forcibly (Fig. 6.20).

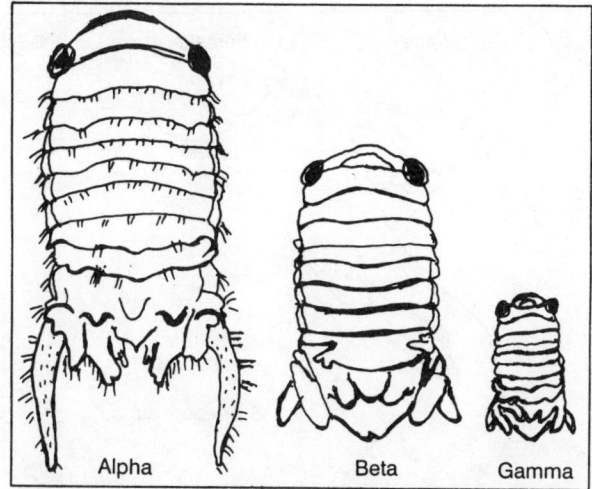

Fig. 6.19. Three different forms of the sponge isopod : The large *alpha* male, the female sized *beta* male and the tiny *gamma* male. Each type not only differs in shape and size, but also uses a different manner of acquiring mates.

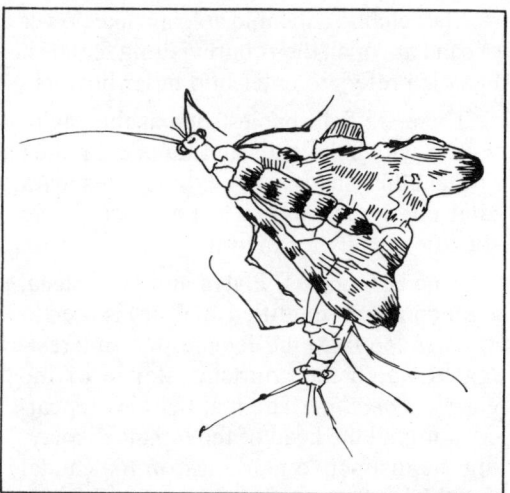

Fig. 6.20. Forced copulation (Rape) in Panorpa scorpion flies occurs when a male without a nuptial gift grabs a female and will not release her until she mates with him.

COURTSHIP AND MATING RITUALS IN VERTEBRATES

The courtship and mating behaviour prepares both the male and female for the act of copulation. Immediately after copulation, behaviour of many species serve to diminish the interest of the male in the particular female. Cases of courtship is rare in fishes, common in birds and mammals and sporadic in amphilions and reptiles.

FISH

Different species of fishes display diverse courtship and mating patterns.

External fertilization takes place in three-spined stickleback fish but elaborate courtship behaviour of this fish is interesting to note. Male fish selects a suitable place and makes a nest of weed. Now he attracts a prospective female and drags her for "*Sigmoid*" or "*S shaped dance*". After some time male stickleback fish muzzles female with his snout at the base of her tail and stimulate her to lay eggs. The female swims away of the nest and the male immediately follows her shedding his sperms on the eggs released by the female (Fig. 6.21).

The brilliantly coloured male of siamese fighting fish Betta swims round the female in a state of excitement. While swimming round the female male fully extends his coloured fins, mouth widely open and the rays protruding out to expose the bright red gills. This stimulates the female who signals her willingness to mate. The male lifts the female by placing his pelvic fins beneath hers. At first the fish swims obliquely side by side towards the surface of water. Later, their position changes and they swim vertically upwards. The anal fins of the two fish together form a gutter into which the eggs and sperms are shed.

The common tragonet, *Callionymus*, also indulges in elaborate sexual display, but the eggs are abandoned after spawning.

Male cichlid fish build volcano like bower of sand in which they court visiting females. Female prefers to enter into taller bowers.

There are fish species such as the angle-fish, in which the male and female threaten one another incessantly (sometimes with fatal consequences) in order to elicit the specific signals for mating.

Among Guppies, Platys and Gambusia, a gonopodium (modified anal fin) is used to transfer sperm to the female. It is interesting to watch the courtship dance of the guppy (*Poecilia*). The male circles repeatedly around the head of the female displaying the distinctive markings on his caudal fins. Male of one species of guppy - *Poecilia reticulata* perform 'Sigmoid' dance. The male holds a position in front of the female and quivers for several seconds. The males have conspicuous markings on the body. A mating attempt by a male swings round and attempts to insert his gonopodium into the genital pore of the female. Thus fertilization is internal (Fig. 6.23). Male platys approach females with a sidling movement and also display patterns of backing towards the female, quivering of the body, and swinging of the gonopodium.

Male Shark has modified anal fin called claspers. Male shark grasp the hind edge of female's pectoral fins, turning her on his back, and insert claspers to transfer sperms.

The courtship and mating behaviour of tropical aquarium fishes has been lucidly described by Barlow and Green (1970). Blackchin mouthbreeders, (*Tilapia melanotheron*) display four courtship patterns. These are :

(i) the *nod* (rapid tilting down and forward),

(ii) *quiver* (a pattern of head shaking),

(iii) *nip* (biting the substrate), and

(iv) *skim* (remaining motionless near the nest).

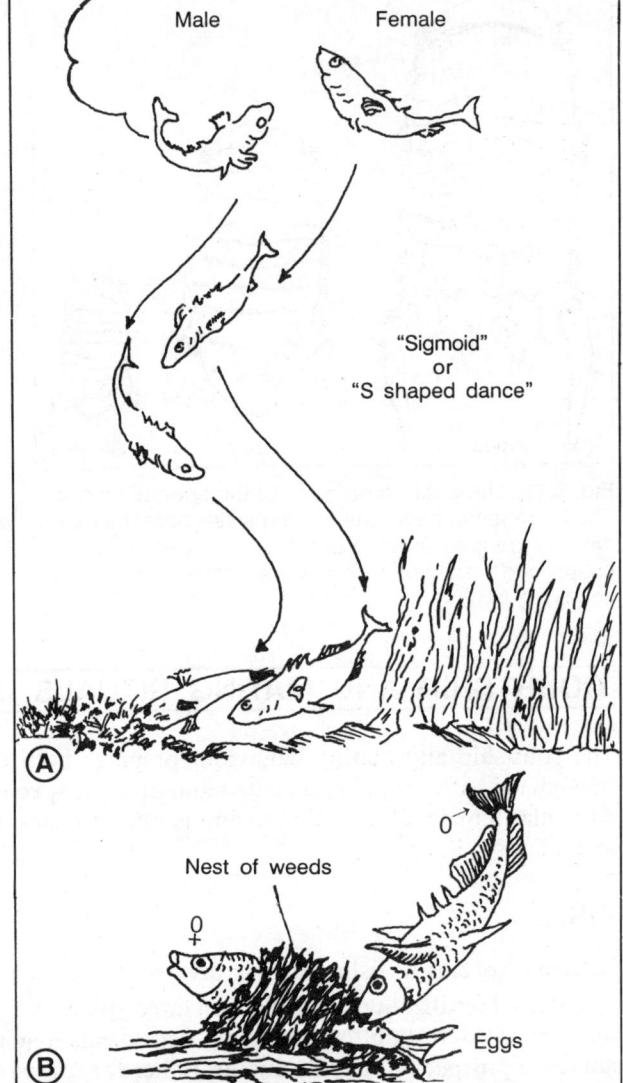

Fig. 6.21. (A) Courtship activities performed by three spined stickleback – Sigmoid dance; (B) Male stickleback muzzles back of female to release ova.

Clark, Aronson and Gordon (1954) observed that male approach female with a sliding movement and also display patterns of backing towards the female, quivering of the body and swinging of the gonopodium.

AMPHIBIA

Very few amphibians exhibit courtship behaviour. Most frogs and toads have external fertilization. Sexually excited bullfrog males produce crocking calls to attract female of that vicinity. Bullfrogs make louder calls from places in ponds where water temperature and vegetation factors are suitable for egg development. Louder calls are more attractive to females and more inhibitory to other males (Fig. 6.24A). Sexually excited females approache to the chorus and move towards a male. Male frog mounts on her back and tightly clasps her. Amplexus usually does not occur until a female actually touches a male, an observation suggests that a female can mate with the individual of her choice. Female prefer to mate and lay their eggs in the territories of large males. Richard Howard has shown that embryo mortality from overcrowding and leech predation is lower in territories controlled by larger males than in sites monopolized by their smaller rivals. Thus by mating with large males, female bullfrog gain material benefits and fitness too. The male's clasp is so tight that it is difficult to dislodge the male from the female during amplexus. Increasing compression on female's body by the strong grasp of the male for a few hours increases the internal pressure in female's body so much that she is eventually forced to shed her ova into water through her cloaca. Simultaneously, the male also sheds its sperms on the spawn to ensure fertilization (Fig. 6.24B).

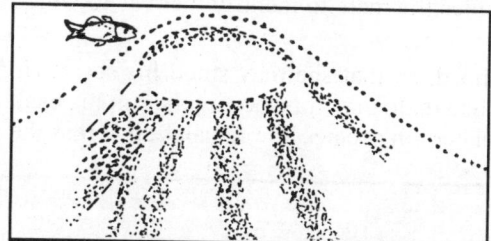

Fig. 6.22. Female Mate Choice in Relation to Bower size in a Cichlid fish.

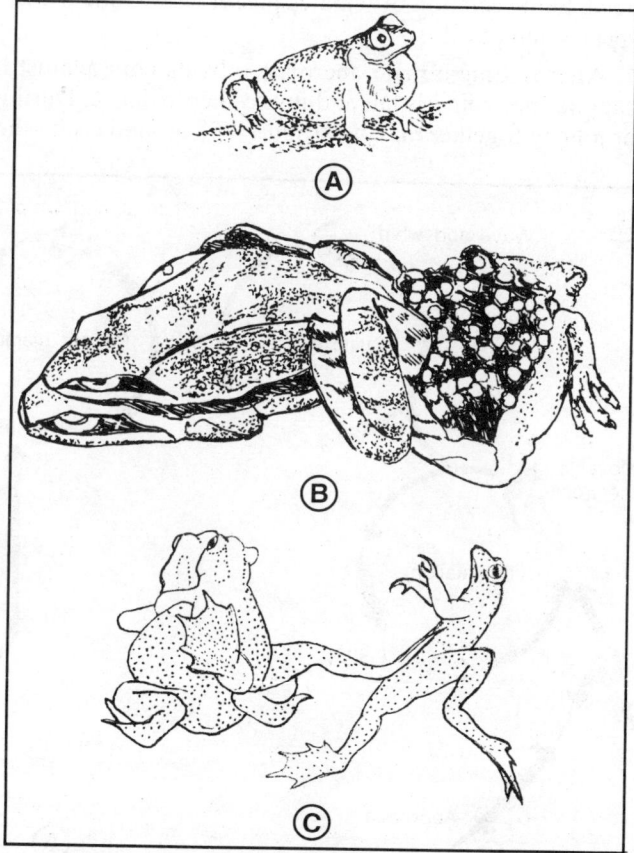

Fig. 6.24. (A) Male frog producing croacking calls; (B) Amplexus; (C) A male toad trying to dislodge the mating male. Copulating male is repelling a rival toad by hind leg.

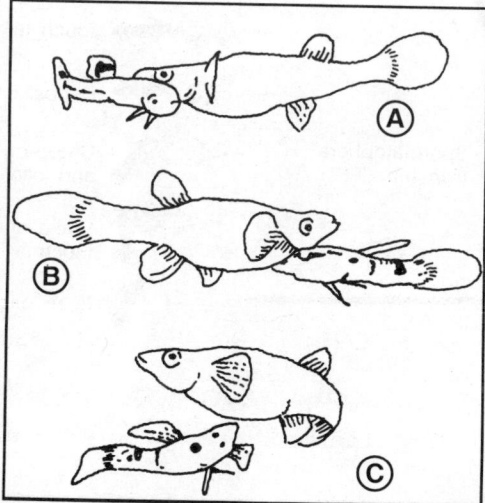

Fig. 6.23. (A-C) Stages in Courtship dance by guppy-*Poecilia.*

Nick Davies and Tim Halliday (1977) observed in toads that the male sit on the back of females for few days before the female lays eggs. Sometimes other male toad try to dislodge the mating male from the female, by pulling him off. But the copulating male repels the rival by hind leg (Fig. 6.24C).

Urodels such as newt (*Triturus*) develops a large crest, black, blue and red spots and an orange belly in the breeding season. Courtship of urodels is peculiar. Male newt performs a specific dance to attract the female. If she follows the male and touches his tail with her snout then he releases spermatophore in water. Females pick up spermatophores inside her genital duct through cloaca, where internal fertilization takes place. Male newt again renews his dance and releases two or three more packages of spermatozoa before his arrival to the surface of water for breathing. Again female newts picks up these packages of spermatozoa in her cloaca. The female thus tests the vigour of the male. According to Halliday the chance of fertilizing the female by the male newt depends on how long he can stay submerged and the number of spermatophores he can produce. As mentioned above fertilization takes place in the oviduct and then eggs are laid separately warapped in leaf (Fig. 6.25A).

In Salamanders scent is the main factor in recognition of own species and opposite sex. Males and females are of different colours and size (sexual dimorphism) and each species has its own peculiar smell. In the males, the "Hedonic glands" are located at the base of the tail and on the underside of the head. Skin secretion of females possesses the odour that enables the male to identify them as to which species and sex it is.

After finding a mate, the male rubs its chin against her head, so that she may smell his scent. He captures her with his tail and invites her to dance. During dance male may transporting her on his back or joining together making a figure of 8 around each other. In certain species, the females sit across the

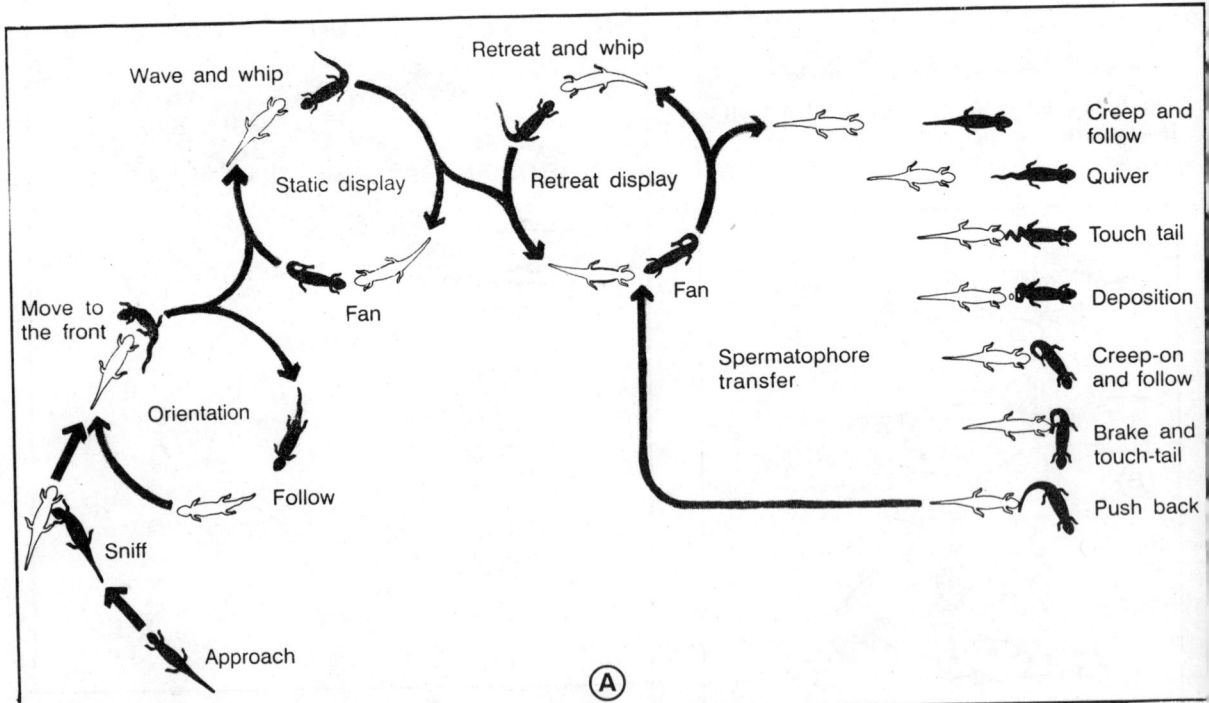

Fig. 6.25. (A) Courtship of smooth newts (*Triturus vulagaris*).

legs of males placing her head on the base of the male's tail and then the two walk with short steps together in this position. The male of two lined salamander, *Eurycea bislineata* applies a secretion from glands on his head on to the female's skin. He then lacerates her skin with two protruding teeth so that the secretion enters her blood stream. In most salamanders fertilization is internal but it is accomplished in manner different from that employed by mammals where the male feels that the female is sufficiently excited. Male salamander deposits a small jelly like spermatophore either on land or in water according to the habit of species. Female comes and picks up one of the package of spermatophore with the lips of her cloaca. It is then placed inside her body in a special receptacle known as spermatheca where the sperms remain stored to fertilize the egg (Fig. 6.25B).

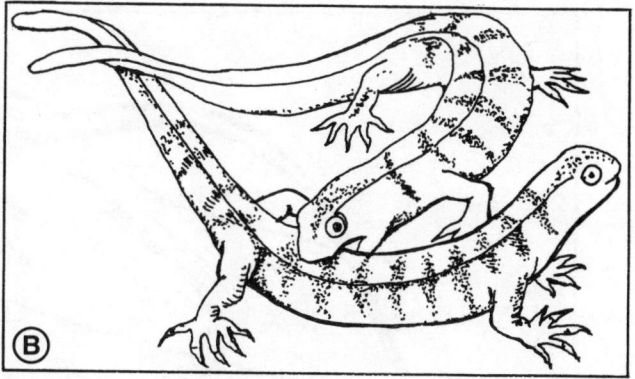

Fig. 6.25. (B) Courtship of two lined Salamanders (Eurycea bislineata) with male lacerating the female.

REPTILES

Many reptiles show well marked courtship behaviour and they display various breeding actions. Fertilization is internal through use of intromittent organ.

The male American Chamelion (*Anolis carolinesis*) displays rhythmical up and down bobbing of his neck to show his dewlap, a bright red spot of skin. As the female approaches, the male twists his tail around that of the female and inserts his hemipenis in the cloaca of female. Wall lizards and Garden lizards also deliver neck trip, twist their tails around that of the female, and insert their hemipenis in the cloaca of female to release sperms.

Courtship in most species of snakes is based on tactile stimulation of the female and olfactory stimulation of the male. The "Courtship dances" which two snakes become closely intertwined have generally proved to be male-male aggressive fight. The general believe that snakes make pair is wrong. The male snake can mate with many females in breeding season.

In turtles and tortoises reproduction is initiated by fighting between males. The males of Harmann's tortoise injure other males quite seriously during such encounters. In case of spotted turtles, when a male spotted turtle approaches a female, the usual response of the female is to make sure that the male is following her.

Sexual maturity of male Estuarine Crocodile (*Crocodylus porosus*) is attained at the age of 16 years (3.2 m length) and in the female in 10 years (2.2 m length). Mugger (*Crocodylus palustris*) is smaller than Estuarine Crocodile or the Gharial in size. Males exhibit a strong dominance hierarchy and the dominant male mates with several females. Mating takes place in water.

LESBIANISM IN LIZARD

Sexual behaviour in parhenogenetic lizards is interesting to note. These lizards are composed entirely of females. If a female is courted and mounted by another female (and females do engage in pseudomale

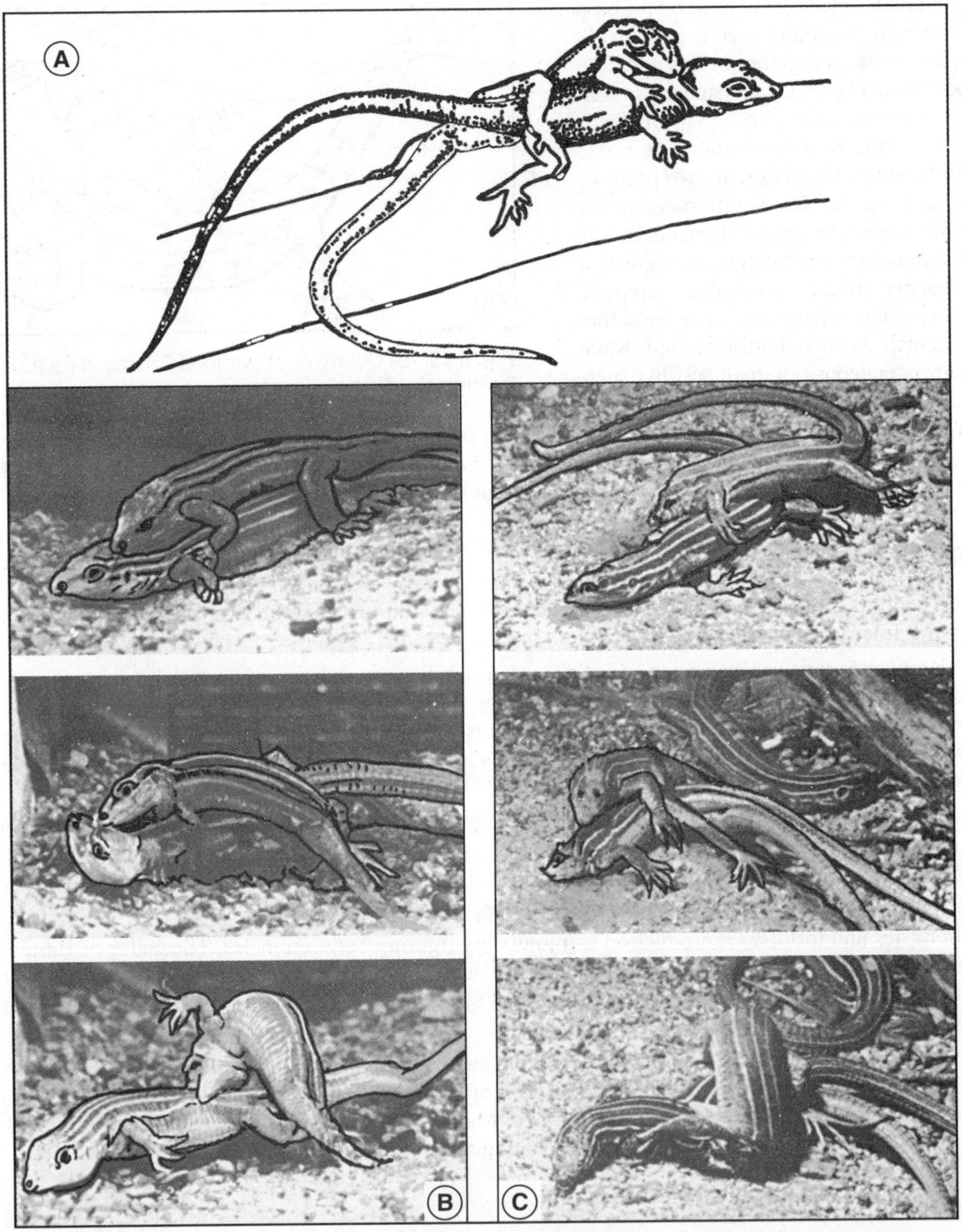

Fig. 6.26. (A) Mating pattern of green anole lizard; (B) Sexual Behaviour in Whiptail Lizards : A male whiptail lizard engages in courtship/copulatory behaviour with a female; (C) Lesbianism in Lizard : Two females of a closely related parthenogenetic species engage in mock mating process.

sexual behaviour for reasons that are not fully known), she is much more likely to produce a clutch of eggs than if she does not receive sexual stimulation from a partner of same sex (Fig. 6.26C).

BIRDS

Courtship among birds has remained a matter of interest since old days because birds exhibit many interesting courtship activities during breeding season. Some male birds simply keep showing of their special brilliant plumage to the females in showy series of posturing and walking in an upright proud way, while some conduct their courtship in a quite discrete manner. In birds phenomenon of courtship attain a complexity incompatible to man. Birds exhibit very elaborate courtship behaviour in general, combined with bright colours, various forms of adornment and many striking songs. Songs are seasonal complex accoustal pattern emitted primarily by males during the courtship and mating and territorial differences with more individual variation. Genetic factors are predominant in vocal ontogeny (Nottebohm, 1972) as seen in domestic fowls and ring doves (Komishi, 1963, Nottebohm and Nottebohm, 1971) where vocal repertoire of the adults develops normally in birds which are raised in isolation from members of their species.

In most of birds species , there is not external genitalia and the sperms are transferred through organs called cloaca-the male expelling sperms in to the female with a cloacal kiss.

Most birds have some kind of courtship display to win the female's heart. Dancing of peacock is a well known example. While courting, male peacock takes numerous forms such as fluffing out of ornamental plumage, fanning and erecting the tail and dancing in front of the peahen. But as soon as peahen comes in front of him, he takes about turn showing his rear portion. Now if peahen is motivated for mating, she will run swiftly around the tail to be able to see it from the front again. The cock responds by rustling his tail feathers. Then he will turn around again and this courtship game will be repeated several times. At last the peahen will lie down in front of him giving signals for mating.

Male robin puffs out its chest in order to show the female robin red colour of the breast feathers. He also spreads his tail and opens his beak wide to display the bright yellow colour of his throat. This attract female robin to surrender for mating.

Male Japanese 'quail' grasps the feathers of the female's neck in his beak, mount her by standing on her back, and orients until the cloacal openings can be brought together.

Parakeets posture and pose ludicrously standing first on one foot and then on the other to attract his sex partner.

A male sparrow adopts special postures to display his black throat which attract female sparrow for mating. House sparrow's mount repetition is maximum in animal world.

Many of us must have watched that male pigeon tumbles and turns somersault in the air before a prospective female.

Only a few birds (Ratites, Ducks and Gees), have a well developed copulatory organ or penis. Ethologists have discovered that male bufallow weaver birds have *orgasm* – an experience apparently denied to other birds. And it is all because of an organ that resembles a penis but has nothing to do with the actual process of reproduction.

Male red billed bufallo weaver (*Bubalornis niger*) possesses a stiff rod of connective tissue, about 2 cm. and situated near the cloaca. This "false penis" contains no ducts, and hence cannot be used for transferring sperms. This bird is native of Namibia and their mating ritual usually occurres deep in the wood and away from the nest. Copulation goes on for half an hour or so, with the male rubbing his false penis against the female cloaca, sperms are deposited only when males reach an orgasm. There is no evidence of females achieving orgasm.

The results indicate that the false penis is a stimulatory organ, designed to encourage the female to take up more sperm, says Prof. Birkhead. "Ten years ago, we all assumed birds were monogamous and mated for life. DNA studies have transformed that view." When the team studied DNA from the buffalo weaver, it was found that about 75% of the broods contained chicks fathered by different males. "When sperm competition is intense, you get anatomical or behavioural changes to try to ensure that males will win, and succeed in fathering offspring," Prof. Birkhead says.

Lsorenz studied various courtship patterns of male ducks. In this grunt-whistle, the male lowers its bill to the water, arching the body upward, flicking the bill, and emitting a loud whistle followed by a grunting sound. The head-up-tail down display is accompanied by a loud whistle. In the down-up display, the breast is dipped into the water and the bill is jerked upward and outward, flipping a column of water.

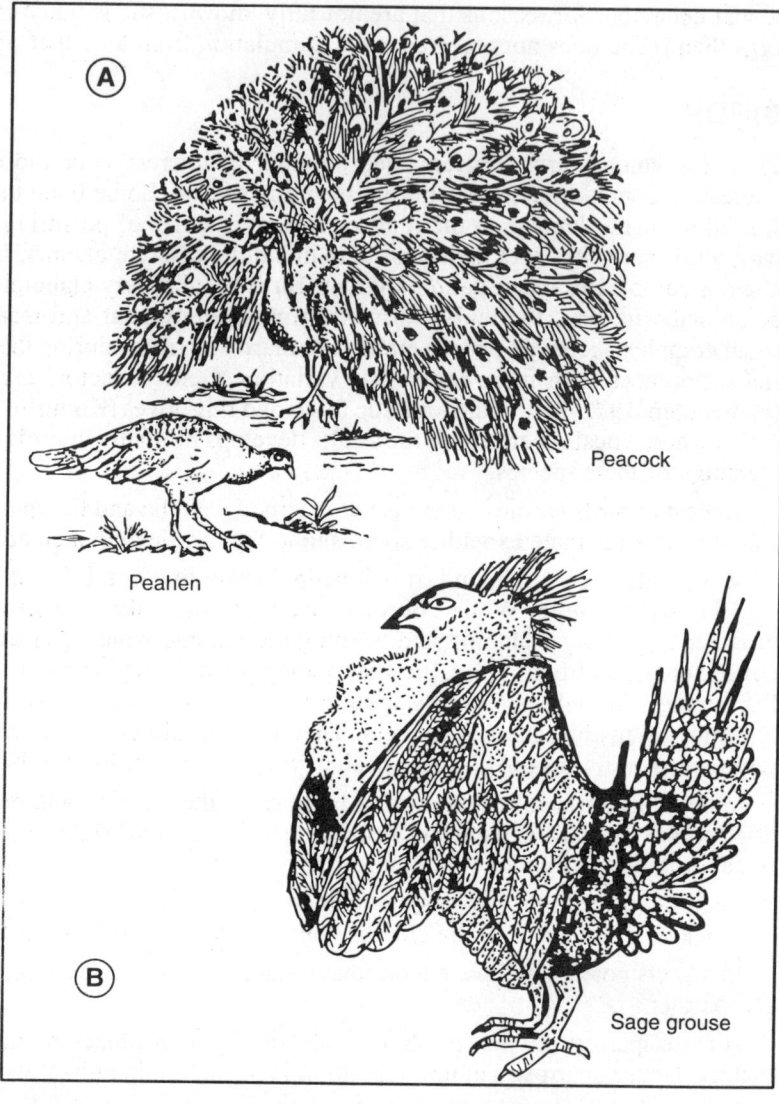

Fig. 6.27. (A) Courtship Dance of Peacock pheasant to attract peahen pheasant. (B) Male sage grouse at the peak of his 'strut' display, used in courtship.

Green herons set up their own territories. The calls of males attract females. Females are initially repelled with full-forward displays, but females persist and courtship is eventually initiated with the appearance of the snap display and the stretch display. After pairing, the two birds fly about the territory, occasionally showing the more intense flap-flight display. Display patterns then become more contact-oriented until copulation takes place (Mey Erriecks, 1960).

Both male and female Avocetes preen their feathers in hasty fashion during courtship (Fig. 6.28 D). After preening the female adopts a characteristic flattened attitude which is the sign that she is ready to mate. Now the male mounts and copulates.

The precoition displays of herring gulls (*Harus argentatus*) is very interesting. Both male and female

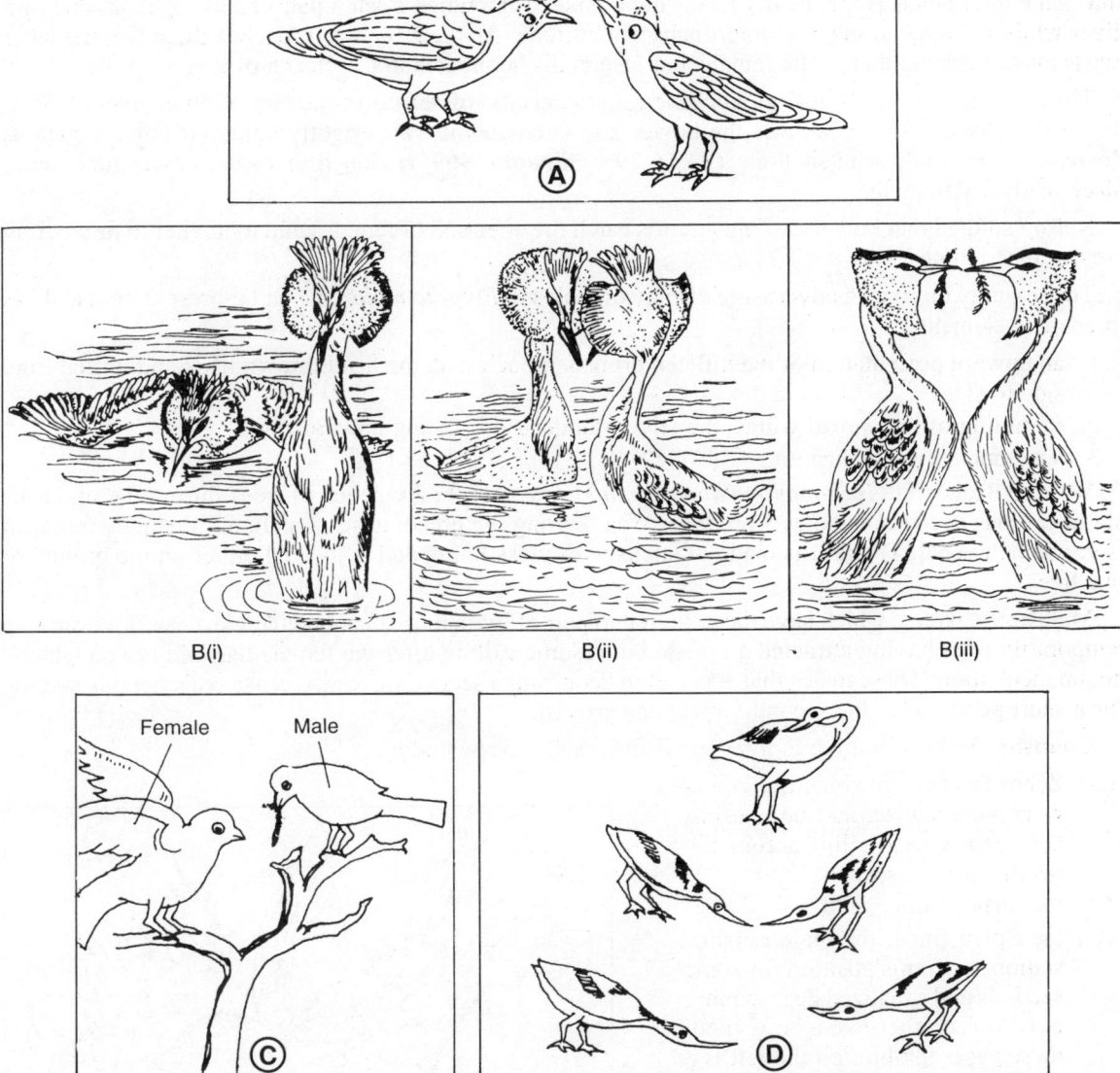

Fig. 6.28. Courtship patterns of four species of birds : (A) Coition display of herring gull (B) Ritualized courtship in great crested greb, (C) Male Kestrel passing prey to female, (D) Displacement preening courtship and group display among Avocetes.

bob their heads upwards uttering a soft melodious call with each bob. After a series of such mutual head tossing the male takes the initiative in copulation and suddenly mounts and mates (Fig. 6.28A)

The largest grebe (a bird similar to a duck but without webbed feet) we have in India is the Crested Grebe (*Podiceps crestatus*). It is known for its spectacular courtship movement and pair bonding which is not found anywhere in the animal kingdom. The courtship ceremony consists of a series of behaviours such as *head shaking ceremony*; *dive and cat displays*; *mutual greeting and cat displays*; and penguin dance (Fig. 6.28B). During head shaking ceremony they raise their conspicuous crest, face each other and shake their heads emphatically from side to side. Sometimes when a pair comes together, one bird dives while the other waits in extraordinary cat attitude. As the female approaches the male, the latter twists his tail around that of the female and inserts his hemipenis in the cloaca of female grebe.

The male satin bower bird (*Ptilonorhynchus violaceous*) of Australia and New Guinea lives along in the forest, clears a space, weaves the bower and decorates it with brightly coloured objects such as flowers, stones, molluscan shell etc. (Fig. 6.29). Gilliard (1969) reasoned that satin bower function in place of showy plumage.

Nelson studied that how male frigate birds catch the attention of females and tempt her to move from present place to nest site.

The sexually motivated advertising display of males in *Fregata minor* is a Gular presentation and has three main elements :

1. an upward presentation of the inflated crimson pouch with the head thrown back and turned from side to side;
2. trembling of the spread wings, the silvery under-sides facing upwards; and
3. accompanying vocalization.

Western Tragopan (*Tragopan melanocephalus*) roosts in the branches of trees during the night. Its alarm call has been rendered as Waa, Waa, Waa. During the breeding season (June), the male tragopan is very much vocal. The nest is made of sticks with grass lining and is located either on the ground or in a tree.

Male house wrens, which have the potential to pair off with more than one female, cease loud singing temporarily after having attracted a female but resume calling after the female has laid her clutch and begun incubation. These males that succeed in acquiring a second mate also cease conspicuous singing for a short period after the second female has arrived.

Courtship by beak-wiping in three grass finches has been studied :

(A) Zebra finches, in which the movement is unritualized and the male just about to wipe his bill across the perch. In both species,

(B) the Striated finch, and

(C) the Spice finch, the male remains stationary in this position for some seconds and ritualized beak-wiping now looks rather like a bow. In all these cases the bird on the left is a female.

The Malabar grey hornbill is sexually dimorphic : the male has a large, bright orange bill and golden brown iris, while the female has a relatively small and pale-coloured bill and dark brown iris. The species is monogamous, the nesting pair usually exhibits high nest-site fidelity, occupying the same nest cavities every year (Kemp 1978, Ali and Ripley 1978, Mudappa and Kannan 1999) . This spe-

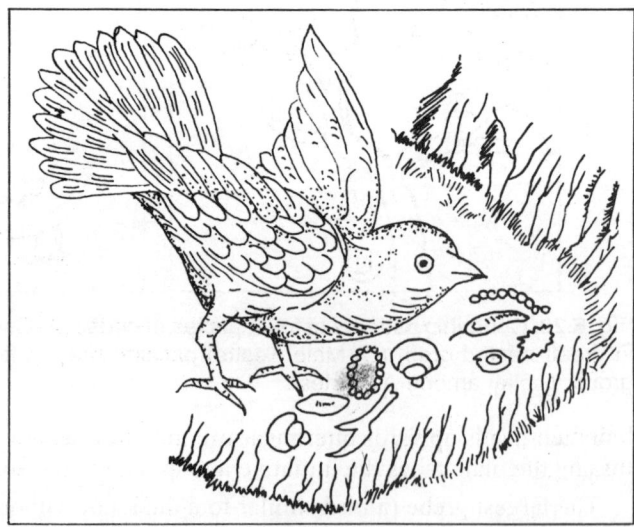

Fig. 6.29. Courtship of satin bower bird : a male Satin bower bird at his bower at a time when a drably coloured female has come to visit the bower and inspect his behaviour.

cies exhibits biparental care like most other monogamous birds with altricial young (Clutton-Brock
1997). While the incubating female is incarcer-
ated, the male provides her with the food.

Nest cavity remains approximately 14 m on the
Artocarpus lakoocha (Moraceae) tree. The cavity
entrance is always almost circular is shape and
orientation towards northwest.

Female enter into a nest cavity in the first week
of February. She clean the nest & widen the nest
entrance. After this a regular movement of the
breeding pair occure in the vicinity of the nest
tree. The male and the female visit the nest 8 times
in 6 hrs. During these visit they copulate. Now
female hornbill seal the cavity entrance, leaving
only a slit, through which the male feed the inmates during the nesting period. Female eject her
faecal matter through this slit.

The males are never involved in nest sealing,
repair, or delivering any kind of sealing material.
Female often repairs the seal with its bill. The female clean the nest-cavity by throwing out a lot of
seeds and woody debris. The female hornbill may
use her own excreta, rich in Ficus seeds, as material for sealing the cavity entrance.

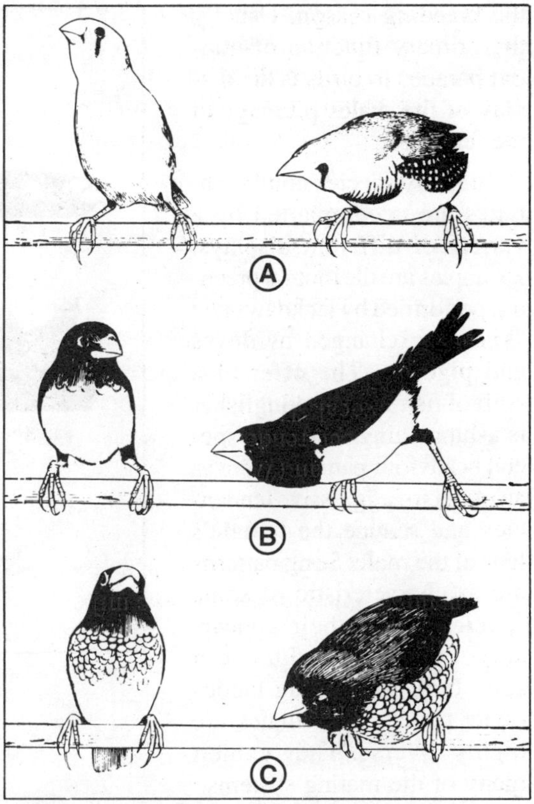

In case of Baya (weaver bird – *Ploceus
Phillipinus*) the act of building a nest is itself a
form of courtship and the female chooses as mate
the male whose nest catches her fancy. Baya also

Fig. 6.30. Beak-wiping during the courtship of three grass finches. (A) Zebra finch, (B) striated finch, (C) spice finch.

make whistle like mating calls in chorus accompanied by flapping of wings while weaving their nest in a colony. Female Baya selects the best woven nest. Selection is done during half woven condition. Subsequently, the sexual activity of the male and female must be synchronized so that the partners are "ready" at the same time.

In the fighting quail, it is the female which performs a parade and calls to attract the males. She mates with several males.

Lorenz studied various courtship patterns of male ducks. The male grunt whistle, lowers its bill to the water, arching the body upward, flicking the bill, and emitting a loud whistle followed by a grunting sound. In the down up display, the breast is dipped into the water and the bill is jerked upward and outward, flipping a column of water (Fig. 6.31).

In a number of large-bodies bird species where there are no great differences between males and females in their plumage patterns, "mutual" nuptial parades are often observed, with the male and female simultaneously performing the same behaviour patterns. This is the case with grey herons, great crested grebes and laughing gulls.

Depending on the species, nuptial parades can take place on the ground, on water or in the air. The contest of the ruff takes place in the middle of an arena on meadow land. The mallard duck and grebes carry out their preludes to mating on the water. The black kite performs spectacular aerial ballets during the breeding season. Usually the primary function of nuptial parades in birds is the display of the males plumage to the female.

In many species nuptial parades are accompanied by a variety of different displays. Examples are the mutual preening performed by jackdaws and "kisses" exchanged by doves and pigeons. The offer of a "gift of fish" among kingfisher is ashtonishing. All these special behaviour patterns serve as an outlet for aggressive tendencies and reduce the female's fear of the male. Song patterns are as characteristic of some species as are their appearance. Dunnock is a European song bird, the mating tactics of its males and females are highly diverse. They exhibit many of the mating systems.

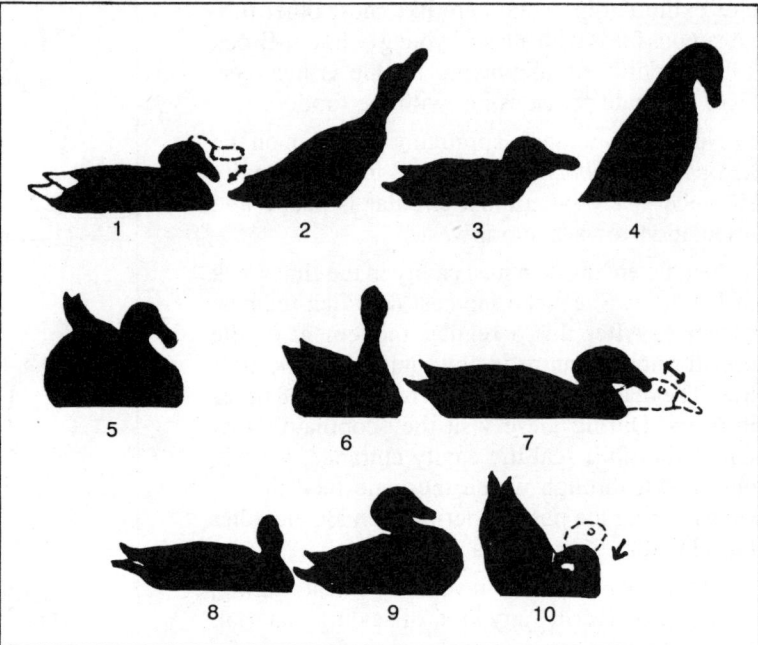

Fig. 6.31. Courtship of male mallard duck.

CO-OPERATIVE COURTSHIP IN BIRDS

Long tailed manakin, a beautiful bird of Central America are among the very few in which males perform a joint venture to attract and court females.

Pairs of males co-operate by loudly whistling, "toe-lay-doe" together as many as 300 times per hour at a display perch. Attracted females fly in and land on a central display perch. In response, the two males dart in the land close to the prospective female. The two partners first perform an astonishing cartwheel display. The male closest to the female leaps into the air and then begins to come down to where his partner is perching. To make room for the descending bird, the other male move in the specified direction in a shy manner as if it does not want to be noticed. It jump quickly back to the

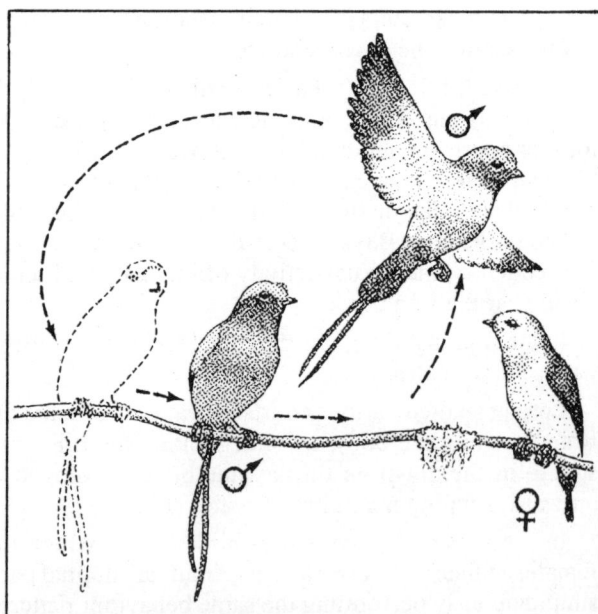

Fig. 6.32. Co-operative courtship of the Long-tailed Manakin. The two males are in the cartwheeling portion of their dual display to a female, who is perched on the vine to the right.

jumping-off point used by his companion, and then leaps up to exchange places. After a series of cartwheels, one male may leap over the head of the female, with the other member of the pair instantly following in order to perform a new run of cartwheels (Fig. 6.32).

Long tailed manakins have other joint displays, including a combined slow fluttering flight like butterfly. Birds that are helicoptering back and forth in this fashion may suddenly switch to the other extremes in which they fire back and forth at top speed over the head of the female. Despite the elaborate and attractive co-operative flight of the males, female visitors only rarely signal that they are ready to mate, by beginning to jump about on the perch. At this cue, one member of the display duly discreetly leaves, while the remaining male stays to copulate. The female then leaves, and the mated male calls for his male partner, who flies back to resume his co-operative calling and courtship duties.

One male is dominant to all others at the site, including his primary display comparison, a *beta* male, which in turn is dominant to a variable number of other part-time co-operators.

MAMMALS

Ewer (1968) observed keenly some courtship patterns of mammals and came of the conclusion that olfaction and tactile contact play major role in the regulation of courtship in many mammalian species. Patterns of anogenital investigation and urine testing are common in horses, zebra, giraffe, lion, dog, fox etc. After smelling a female, the males of many mammalian species display a Fehmen response, in which the neck is extended and the upper lip is curled. This pattern appears to function more in facilitating perception of the odour than as a display. The secretions produced by a bitch in heat attract all the male dogs in the neighbourhood, whereas they show no interest at all if her odour is some how suppressed. In the past, horse-thieves used to employ a sponge soaked in urine from a mare in heat in order to attract stallions that they wished to steal from a meadow. In rabbits, the male excites the female by leaping over her while spraying her with a stream of urine. It is the combination of these two stimuli which renders the female receptive to the male for mating.

Female mammals often solicit mounting, sometimes by approaching a male, nuzzling and licking him, and often by darting from him. Much of the running from the male done by females appears more as solicitation behaviour than escape.

HERBIVORES

In the large herbivores, a male will perform in front of the female a series of movements which will allow her to recognize him as a member of her own species and also make her receptive. This kind of behaviour has been particularly well observed with large African antelope species, in which it is very ritualized. Commonly males allure female for mating but exception in courtship behaviour in mammal is black buck where female black buck allure males to mate.

Male uganda Kob, exhibit visual signal to allure female for mating. As soon as a female Uganda Kob approaches the territory of a male, the latter begins to paw the ground, displaying the black stripes which are present on the forelegs, and then raises his head so that the female can see the white patch on his chin. Subsequently, the male excites the female by touching her repeatedly with one of his forelegs. If the female moves off, the male will follow her to his territorial boundary, but not go beyond the territory. In all ungulates (hoofed mammals), the ritualized nuptial parades are performed to emphasize secondary sexual characters such as coloured patches, stripes of varying intensity, markings on the rump, tufts of hair, tail tufts, horns or antlers.

Male deer live together peacefully for much of the year but they split up and behave aggressively towards each other at the beginning of the breeding season in order to acquire and defend territory necessary for their mating performance.

In the large herbivores, a male will perform in front of the female a series of movements which will allow her to recognize him as a member of her own species and also make her receptive. This form of behaviour has been particularly well observed with large African antelope species, in which it is very ritualized.

The female red deer frequently runs away when approached by the male red deer (stag) but she soon stops and waits for him like heroin of hindi films. Female licks him and then runs again only to wait once more for his approach. Thamin (*Cervus eldi eldi*) is endangered species among deer. It is found only in Loktab lake Keibul Lamjao National Park (Manipur). Local people call it manipur deer or laxk;. Hindi name is Thamin but known as Dancing deer or brow antlered deer. The upper skin bear rough fur. The fur of male become dark brown in winter and almond coloured in summer season. Male thamin dance like a specialist dancer in breeding season and allure female thamin by their spectacular dance. The big chunk of Lamjao National Park float in the lake and hence this park is known as floating park. This park contains a special type of grass called 'Fumudi'. This grass is main food of thamin and hence this deer is found only in Lamjao National Park, Manipur.

HYENA

People of different parts of the world wish their relatives with various ways when they meet them after a temporary separation. We wish our relatives with folded hands. But spotted hyena greet their clan members by a very peculiar way. They greet their clan members by creeting their penises when some clan members rejoin their groups after a temporary separation. It may be surprising for you to know that female spotted hyenas participate fully in this activity, for they too have something that looks exactly like a penis called pseudopenis. This pseudopenis is elongation of clittoris in female hyena. The "penis" sniffing rituals of hyenas is OK for social behaviour but imagine about their copulation. How a male penis will penetrate into a pseudopenis of female hyena. The copulation in hyenas gives the appearance of being difficult to achieve. It is funny to observe the mating of hyena because male penis is inserted into pseudopenis of female (Fig. 6.33).

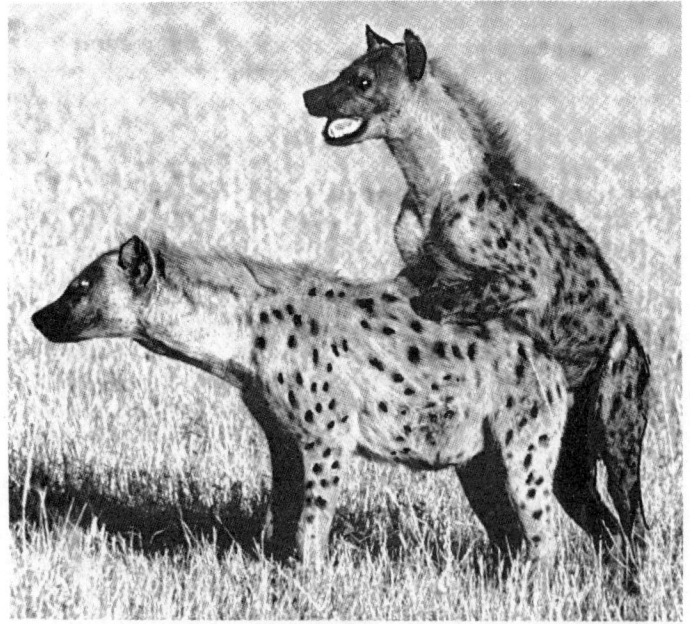

Fig. 6.33. Copulating hyenas. In order to mate, a male insert his penis through the narrow tubular clittoris (pseudopenis) of female hyena.

RATS & CATS

Mating behaviour of rats, (*Rattus norvegicus*) has been studied in laboratory in detail. If a receptive female is introduced into a cage containing a vigorous male, a predictable sequence of events ensure. After initial courtship behaviour (sniffing, chasing, soliciting by the female), the male pursues the running female. As the male mounts the female from behind, the female adopts a stereotyped posture termed as "lordosis". Same posture is observed in cats during copulation.

In rats and cats mating takes place in a stereotyped fashion called "intromission". The male's penis is inserted into the female's vagina for a period of about ¼ second before the male displays a rapid dismount. Although there may be extravaginal pelvic thrusting by the male prior to insertion but there is no intravaginal thrusting. After about ten such brief intromissions spaced about a minute apart from each other, the male displays a different pattern called "ejaculation". The male shows a kind of convulsive thrusting during ejaculation and clasps the

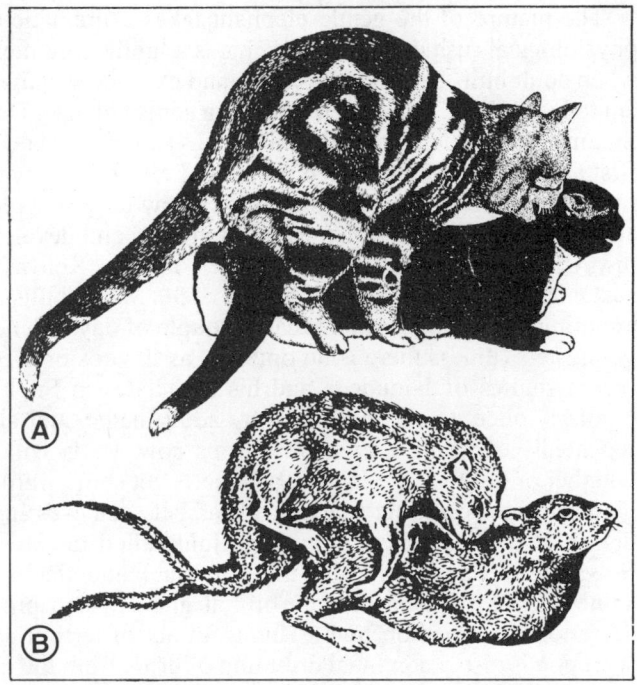

Fig. 6.34. Female cat & Female rat showing a characteristic posture called "lordosis" during mating.

female for a few second before he dismounts. A complete group of intromissions ending with an ejaculation is termed a "series". Ejaculation and the associated sperm transfer never occurs without prior intromissions (Fig. 6.34).

Ejaculation is followed by a temporary cessation of sexual activity. After a lapse of about 5 minutes, mating activity again resumes and a second series occurs. Usually rats perform about seven ejaculatory series before they attain satiation.

ELEPHANT

Naturalists such as Dr. Joyce Poole (who has been in Kenya for over the last two decades) and Dr. R. Sukumar of the Indian Institute of science, Bangalore, have made elephants their special subject of study. Rob Stotow and Gus Van Dyte studied in detail the courtship and mating patterns of elephants. These pachyderms do not go about mating with brutish behaviour. It is rather a courtship of affection, tenderness, joy and playfullness. The "bull" and "cow" elephants pair up well before the cow becomes oestrous, and stand apart from the herd.

They walk and graze together, stroke each other and entwine their trunks into a double helix, nudge each other teasingly – a picture of romantic engagement before mating. Bull elephants are tender lovers. The mating act itself is over in no more than ten seconds but the foreplay and after play last for many-many minutes.

Rivalry between suitor males is also a stylized affair, a trial of strength by locking forehead to forehead, and the defeated bull elephant quietly bows off. The female for whom they are competing waits grazing near by. She walks off with the winner.

The picture of the gentle elephant takes a dramatic turn when the male elephant experiences the physiological rush called *musth*. This is a hindi word meaning elation, rapture, intoxication. It is a time when adult bulls become aggressive and extremely dangerous. Even tamed elephants become disobedient to his mahout. It has been studied in some detail by Dr. Joyce Poole in African elephants, and by Dr. Sukumar in the elephants of south India. It appears related to the coming of age or adulthood, coming on first around the age of 15. It is an annual event or many occur even as many as three times a year. This rutting behaviour may last as short as a few days or as long as several months at a time. The duration and severity of *musth* varies with individuals and develops progressively with age. Dr. Poole, studying the African elephants in the Amboseli Park in Kenya, found that the males there enter a period of sustained *musth* only beyond the age of 30. While bulls as young as 15 may start *musth*, the symptoms are minimal, lasting no more than a couple of days. Generally females do not prefer to mate with these youngsters (unless there is no option – as in zoos or breeding stations), but go for the older ones. The recent studies of Jainudeen and his associates in Sri Lanka have shown that *"musth"* occurs fairly regularly once a year in all healthy adult males, and although it may be brought on prematurely by repeatedly exposing a bull to oestrous cow. Bulls will mate at any time of the year, irrespective of whether or not they are in *musth*. Experts get some warning of impending *musth*, because the temporal glands located on either side of his head between eyes and the ear, starts to swell. Eventually it begins to discharge a strong-smelling watery fluid called the *musth fluid* down the side of the face. This fluid flows on for days, and stains the skin black and smells like coaltar. As it dries up and crystallizes, it shines. Male elephant bear an orbital gland which produce a copious secretion during musth. This secretion is rubbed on trees. This is an act of territorial marking. Accompanying the temporal gland secretion is also a continual dribbling of urine from the tip of the penis. The composition of the urine is yet to be fully analysed, as also the significance of such a great loss of water from an animal which spends most of its time seeking water sources. It is very likely that, like the *musth fluid,* the *musth urine* also contains substances that signal potential mates (invitation) as well as potential competitors (warning to bull elephant not to enter his territory).

It is fact that *"musth"* is associated with an enormous increase in the blood testosterone level which may account for the aggressive behaviour, but there is little information about the behavioural significance of *"musth"* in elephants in the wild state. African elephants, which in many ways are so similar to their Asiatic cousins, do not show *"musth"* & their temporal glands secrete copiously irrespective of age, sex or season.

Male and female elephant herd are separate. Male herd walk away from female herd. Catti Payan discovered that female elephant call male *musth* elephant through *infrasonic sound signals* during breeding season. O'Cannel Rodwell observed that seismic signals play a role in elephant reproduction. Elephants send out seismic signals to potential mates far away. High ranking males leave the herd and compete for oestrous females. Only one male from any one bull groups is in

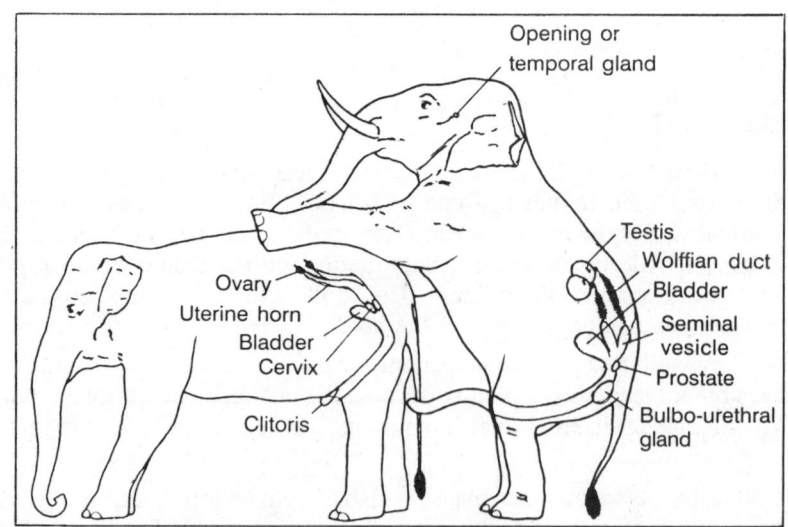

Fig. 6.35. Mating Posture of Asiatic Elephant.

musth at any one time so that direct sexual competition occurs between *musth* males from different herds. The highest ranking male elephant mates with the oestrous female. Elephant pair copulate back to back (Fig. 6.35).

CETACEA

Ethologists have also taken strain to observe the courtship behaviour of large marine mammals belonging to order cetacea. Courtship in bottle-nozed dolphins entails vocalization, kissing the partner, licking and nuzzling of the partner's genitalia, rubbing of bodies, stroking with flippers, displaying of white underside, leaping, chasing and head butting. The females then choose a male partner and rest of the males are disappointed. Here male dolphins do all acts like a typical hindi movie hero and female selects a mate on the line of ancient Indian *Swayambara*. The spectacular ballet of dolphins was studied by Puente and Dewsbury (1976). Unfortunately, observation of mating displays of the aquatic and nocturnal habits of most mammals is extremely difficult. It is for this reason that such behaviour has been more studied in terrestrial mammals.

PRIMATES

Courtship and mating behaviour of primates is something different than non-primates. The female primates differs from the females of other mammals by not showing a sharply circumscribed period of heat during the reproductive cycle. Although monogamy is not common among mammals, it does occur in more than 14 primate species (Clutton Brock and Harvey, 1977). Courtship among primates can be marked easily. Both female and male may show many postures of appeasement. Kissing is one of the most frequent behavioural exchanges between courting human. Opposite sex involve close physical contact and sexual stimulation. The display of the erect penis/vulva are common act in primates.

Phallic displays are very common among male primates. Squirrel monkeys threaten one another by displaying erect penis. Sentry males of monkeys and baboons often sit with their legs open and have partial erection. When an intruder approaches, the penis of sentry becomes fully erect and often bobs up and down as, a gesture of threat. In many cases, the genitals of these animals are of a different colour from the rest of the body and this contrast increases the conspicuousness of phallic display. Male Mandril baboons have red, blue and yellow genitals, and male Vervet monkey have red, white and blue genitalia.

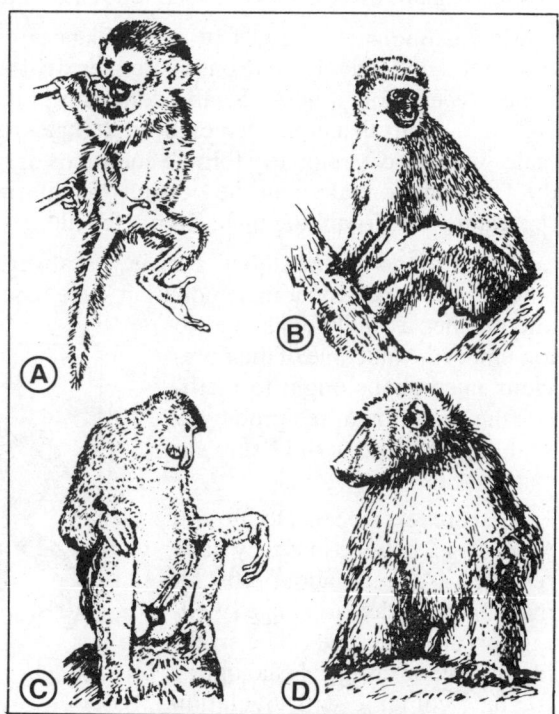

Fig. 6.36. Genital display of male Primates : (A) Squirrel monkey (*Saimiri*); (B) Velvet monkey (*Ceropithecus*); (C) Proboscis monkey (*Nosalis*); and (D) Baboons (*Papio*).

MONKEY

A dominant male monkey is more able than a subordinate one to mate with an attractive female. A female monkey may form a sexual consortship with a dominant male and she then becomes his equivalent in rank, but only for as long as their partnership endures.

BABOON

In baboons there are several paths to sexual success in addition to securing high male status. Males can and do develop "friendships" with particular female, relationships that do

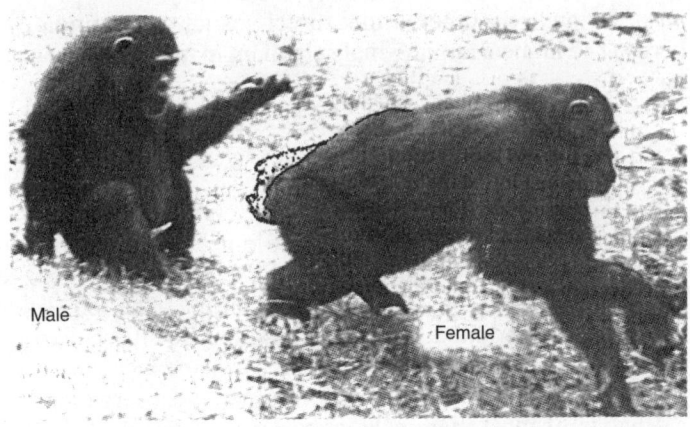

Fig. 6.37. Sexually aroused female chimpanzee greet male chimpanzee by exhibiting her swollen genital area.

not depend on physical dominance but rather on the willingness of a male to protect a given female's offspring - even if the younger is not his own. Once a male has demonstrated that he is willing and able to provide protection for a female and her infant, that female may seek him out when she enters into oestrous again, even if he is not the top male in the social hierarchy of her troop.

Male baboons also regularly form alliances with other males. Through these friendship, they can sometimes collectively confront a stronger rival that has acquired a partner, forcing him to give up the female, even though he is socially dominant in one-on-one encounters. Noe found that in one band of yellow baboons that contained eight adult males, three low-ranking individuals - fifth to seventh-ranked males in hierarchy regularly formed coalitions of two or three males to defeat single high-ranking males, the fifth-ranked male won the oestrous female in 17 or 18 cases in which the partners succeeded in separating a high-ranking male from a female.

Packer found that a "stolen" female was always claimed by the male that has solicited the support of a helper. He argued that male coalition were based on reciprocity. The ability of baboons to recognise one another as individuals and to remember the outcome of their previous interactions ought to facilitate the evolution of reciprocity by enabling males to avoid being socially ahead.

Researchers, Leah Domb and Mark Pagel believe that they have resolved a dispute about why female baboons develop huge swellings on their rear ends. The swellings have long intrigued ethologists, for they coincide with ovulation and are a clear signal to male baboons about the female's fertility. But what the signal exactly is has been strongly debated. For some

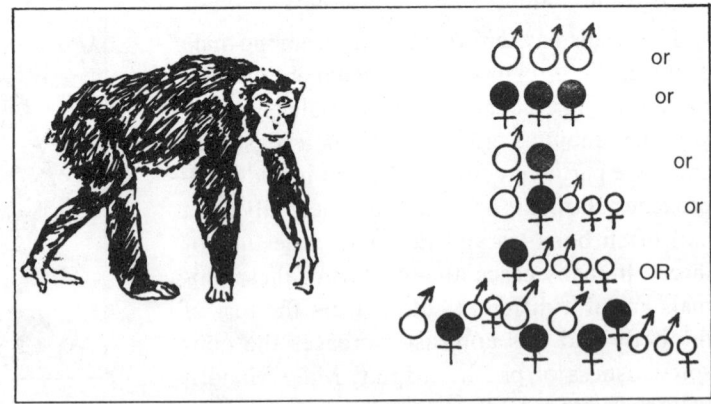

Fig. 6.38. Chimpanzees form temporary groups having all males, all females, adult females and their infants or combination of males and females.

ethologists, the swellings are intented to attract males to join groups of females and their young to provide a defence against predators. For others, the swellings aim at provoking males into a competitive frenzy, enabling the female to stop the strongest one and select him for her mate. But Leah Domb and Mark Pagel are, convinced that the swellings in fact are a sign of the female's genetic potential.

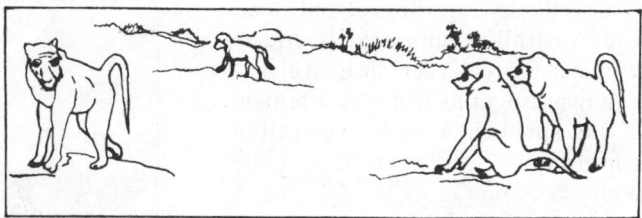

Fig. 6.39. A baboon Coalition. The two males on the right have formed an alliance to defeat the male on the left in dispute over possession of an oestrous female. Only one of the two males will copulate with the female. According to Packer male coalition is based on reciprocity.

BONOBO

Bonobo's sex life is richer than prosaic couplings of chimpanzees and gorillas. Bonobo females remain in oestrous for most of their 46 - day cycle, signalled by their swollen pink rumps, and were eager to mate almost all the time. Chimpanzee females, in contrast, were interested in sex for only ten days each monthly cycle.

Bonobos frequently mate in the face-to-face position, whereas chimpanzees almost exclusively mate in the belly-to-back positions.

A Japanese researcher Kano (1972) observed that whenever tension arose among the bonobos they calmed each other with sex in a variety of postures. They are truly the great apes that make love, not war. In any event, bonobos are promiscuous, like chimpanzees. Each ape mates with many partners and Kano even saw young females soliciting juicy sugar cane stalks from adult males, offering sex in return. The bonobos have at least 20 mating gestures and call, such as feverish hooting, the displaying of their bodily charms and the proffering of food.

De Weall once observed a young bonobo female approach a male who held an orange in each hand and offer to mate with him, when they finished, she took one of oranges and walked away.

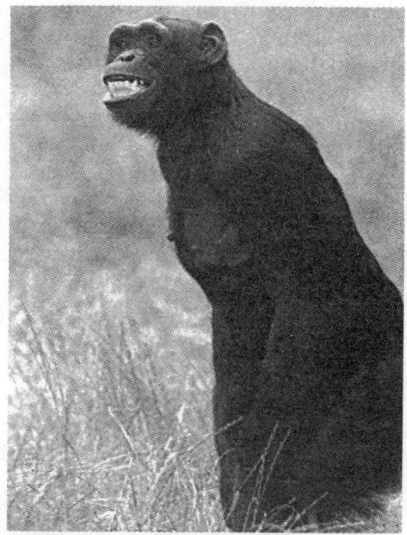

Fig. 6.40. Bonobo (A pygmy chimpanzee) have at least 20 mating gestures and calls.

INDISCRIMINATE SEXUAL BEHAVIOUR OF MALES

When the sexes differ in their potential reproductive rate, one sex will become a scarce commodity for the other. Since female have a lower potential rate of reproduction, which will be limited by the time required to secure resources for production of large gametes. As a result, there will be fewer receptive female than sexually active male at any one time leading to competition among males while providing the opportunity for females to choose among potential males. This situation sometimes creates indiscriminate sexual behaviour of males. For example, male elephant seals are so eager to copulate that they will readily pursue an artificial model female (Fig. 6.41).

Copulatory eagerness of male toad and Australian buprestid beetle is shown in Fig. 6.42. A male toad clasps a human finger as if it was a female of his species. A male Australian buprestid beetle attempts to copulate with a beer bottle.

INFANTICIDE

Killing of own progeny by male is a routine matter of some mammalian species. Many cases of infanticide by males in mammals and birds is reported. The act occurs under thoroughly 'natural' conditions. For example infanticide in lions predictably occurs when a male lion successfully takes over a harem of female. The incoming male hunt down cubs and try to kill them, although lioness tries her best to protect her cubs. Lioness unable to prevent infanticide resume sexual cycling and mate with the killer of their offspring. Since a male can expect to remain in a pride and have

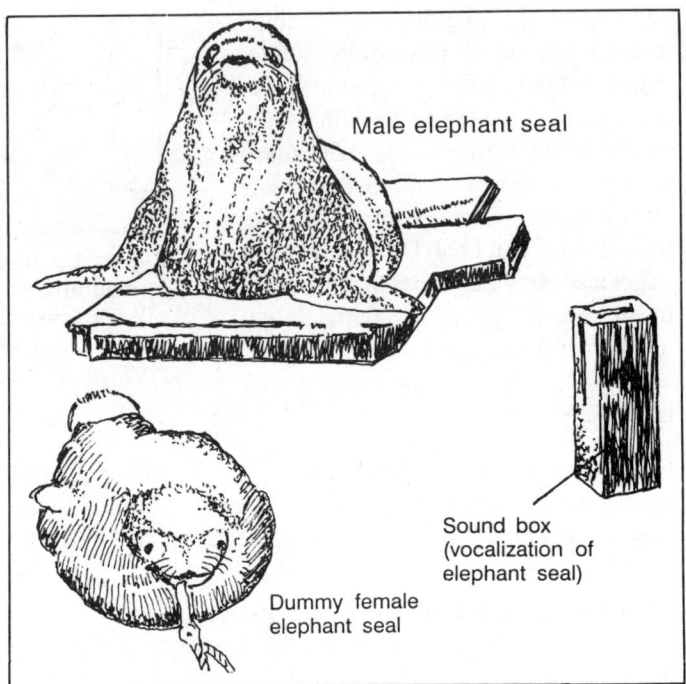

Fig. 6.41. Male copulatory eagerness in elephant seal. A dummy female elephant seal attract a male of her species.

access to its females for just 2 years on average, the reproductive benefits of infanticide from the male's perspective are evident. It may not be surprising, therefore, that male lions are responsible for about a quarter of all the deaths of cubs in at least some populations. Like lions, cats and langurs also commit infanticide frequently under natural conditions.

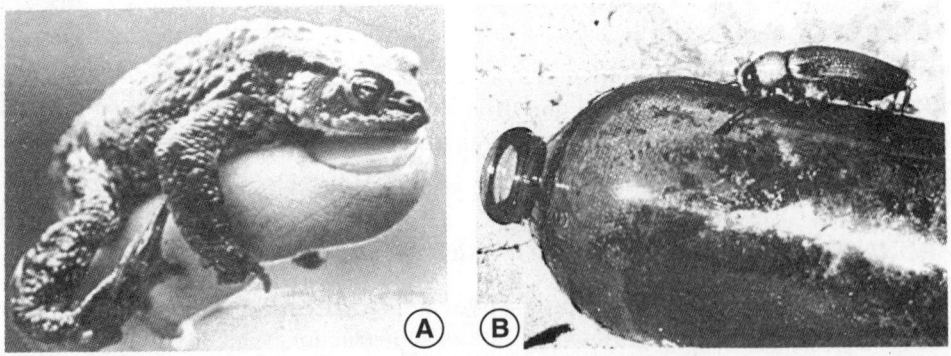

Fig. 6.42. Indiscriminate sexual behaviour of males. (A) male toad clasps a human finger as if it were a female of his species. (B) A male Australian buprestid beetle, attempts to copulate with a beer bottle.

Infanticide is due to sexual competition. This hypothesis gains additional support from some experimental studies of birds, including one involving jacanas. In these water birds, the typical sex roles are reversed, with female defending "har-ems" of males that care for their off-spring. Emlen and Demong arranged to have some females experimentally removed, freeing their several mates for take over by neighbouring females. These neighbours did move into the vacated territories and, in three or four cases, killed the baby jacanas. Within 48 hours the males that had lost their offspring were involved in sexual re-lation with the infanticidal females. By committing infanticide, these females had gained caretakers for their future clutches of eggs sooner than if they had waited for the males to finish rear-ing their current broods.

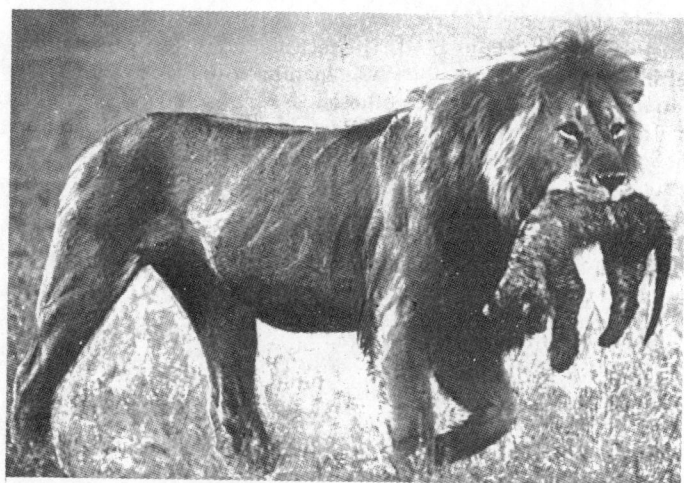

Fig. 6.43. Infanticide by a male lion.

Among hanuman langur (*Presbytis entellus*) strange males may take over a group, driving out the resident male. The new male may then kill the young sired by the previous male (Hrdy, 1977). Females who have lost their young soon become sexually receptive, and the new resident male can inseminate them. Infanticide by adult males thus may be viewed as a "remator male" adaptation.

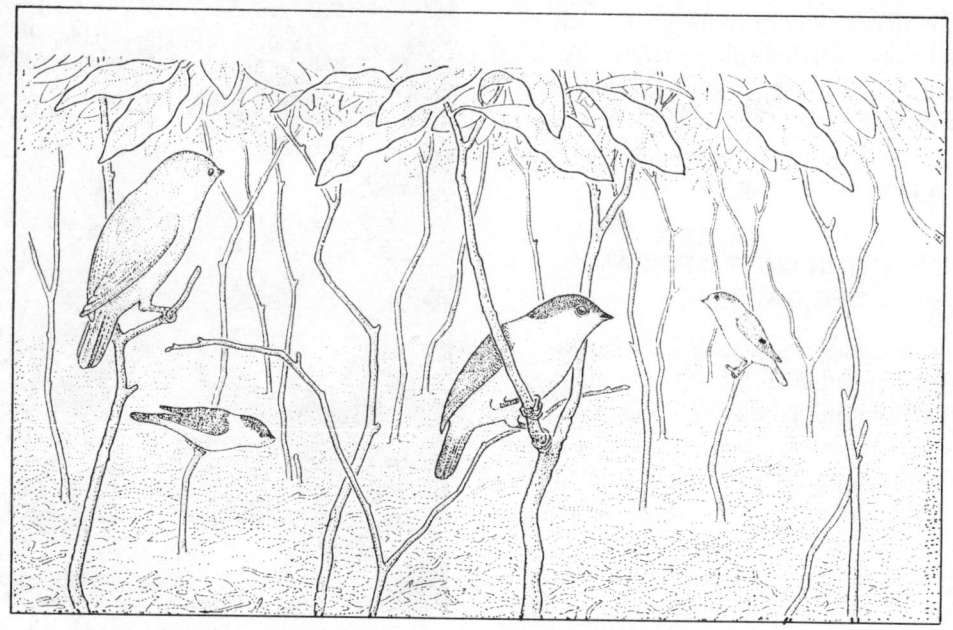

Fig. 6.44. Lek polygyny in the white-beared Manakins. Males defend tiny territory. A female visits the lek to select a mate from among the several males present.

LEK POLYGYNY

Lek polygyny is a kind of mating system exhibited by polygynous males. Males own a very small territory. Territory contain no clusture of mates nor any resource of value to potential mates. Females visit these "symbolic" territories (traditional display area or lek) just to select a mate ; after copulation, the female departs and may never see the male again.

LEK POLYGYNY IN BIRDS

Lek polygyny is found in the white-bearded manakin. Each male's territory consists only of a tree or two in the forest and a bare patch of ground underneath the perch site, which the bird clears of leaves and debris to make a display court ; the site contains nothing of value to the female. There may be as many as 70 display courts in an area only 150 to 200 meter square. The male begins his display routine with a series of rapid jumps between perches, loudly snapping his club like wing feathers together in flight. The male then pauses with body tensed before jumping to the ground with a snap and immediately back to the perch with a buzz, and then back and forth "so fast he seems to be bouncing and exploding like a firecracker."

The arrival of a female at the lek delights males to display, courtship behaviour. They produce an uproar. If the female is receptive and chooses a partner, she will fly to his perch for a series of mutual displays, followed by copulation.

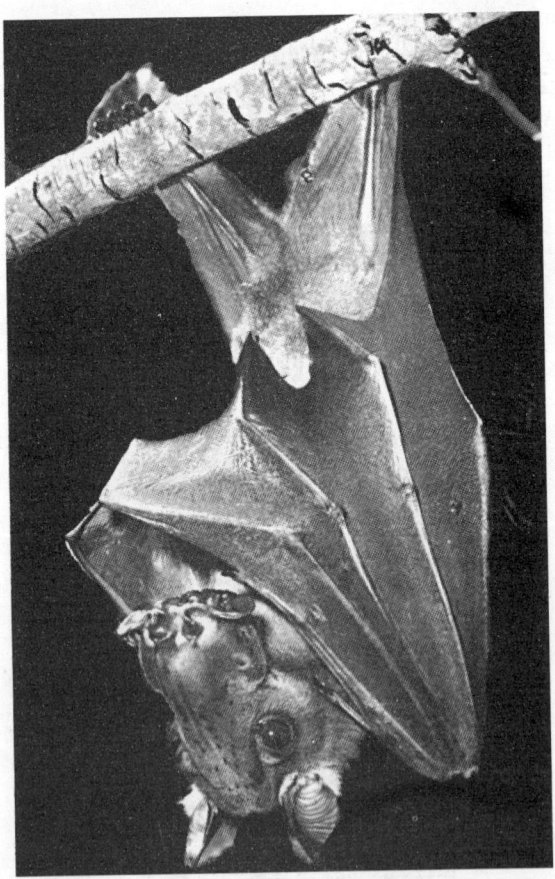

LEK POLYGYNY IN FALLOW DEER

Male fallow deer gather in areas where each male establishes a small display territory. Females visit the lek, inspect males, select a partner, mate with the selected male and leave. Females choose certain dominant males much more often than subordinates.

LEK POLYGYNY IN WEST AFRICAN HAMMER HEADED BAT

During the breeding season, males of hammer headed bat gather in the evening along river edges at traditional display areas. Each bat defends a territory that is 10 meters in diameter while he hangs from a perch high in the tree. Males produce loud sound. Receptive females fly to the lek and visit several males, each of which responds with a violent expression of wings-flapping displays and vocalization. Only about 6% males at one lek are successful for 80% of all matings.

Fig. 6.45. Hammer headed bat of West Africa exhibit lek polygyny.

EXERCISE

1. Define and explain sexual behaviour in animals.
2. What do you mean by sexual selection, Describe in 200 lines about intersexual and intersexual selection.
3. What do you mean by breeding season ? How season help in inducing sexual behaviour.
4. What do you mean by territory and aggression ? Describe territory and aggression in some mammals and birds.
5. Define courtship. Describe some important courtship behaviour of birds.
6. Define mating. Describe some important courtship behaviour of primates.
7. Describe at least five significant courtship behaviours among birds.
8. Describe courtship and copulation behaviour among members of arthropoda with special reference of scorpion, spider, honeybee, dragonfly and fruitfly.
9. Describe territory and aggression behaviour among different mammals.
10. Define mating. Describe mating behaviour in some mammals.
11. Courtship diffuses aggressiveness among many animals. Explain it with suitable examples.
12. Describe courtship and reproduction in palolo worm and Nereis.
13. Describe mating strategies of marine isopod (*Paracerceis sculpta*) and scorpion.
14. What do you mean by co-operative courtship. Describe it taking the case of long-tailed mannakin (a bird of central America).
15. What do you mean by Infanticide ? Describe this in context of some bird and mammalian species.
16. Define Lek polygyny. Describe Lek polygyny in white-beared Manakins, fallow dear, and West African hammer headed bat.
17. Describe indirect method of transfer of sperm by insects into genital tract of females.
18. What do you mean by sperm competition ? Describe it giving suitable examples.
19. Define sex dimorphism. Describe sex dimorphism in vertebrate series giving suitable examples.
20. Describe Lesbianism in lizard, Co-oprative courtship, genitalia of hyena and indiscriminate sexual behaviour of sexually aroused male toad and Australian buprestid beetle.

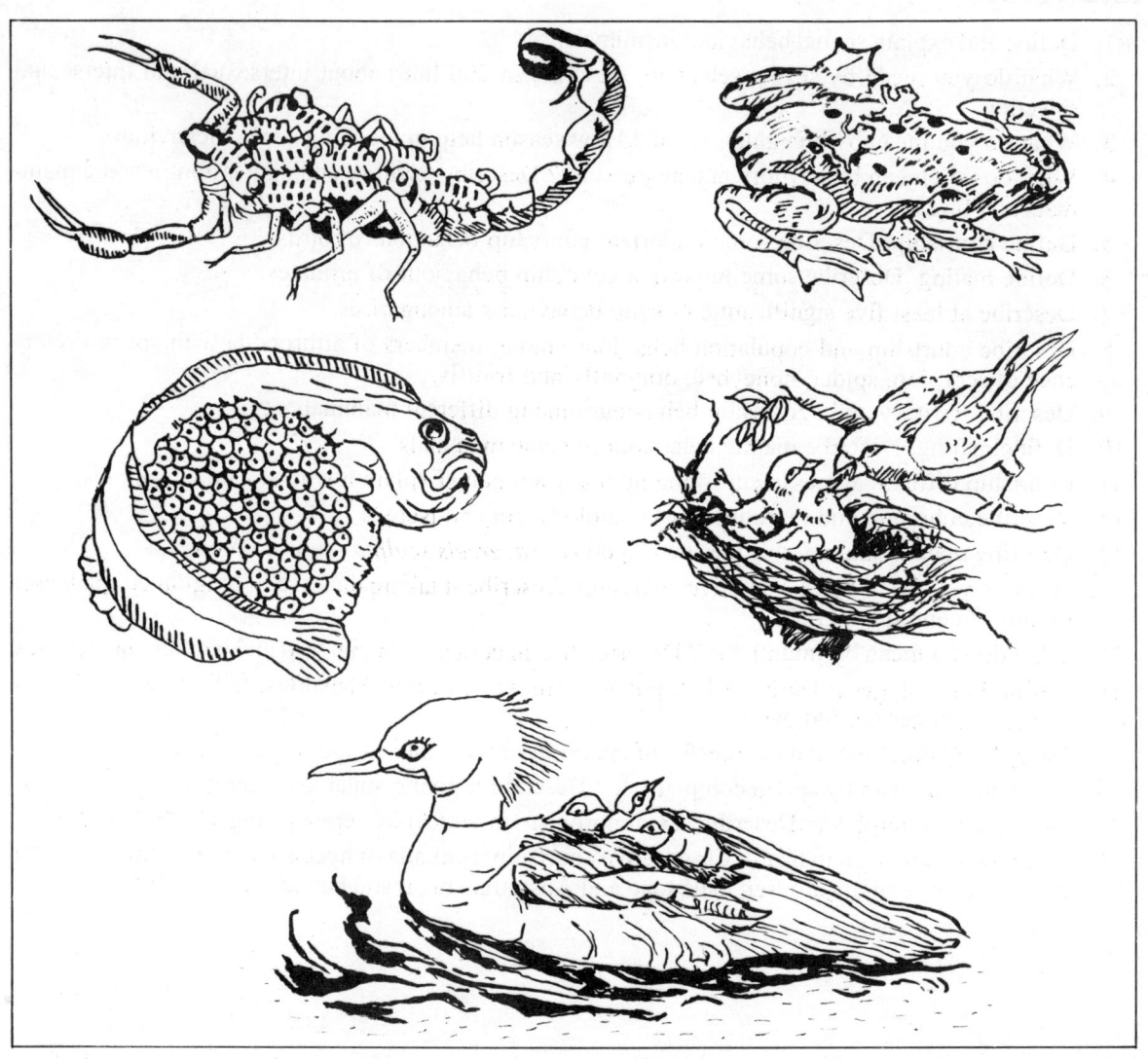

*W*hy birds sit on eggs? Why parents protect their children and feed them? The answer is "instinct of parental care force them to do so". Parental care occurs in many lower animals and almost all higher animals. Period of parental care in insects, fishes, amphibians, and reptiles is usually limited to protection of eggs and young by their parents. But the period and degree of parental care gradually increases in birds and mammals. In this chapter we shall examine different aspects of "Parental Care" in parental species specially arthropods, fishes, amphibians, reptiles, birds and mammals.

PARENTAL CARE 7

INTRODUCTION

Protection and care taken by parents to their offspring for successful continuation of race is known as parental care. Parental care is instinctive behaviour and it is species specific. Parental care is a form of altruism in which a parent contributes his or her genes in their offsprings and spend time and energy to secure survival of their broods at their own cost. The degree of parental care differs in different species. Evolution of parental care has occurred in different groups that balances minimum cost suffered by each parent during act of parental care and maximum protection to the brood for survival. To ensure maximum care to the brood, the different groups of animals have evolved "evolutionary stable strategy" that also guarantees maximum protection to the genes of parents.

The instinct of parental care is so strong that parents protect their offspring very aggressively. The aggression shown by parents to any stranger which attempts to their offspring has also been the subject of study. Such aggression can sometimes be extremely violent, even when the parent is quite small and is attacking a member of a larger species. The famous animal's photographer Eric Hosking was attacked fiercely on one occasion when trying to photograph some young birds of prey in their nest. The mother bird attacked him so fiercely that she blinded him in one eye. Even the female of the relatively small eared owl will not hesitate to attack a human being to protect her clutch.

In one of his books, Konrad Larenz tells a strange story about a case of animal savagery. A female shelduck walking along with her ducklings spotted its owner holding in his hands a tiny, freshly - hatched mallard duckling which was uttering distress calls. Leaving her own ducklings, she rushed towards the man and attacked him so courageously that he was forced to drop the mallard hatchling. A thing that happened after is even stranger. The young mallard mingled with the shelduck's offsprings and the female then attacked him so fiercely that he would have been killed on the spot if the owner had

185

not intervened in time. Naturally, Those watching this sequence of events, who has been admiring the female shelduck's initial response, were quite perplexed. What has happened? "The explanation of such apparently contradictory behaviour is quite simple, "writes Lorenz". The distress calls of the mallard hatchling are almost identical to those of a young shelduck and the defensive response of the female is therefore stimulated automatically. But the plumage of a young mallard is quite different from that of a shelduck, so it is identified as a stranger and this evokes another automatic aggressive response, that of protecting the clutch against the intruder. Thus, the young mallard which at one point was a lost infant in need of help an instant later become an intruder to be chased away.

Instinct of *parental care* is found in numerous species, but instinct of *parent's care* is not found in any species not even in humans. Our children take our care not by virtue of instinct but due to social learning and high grade of reasoning. Other factors such as long association with parents, imprinting, feeling of obligation, transmission of cultural learning etc. force them to take care of their parents.

PARENTAL CARE IN ANIMALS WITHOUT BACKBONES

It is unfortunate that ethologists have shown more interest in studying parental care of animals with backbones than animals without backbones. However, some information about parental care in animals without backbones is given below.

GIANT WATER BUGS

Female of large aquatic water bug, *Lethocerus medius*, lay their large, mottled eggs on branches of plants well out of the water. Males leave the water to perch over them (Fig. 7.1A).

After mating female giant water bugs donate sequential clutches of eggs to several different parental males. Male giant water bugs participating in mating show more curiosity in receiving eggs from his partner and permits his mate to glue her eggs on his back. The male bug will carry eggs till they hatch. If one female cannot use up the male's breeding space, he will accept additional eggs from other females (Fig 7.1B).

BEETLE

Ladybird beetle (*Harmonia axyridis*) is a small beetle. The colour of this beetle is bright and the body bear dots and hence called lady. Since it can fly called bird. This beetle is great friend of farmers because they eat up pests of corn, cotton and citrus plants. Ladybird lay their eggs inside

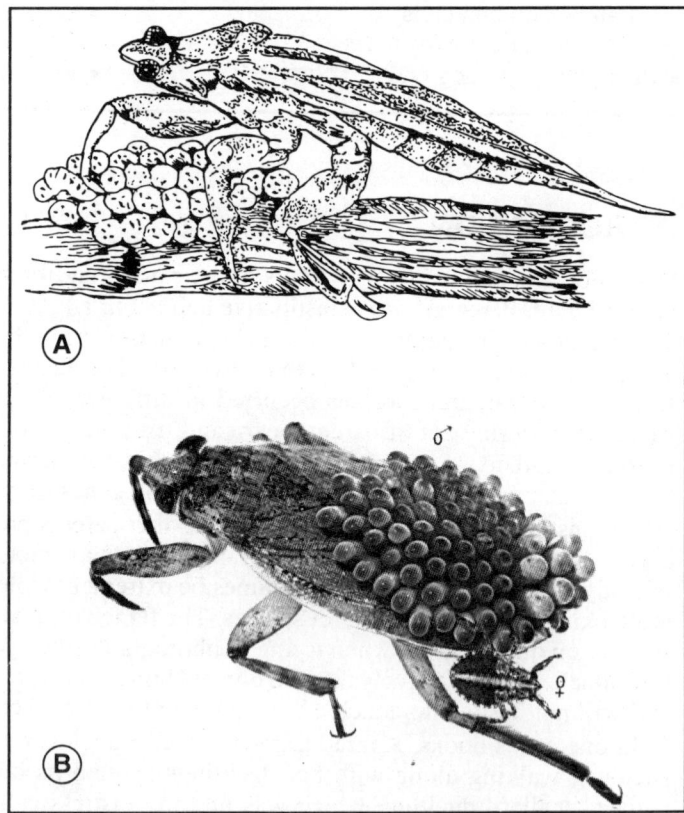

Fig. 7.1. (A) Female of large aquatic water bug, *Lethocerus medius* arranging her eggs on the branch of a plant. (B) Male water bugs carrying eggs, glued on their backs by his female partner.

the leaves of host plants and before leaving the place, keep there a lot of insects. Young beetles emerging from eggs eat up insects provided by their parents (Fig. 7.2A).

Males of certain species of burying beetles regularly cooperate with a female in burying a dead mouse of other small animal and constructing a "brood ball" of flesh. The beetles treat the dead and decaying flesh with chemical secretions in order to hide the material by other consumers. The female lays a clutch of eggs near the brood ball, and when the larvae hatch out they move onto the treated flesh. There they are fed flesh taken from the dead body by the female and sometimes by a parental male if he has remained with his mate (Fig. 7.2B and C).

Dung contains volatile substances. Dung beetles quickly take to the air when they smell far off faeces and fly zigzagging up the odour trail to them. A male and female beetle cooperate in rolling away a ball of dung. The female lay an egg on the dung ball after the pair have buried it underground. The resulting grub will feed on the food kept by their parents (Fig. 7.3).

WASP

Female great golden digger wasps (*Sphex ichneumoneus*) lay their eggs in under ground burrows that they have provisioned with katydids (long-horned grass hoppers) as food for the larvae. Jane Brockmann and Dawkins, (1979)

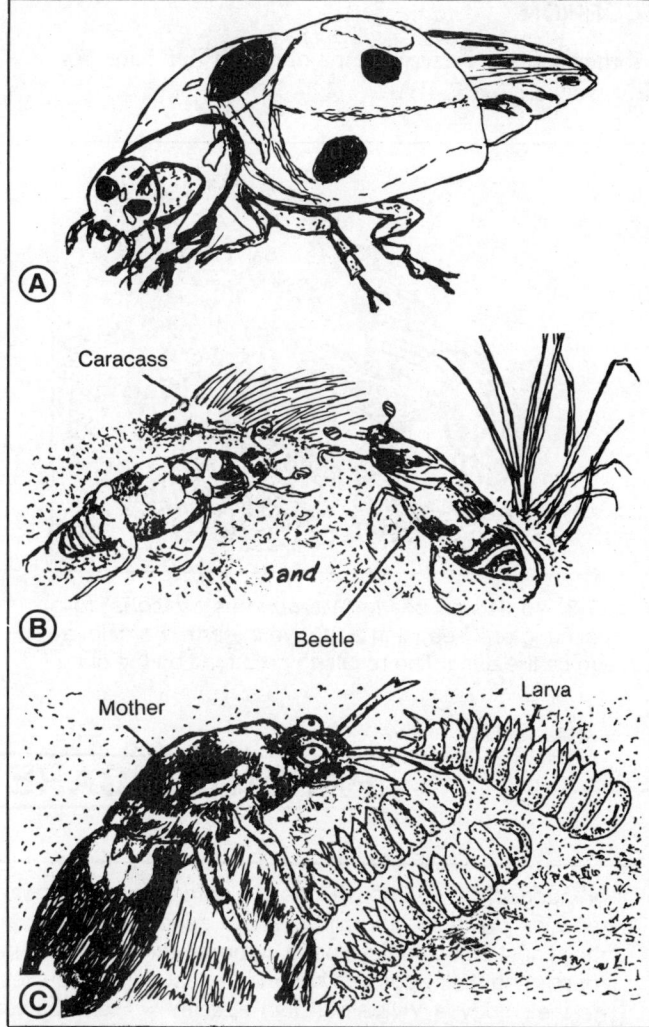

Fig. 7.2. (A) Ladybird beetle lay eggs inside the leaves of host plant and provide lots of insects for young beetles. (B) Burying beetle, *Dendroctonus pseudotsugae*, recycles a dead mouse or other small animals by laying eggs near its body. (C) Mother beetle then feeding larvae bits of regurgitated caracass.

studied the parental care behaviour of female wasp in detail. They studied the nest-related activities of 68 individually colour marked female at three different fields sites over a total of six breeding seasons. They observed that the female obtain a burrow either by digging or by entering on already dug burrow. She then provisions it with paralyzed katydids, lays a single egg, and seals up the burrow prior to starting the cycle again. There is 5 to 15 percent chance that her burrow will be entered by another female wasp, who also provisions the burrow. Both wasps will be engaged fully in provisioning the same burrow and will not have another burrow open at the same time. Because both wasps spend most of their time hunting, it may be some time before they meet. When they do meet they fight and one wasp is usually driven away. Only one wasp eventually lays an egg in the brood chamber (Fig. 7.4A).

SCORPION

Mother scorpion carry their young on her back for few weeks.(Fig. 7.4B).

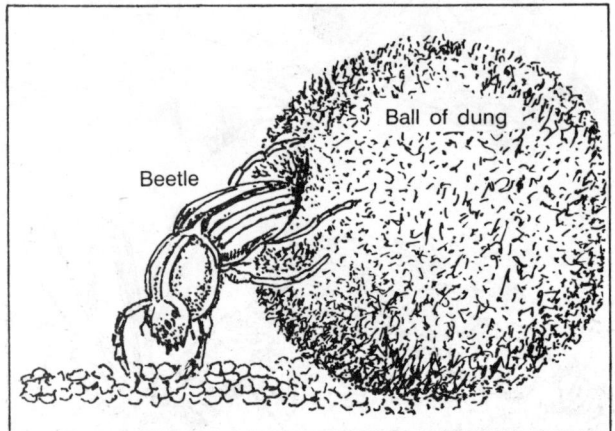

Fig. 7.3. An African beetle (*Nicrophorus orbicollis*) rolls animal dung and keep it in a groove in earth. Female lay an egg on the dung. The resulting grub feed on the dung.

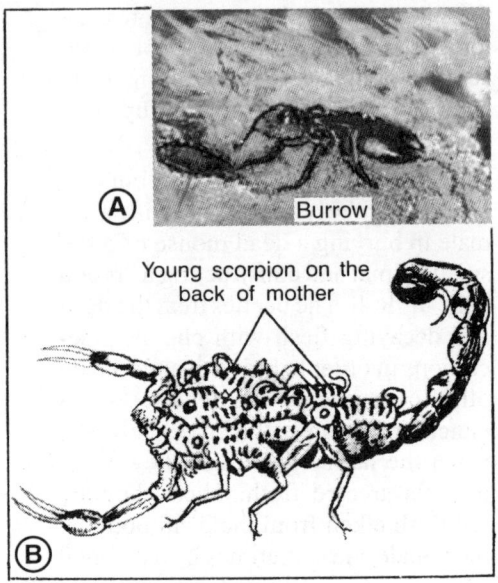

Fig. 7.4. (A) A female digger wasp, (*Sphex ichneumoneus*) at the entrance to its burrow. (b) A mother scorpion carrying her young ones.

PARENTAL CARE IN FISHES

• Introduction • Various kinds of Parental care in fishes • Various methods of Parental care • Fish species which do not build nest but deposit their eggs in safe places • Fish species which do not build nest but have developed some design of depositing their eggs in suitable forms • Fish species depositing their eggs into self-made nest • Fish species keeping their eggs and young both or one in their body • Viviparous fish species • Fish species taking care of independently swimming young ones.

INTRODUCTION

Most species of fish do not take care of their eggs and fingerlings. The fish species lacking parental care behaviour is compensated by the production of great number of eggs. For a fish egg, the odds against survival can be as high as a million to one. That is why some fish lay over 300 million eggs at a time. Marine fishes rely simply on safety in groups. Many marine fish species lay planktonic eggs which float near the surface of the sea. The cod fish whose eggs are scattered at random in the open sea produces over nine million eggs. The carp lays two to four million eggs at random in fresh water and in the neighbourhood of vegetation.

Some species of fish produce limited number of eggs and have evolved various grades of parental care behaviour from random spawning to internal fertilization, from oviparity to viviparity; and from the deposition of large number of uncared eggs to the protection of young. Thus fishes have developed various methods to ensure proper protection of the eggs and young ones by one or both partners.

VARIOUS METHODS OF PARENTAL CARE IN FISHES

   I. Fish species which do not build nest but have developed some design of depositing their eggs in suitable places or suitable forms.
  II. Fish species depositing their eggs into self made nest.
 III. Fish species keeping their eggs and young ones in and on their body.
 IV. Viviparous fish species.
  V. Fish species which take care of independently swimming young ones.

Various grades of Parental care in fishes is described here one by one.

I. FISH SPECIES WHICH DO NOT BUILD NEST BUT HAVE DEVELOPED SOME DESIGN OF DEPOSITING THEIR EGGS IN SUITABLE PLACES

There are many species of fishes which do not build nest but have developed some very interesting design of depositing their eggs in suitable forms in order to insure proper protection to their eggs.

1. Scattering eggs over aquatic plants

In some fishes (*Pikes- Esox lucius; Carps- Eyprinus carpio, Carrassius auratus*) eggs are layed usually over aquatic plants to which they remain attached.

2. Laying of eggs at suitable places

Salmo solar, Acipenser, Oncorhynchus etc. lay their eggs in suitable spawning grounds. These fishes exhibit anadromaus migration for depositing eggs at suitable places. The sand gobi *Pomatoschistos minutus* lays its eggs in some protected area where they are guarded by the male who also aerates eggs by movement.

3. Depositing eggs in sticky covering

Yellow perch (*Perca flavescens*) deposit their eggs in single mass in hollow rope like structure. The eggs are held together by membrane and form long floating bands (Fig. 7.5 i a). In many cyprinids (carps etc.) eggs are usually laid with some special sticky covering by means of which they are attached to each other and to the bottom of stones, weeds etc.

Similarly the eggs of the Anglar fish (*Lophius*) are invested by a gelatinous outer coat and remain together to form a transparent mass of enormous size (Fig. 7.5 ib). The Lumpsucker (*Cyclopterus*) deposit their eggs in the form of spawn in the cervices of rocks above the level of the water at spring tides. One spawn may contain even more than one million eggs. Time to time Cyclopterus presses her head into the spawn insuring proper aeration of eggs.

Skippers, garfishes and flying fishes secrete a sticky thread from their kidney. Eggs remain attached with sticky thread. One end of the thread adhere with any aquatic substratum while the other end of the thread remain free [Fig. 7.5 (ii)].

4. Deposition of eggs in dead shells of mussels and oysters

Some fishes such as members of cyprinid family deposit their eggs in the dead shells of mussels and oysters.

Eggs of Bitterling (*Rhodeus*) are deposited in the mantle cavity of fresh water musels by the female whose oviduct is drawn out in the form of a long tube acting as an ovipositor. After oviposition male *Rhodeus* fertilizes the eggs and guard them. Here one thing is very interesting to note that the male *Rhodeus* is sexually excited not by the presence of female of its own species but by the sight of the shell of the mussel in which the eggs have been deposited. According to Canningham it is an interesting case of *adaptation of sexual instinct* [Fig. 7.5 (iii) & (iv)]

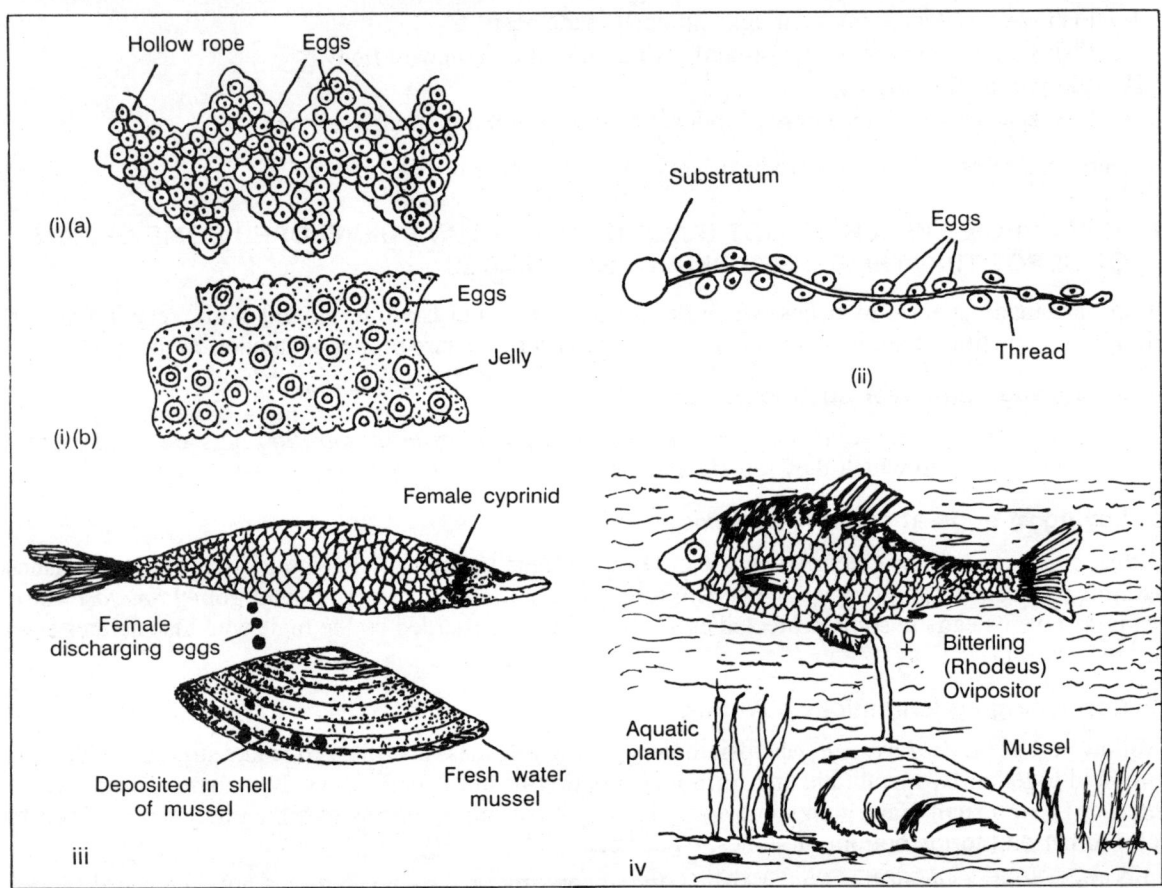

Fig. 7.5. Fish species depositing their eggs in safe places, (ia) Yellow perch fish deposit their eggs in a rope like structure. (ib) Eggs of Anglar fish deposited in a gelatinous outer coat. (ii) Skippers, garfishes and flying fishes secrete a sticky thread from their kidney. Eggs remain attached with this thread. (iii) & (iv) Female Cyprinid and bitterling (*Rhodeus*) deposit their eggs in dead shells of mussels and oyster respectively.

II. FISH SPECIES DEPOSITING THEIR EGGS INTO SELF MADE NEST

Parental care in a few fishes is performed by the formation of different types of nests for the safe deposition and protection of eggs. The nest provide suitable and safe place for the development of their young ones. In the formation of nests only male or both sexes participate. For the formation of nest they use various kinds of materials such as pebbles, aquatic vegetation, secretion of their body etc. Various kinds of nests build by different species of fishes are as follows :

1. Basin Like nests

During spawning season the male Darter (*Etheostoma congregate*) selects a suitable place called domain, repelling with vigour any attempt by rival male to dispute its claim. Any female Darter entering the territory is allowed to remain there. Now female Darter makes a basin like depression for releasing eggs. She sinks in basin like nest where eggs are deposited. The eggs are promptly fertilized by the males and are being covered by the sticky secretion secreted by the kidneys of the male fish. These sticky eggs remain attached to the stone till hatching (Fig. 7.6 i).

Fresh water sun fishes (belonging to family-Contrachidae) scoop out a shallow basin like nest at the bottom of the water. Pebbles are carefully removed leaving behind the large stones. A layer of fine sand of gravel remain attached with the eggs. Male Sun fish guard the eggs till the hatching of the young. Many Cichlid fishes (*Haplochromis burtoni*) build basin like nest, where both parents take up the task of guarding eggs. In some species of North American catfishes (belonging to family-Amiuridae) both male and female prepare a crude nest in the mud for egg laying. American cyprinids (*Chubs* and *Shoiners*) make a nest composed of large heaps of stones but the eggs are left uncared. African osteoglossids usually make nest by cleaning the space among vegetation and lay their eggs.

Bluegill sunfishes become social during the breeding season. Groups of 50 to 100 males build their nests depressions in a sandy lake bottom–side by side.

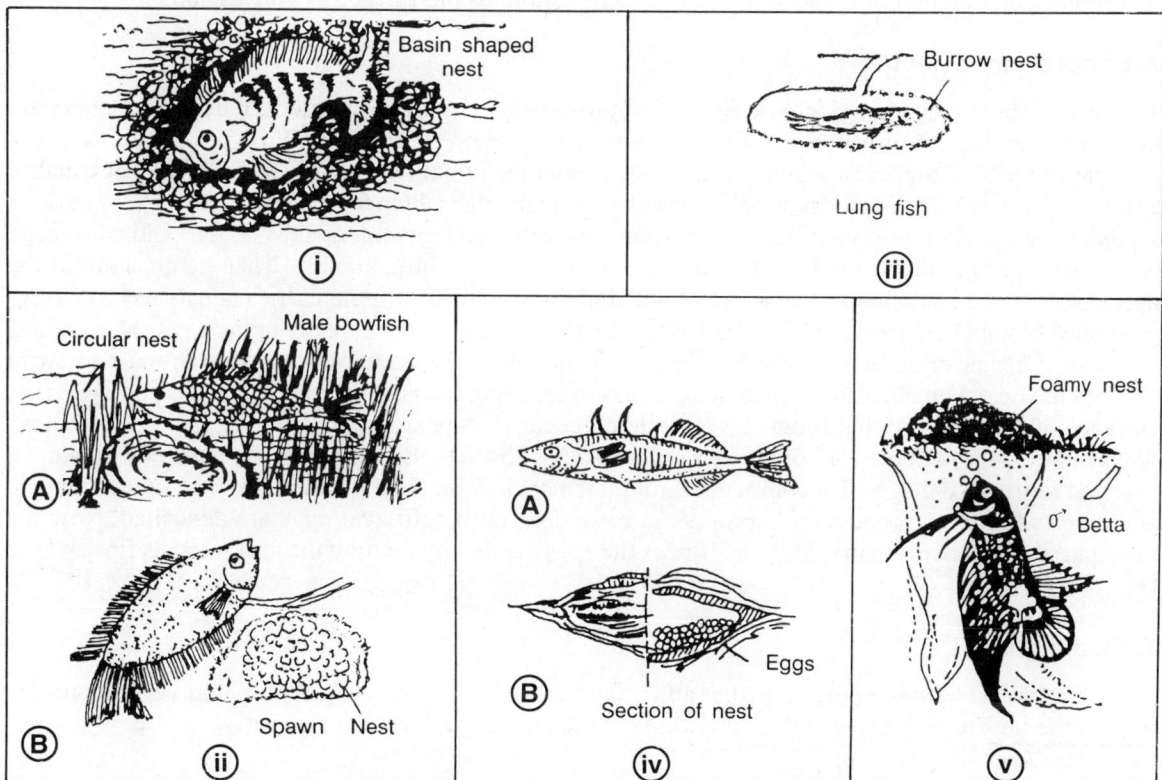

Fig. 7.6. Fishes species depositing their eggs in self made nest. (i) Basin like nest of Darter fish; (ii A) Circular nest of *Amia calva*; (ii B) Circular nest of Siamese fighting fish; (iii) Barrel shaped nest of Lung fish–Protopterus; (iv A&B) Barrel shaped nest of three-spined stickle back fish. (v) Foamy nest made by male fighting fish Betta.

2. Circular nest

Male bow fish (*Amia calva*) construct a crude circular nest at the end of the lake using aquatic vegetation (Fig. 7.6 ii A). One or more females attend the nest to lay her eggs. The male fertilizes and guards the eggs till hatching. The young leave the nest under the protection of father. Male Siamese fighting fish make similar kind of nest and defend its nest vigorously.

Both the partners of cat fishes of America (*Arius*) build a circular excavation at the bed of the river. The diameter of the nest is about 50 cm. The fertilized eggs are covered with large stones and are left uncared.

3. Hole or burrow nest

Lung fishes (*Protopterus, Neoceratodus* and *Lepidostren*) usually make nest in the mud of a swamp (water reservoir). Protopterus scoops out a hole in mud in swampy places along the river banks. The male *Protopterus* prepares the nest. Its nest is surrounded by long aquatic weeds and grasses. The male fish usually provide constant aeration to the eggs of nest by the movement of their fins. [Fig. 7.6 (iii)].

The nest of Lepidosiren is in the form of burrow in the bed of swamp varying in length from 1 to 2 meters. The nest consist of short vertical and much larger horizontal partition in which eggs are deposited. Males take care of eggs. During care of eggs male develops a long red filament from the pelvic fins, performing the function of aeration without coming out on to the surface to gulp the air.

4. Barrel shaped nest

The male "Three-spined stickleback fish" (*Gasterosteus aculeatus*) construct a much more elaborate nest. The construction of nest is completed before the initiation of courtship. First of all male selects a suitable site in shallow water where water flows continuously but not swiftly. Male stickleback makes a shallow pit in the sand, collects small pieces of weeds and glues them together with the help of a sticky secretion, secreted by its own kidneys. When the nest assumes a considerable size, it moulds the shape of a tunnel. For moulding the nest, the male passes through the nest forcibly. Then he goes out of the nest in search of a mate. Finding of a female with bulging abdomen stimulates the male to perform a zig-zag dance around her, displaying his red spot under side. If the female is ready to lay eggs she responds by curving her head and tail upwards. The signal shown by the female stimulates the male to swim towards the nest. Female also reaches to the nest. On reaching the nest the male stretches and opens the entrance of the nest with his snout. The female proceeds to deposit two or three eggs within the nest. She swims off through the wall of the nest on the side opposite to the entrance. The male enters into the nest and fertilizes the eggs. He comes out through the back door. Next day he seeks out another female and repeats the same process. This process is carried on until sufficient eggs are deposited. Now the male guards them persistently. Male fish keeps the eggs aerated by fanning the nest with his fins and tail [Fig. 7.6 (iv)].

5. Floating nest

The Mormyrids (*Gymnarchus*) construct a floating nest of large size using the aquatic vegetation. The wall of the nest remain projected several centimeters above the surface of water.

6. Foamy nest

The male fighting fish (Betta) and many other Labyrinth fishes belonging to the family anabtidae prepare a foamy nest by blowing bubbles of air and sticky mucus. Bubbles adhere together to form a floating mass of foam. This nest is dome-shaped. After nest formation the male collects the fertilized eggs in his mouth, gives them a coating of mucus and finally sticks them to the under surface of the foamy nest (Fig. 7.6 v).

Paradise fish prepare identical foamy nest, where the eggs being lighter rise up to the level of water. Nest float freely without being carried by the male.

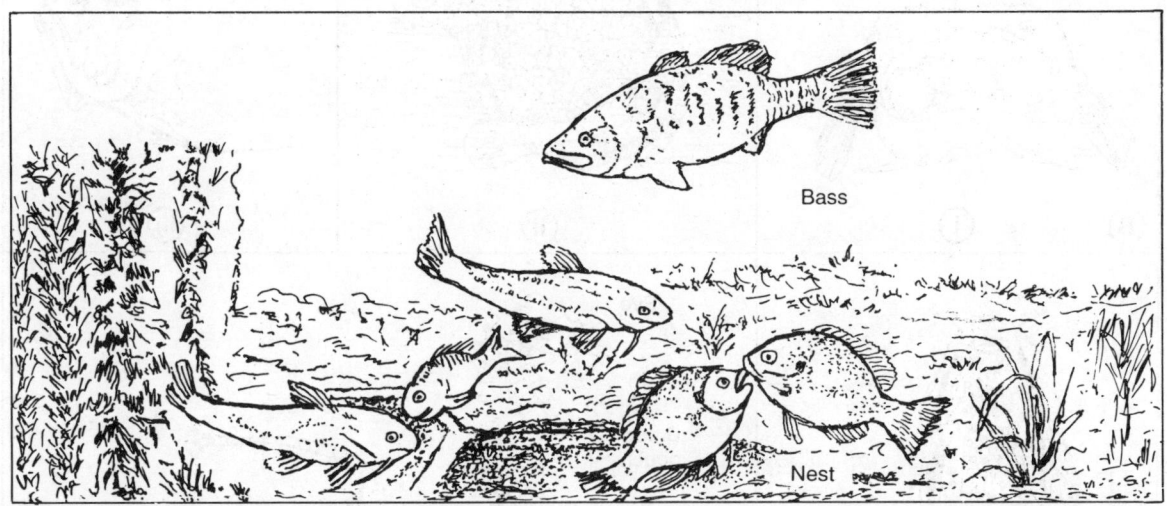

Fig. 7.7. The bluegill fishes nest in groups, with each male defending a territory bordered by the nest sites of other males, and trying to protect his nest against bass (above) bullhead cat fish (left), pumpkeen seed sunfish (right).

III. FISH SPECIES KEEPING THEIR EGGS AND YOUNG ONES IN OR ON THEIR BODY

There are many species of fishes which have developed many structures in their body to safeguard their eggs.

1. Mouth cavity as shelter

Female Cichlid fish (*Tilapia*) protect their eggs by carrying them in her mouth. Males of most of the marine cat-fishes (*Arius*) and cardinal fishes have similar habits of carrying the eggs and youngs in oral cavity until hatching. The male of a Brazilian cat-fish (*Loricaria typus*) develops an enlarged lower lip forming a sort of pouch in which labial incubation takes place. This phenomenon ensures safety and provide perfect aeration. These fishes swim upward to provide mucous to eggs which help in sticking the eggs to the mouth. The male fish do not take food during the act of parental care. Even after hatching the young ones remain near the father and if there is any disturbance they enter into the buccal cavity of father for shelter (Fig. 7.7 i A & B).

2. Formation of egg ball

In Butter fish (*Pholis*) the eggs are rolled into a round ball. One of the parents, often the male, guard the egg ball till hatching of young (Fig. 7.8 ii).

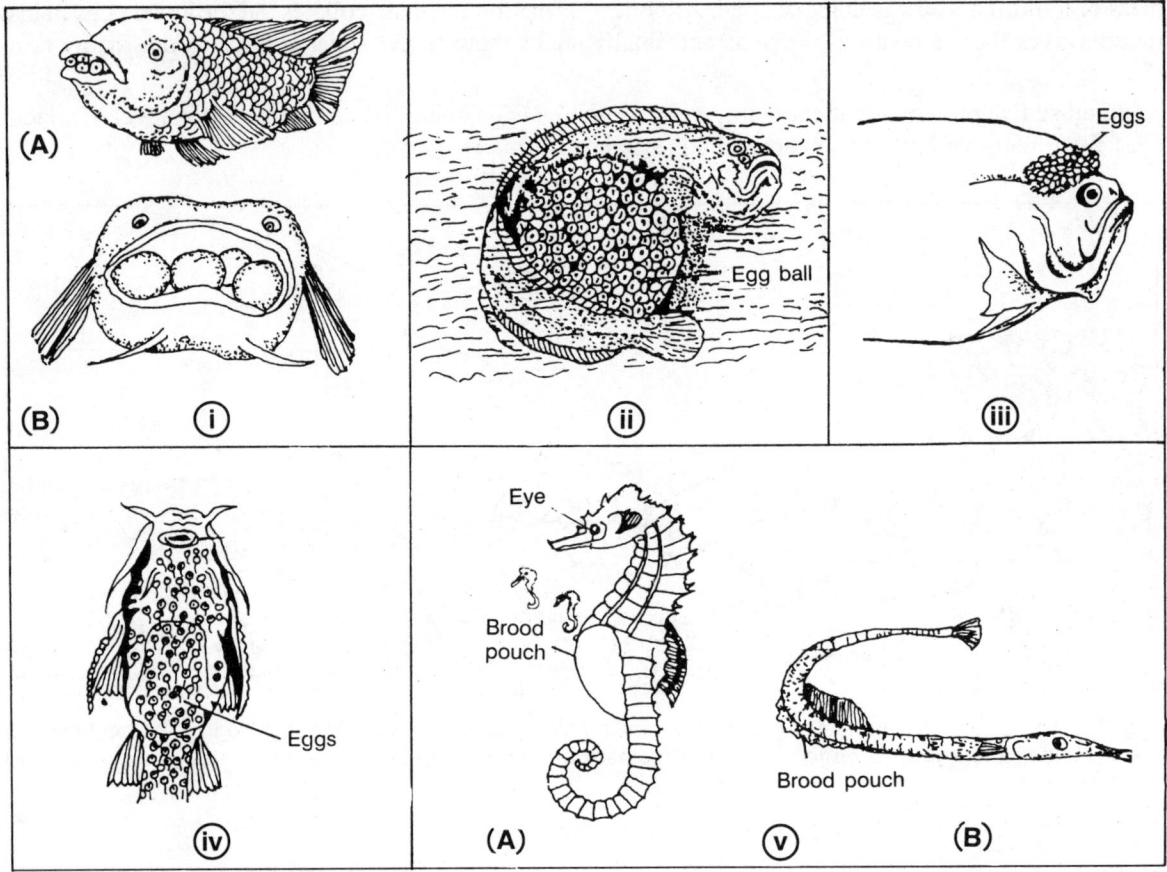

Fig. 7.8. Fish species carrying eggs on / inside body. (i A.) Tilapia carrying eggs in her mouth (i B) Brazilian cat fish keeping eggs in a pouch made inside the lower lip. (ii) butter fish (Pholis) Carrying egg ball (iii) Kurtus carry eggs on forehead. (iv) Cat fish (*Platystacus*) bear eggs in integumentary cups (vA) Brood pouch in male sea horse (vB) Brood pouch in *Sygnathus* male fish.

3. Eggs attached with bony hook

The male New Guinea fish (*Kurtus*) bear the mass of eggs on forehead (Fig. 7.8 iii).

4. Formation of integumentary cups

In the cat-fish (*Platystacus*) the skin of the lower surface of the body of the female becomes soft and spongy during breeding season. No sooner the eggs are fertilized the female presses her body against the eggs in such a manner that each egg becomes attached to the spongy skin in the form of a small stalked cup. It remains in this position till hatching of young (Fig. 7.8 iv).

5. Placement of eggs in brood pouch

Males of the Pipe fish (*Syngnathus typhle*), the sea horse (*Hippocampus*) and sea dragon receive eggs from females, which place them in the male's brood pouch. Brood pouch are found on the lower surface of the abdomen of the male. During the male's "pregnancy", he provides nutirients and oxygen to the fertilized eggs for several weeks, requiring longer to rear the clutch than females need to produce a new batch of eggs. Moreover, a single large female generates enough eggs in one cycle to fill the brood pouch of nearly three large males. Since the sex ratio is 1:1, male pouch space is in short supply, and as expected, males exhibit active mate choice. In this case males discriminate against small, plain females in favour of large, ornamented ones, that can fill their brood pouch with eggs quickly (Fig. 7.8 v A & B) and sufficiently.

In the family Solenostomidae, pelvic fins of females form the brood pouch. Inside the brood pouch numerous long filaments remain present which keeps the eggs in proper position.

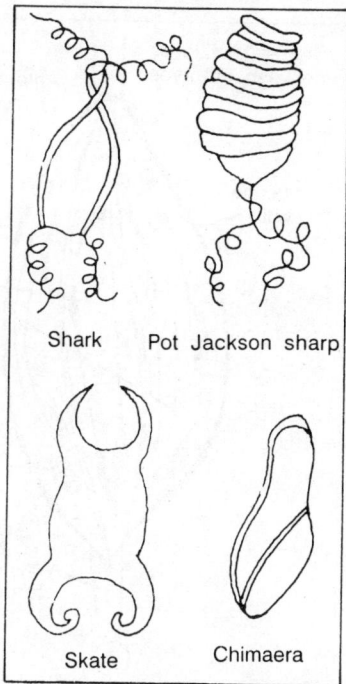

Fig. 7.9. Different Type of Mermaid's Purse : Shark, Pot Jackson shark, Skate and Chimaera.

6. Mermaid's purse

Some of the Sharks and Rays produce a special type of leathery case called mermaid's purse. It is a shell secreted by the shell glands of oviduct. The shape of the purse varies in different groups but the function remains the same, that is, protection of eggs. The corners of the shell are drawn out into four long elastic filaments which serve to attach the purse to sea weeds. The development of eggs is completed within the purse (Fig. 7.9).

IV. VIVIPARITY

Some fishes have evolved internal incubation and they give birth to young ones. Sharks, Surf perch, Cymatogaster, Sculpines and Carps do not lay eggs, rather they directly give birth to their young ones in order to provide absolute protection of eggs. Among the sharks, live bearing has been noticed in more than dozen families, where the development of eggs take place in uterus. In some species uterine wall secretes either embryotrophe or uterine milk. In two orders of teleosts Cyprinnodonts and Perciformes, some species (*Zoarces, Gambusia*-Mosquito larvae eating fish and *Poicilia*) show internal fertilization and the young ones develop within the ovary. The embryos develop freely in a sac inside ovary feeding upon an "embryotrophic" material, apparently produced by the discharged ovarian follicles. The sac becomes highly vascular. Eggs remain present inside the sac throughout the several months of pregnancy.

In shiner-perch (*Cymatogaster aggregata*) the eggs are fertilized in the ovarian follicles but are soon released into the ovary cavity and are nourished by a secretion from the ovary. The young are retained in the ovary until they become sexually matured. The yolk sac forms placentae like sharks.

Among bony fishes, viviparous forms are comparatively rare. In the Culpins and the Carps viviparity is only confined to a single genus each, Comphores and Barbur respectively, where the development of eggs takes place in ovaries. (Fig. 7.10).

V. PARENTAL CARE TO YOUNG ONES

Parental care in fishes does not stop at caring for the eggs only. Members of some families such as Gasterosteridae, Centachidae, Ictaluridae defend their young very actively. These fishes defend their

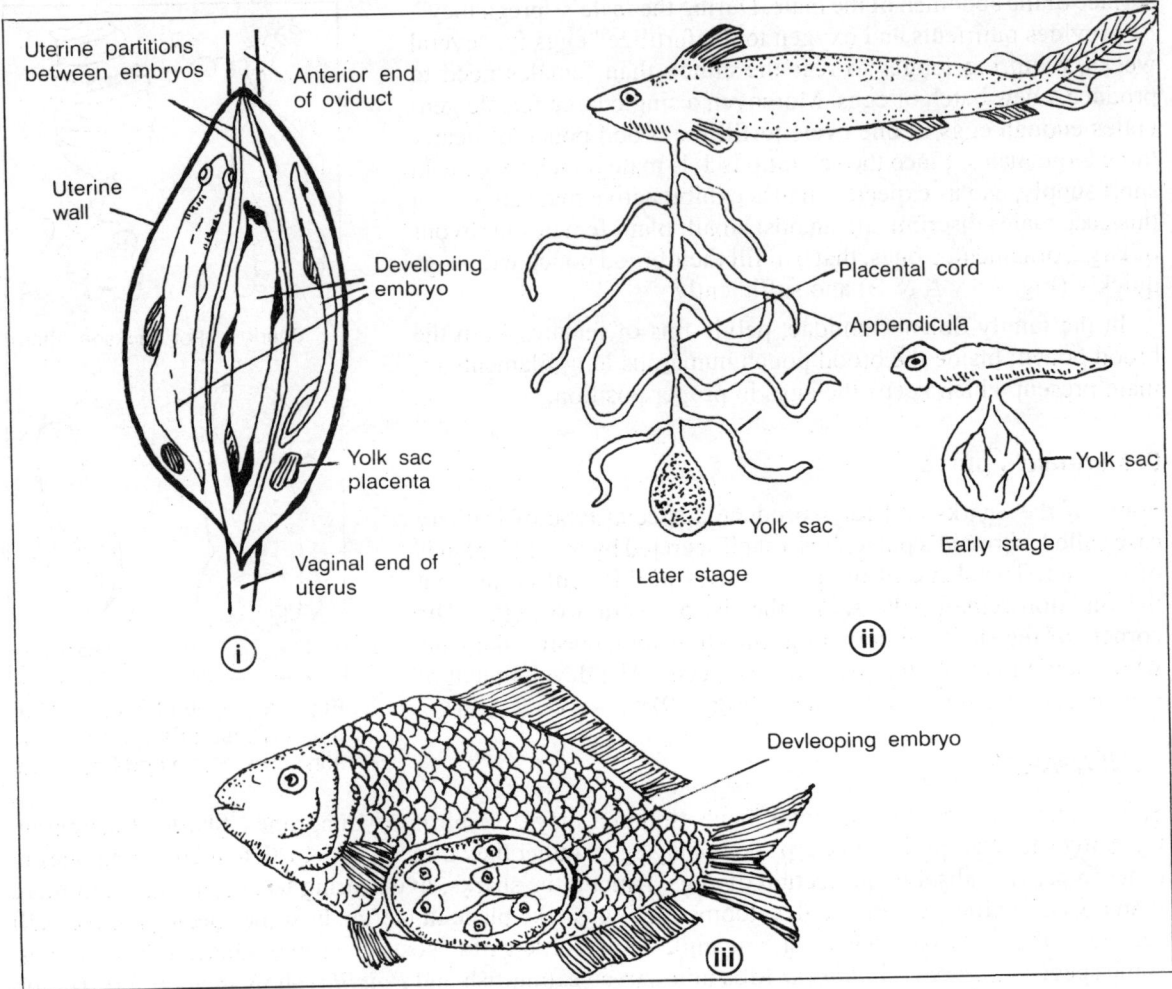

Fig. 7.10. Viviparity in some fishes (i) L.S. of uterus of Shark female (ii) Yolk saa placenta in Shark. (iii) Developing eggs in bony fish carp.

young ones by placing them to safe places and away from the predator and enemies. The hatchings of Tilapia and Pipe fish are protected by their parents. They are protected in mother's oral cavity and father's brood pouch respectively.

Both males and females of cichlid fish secrete a nutritious substance that their young can glean from a parents body. (Fig. 7.11).

ADOPTION IN FATHEAD MINNOW

Fathead minnow is a fish species in which males care for the eggs at their nest site, made at the under sides of rocks in a stream (Fig. 7.12). Appropriate nest sites are in short supply, and males compete for them, sometimes evicting an egg-tending rival in the process. In this circumstance, the victorious males will "adopt" the eggs already present at the nest, even though they have been fertilized by the previous owner. Craig Sargent determined that female fathead minnows find males guarding eggs more attractive than males without eggs. Thus, a male's chance of acquiring his own mate after a takeover is enhanced if his nest has eggs in it, even if he has not fertilized those eggs,

WHY ARE MALE FISHES SO OFTEN PARENTAL?

While going through the parental care of fishes we have observed, male fishes provide many exceptions to the rule that females are more likely to provide care for their offspring.

Parental male fishes are territorial, defending a site that females visit to mate and lay their eggs. By guarding a territory, they also guard the eggs they have fertilized; the territory and the presence of eggs make the males attractive to additional females, increasing male mating success. This creates a very favourable benifit-to-cost ratio for male parental care.

Parental care by female fish may reduce her growth rate because she cannot feed sufficiently while caring for her current offspring. Loss in growth due to parental care, a female pays heavy price in the loss of egg production. Males that are parental grow slowly, but since they are territorial to attract females, the decrease in growth resulting from parental care is negligible. Thus, in fishes, male parental behaviour is probably the evolutionary result of males paying a lower price for parenting than females do.

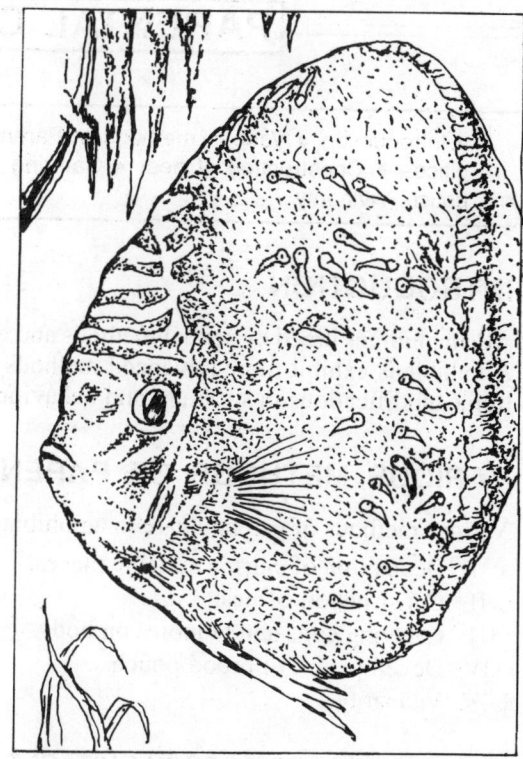

Fig. 7.11. Young of Cichlid fish taking nutritious food secreted from parent's body.

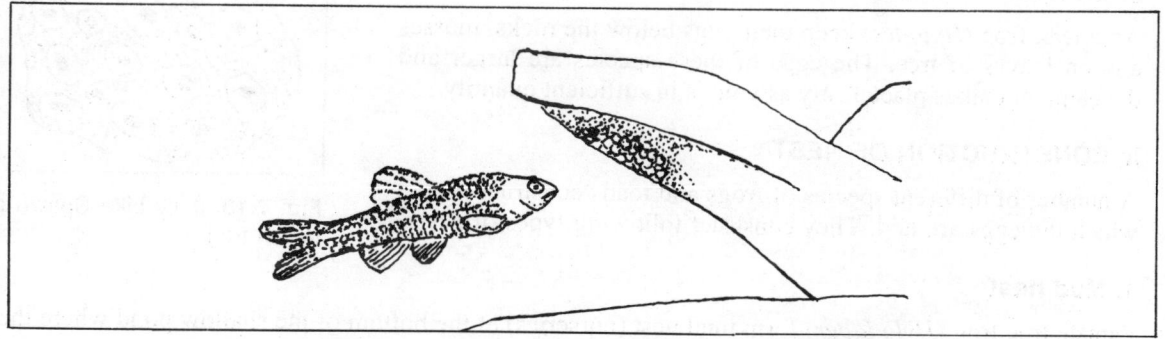

Fig. 7.12. Adaptive Adoption in Fathead Minnow.

PARENTAL CARE IN AMPHIBIA

● Introduction ● Various methods of Parental Care in amphibia ● Deposition of eggs in suitable places ● Construction of nest ● Carrying eggs and tadpoles on body ● Development of brood pouch. Viviparity.

INTRODUCTION

All amphibians breed by sexual methods and each group of amphibians show instances of parental care. Amphibians exhibit more advanced methods of parental care than fishes. For parental care many extreme modifications in structure and behaviour of amphibians have been observed.

VARIOUS METHODS OF PARENTAL CARE IN AMPHIBIA

Various methods of parental care in amphibia may be kept into following five categories.

   I. Deposition of eggs in suitable places.
  II. Construction of nest.
 III. Carrying eggs and tadpoles on body.
 IV. Development of brood pouch.
  V. Viviparity.

I. DEPOSITION OF EGGS IN SUITABLE PLACES

A number of different species of frogs lay their eggs in a suitable place either in water or a land near the water.

1. In water

Rana tigerina (Indian frog) lay eggs in pond water in a jelly like spawn (Fig. 7.13).

2. On Trees or moss away from water

American frog (*Hylodes*) keep their eggs below the rocks, mosses and on leaves of tree. The eggs of these species are larger and development takes place fastly as yolk is in sufficient quantity.

II. CONSTRUCTION OF NEST

A number of different species of frogs and toads construct nest in which the eggs are laid. They construct following types of nests.

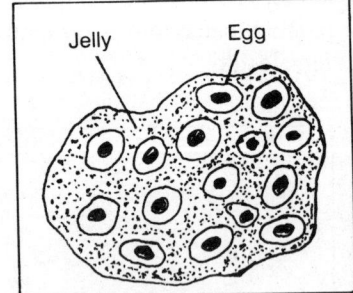

Fig. 7.13. Jelly Like Spawn of Indian frog.

1. Mud nest

Female tree frog (*Hyla faber*) form mud nest (nurseries) at the bottom of the shallow pond where they take care of eggs. They construct 7-10 cm. deep hole in the mud in shallow water. She lays eggs in it after 2 days of nest building. Male discharges sperms there to fertilize eggs. Eggs and young ones are saved from predator (Insects and Fishes) by parents (Fig. 7.14A).

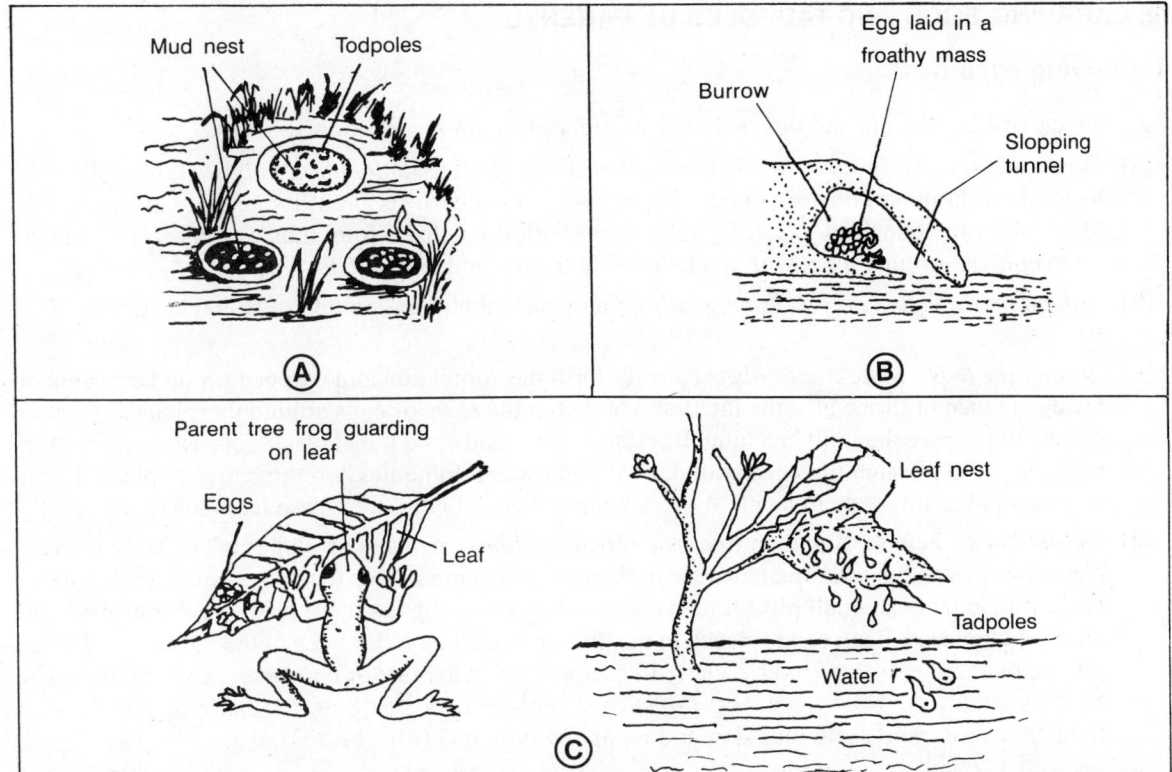

Fig. 7.14. Nests of Hyla And Phyllomedusa : (A) Mud nest of Hyla faber. (B) Burrow nest. (C) Leaf nest of Phyllomedusa.

2. Tunnel nest

Female Japanese tree frog (*Rhacophoras ocellatus*) makes a spherical hole of 6-9 cm wide in mud at pond banks. Both male and female sinks in the hole embraced with each other. They make the surface of the tunnel smooth while sinking. Finally they close the mouth of tunnel. Female emits a spongy ball from her cloaca, laying eggs on it. Eggs become entangled with frothy bubbles. Now male discharges their sperms on the frothy bubble fertilizing the eggs (Fig. 7.14B).

3. Leaf nest

Tree frog of South America (*Phyllomedusa*), India (*Rhacophoras malabariens*) and Africa (*Chiromatis*) lay their eggs on rolled up leaves hanging above water. The nest is covered by many other leaves. Eggs develop into tadpoles. The tadpoles directly fall into the water. Further metamorphosis of larva take place in water. Female glass frog of rain forest of Costa Rica lay her eggs on leaves of tree. Males take care of eggs. After 2 to 3 weeks tadpoles fall into the water (Fig. 7.14C).

4. In gelatinous transparent bag

Female *Phyrynixallus biroil* secrete a transparent bag and keep their fertilized eggs in it. The transparent membranous bag is left in water current of hill stream. Entire metamorphosis occurs in the bag. Small frog come out of this bag after maturation.

III. CARRYING EGGS AND TADPOLES BY PARENTS

1. Carrying eggs

Eggs are carried by parents and this is done by numerous methods mentioned below.

(a) *Eggs are protected by covering them with their body* : Male *Mantophryne robusta* covers the eggs by elastic gelatinous covering in row. Their number in one row is about 17 and they form a bunch. Male sit on the bunch of eggs and holds them with the help of forelimbs. Limbless amphibians (*lcthyophis*) surround eggs with the help of their own body (Fig. 7.15 A).

(b) *Around the head and neck* : *Desmognathus fucus* carry their eggs around neck and head. (Fig. 7.15 B).

(c) *Around the legs* : Male *Alytes obstricans* perform the copulation and oviposition on land. Female lay eggs twice or thrice at some intervals. Male rap the rows of eggs around their legs and pelvic region and carries them till hatching. It rests in some shady and moist places, occasionally coming out at night to moisten the eggs with dew or pond water and quickly returns to safe place. Lastly when tadpoles are ready to hatch, it takes a dip in nearest pond to release tadpoles (Fig. 7.15 C).

(d) *On the back* : Female Brazilian tree frog (*Hyla goeldie*) carries eggs on her back. Male helps to place the eggs on her back. Female toad of Surinam (Pipa pipa*)* keep their eggs and tadpoles on her back. Pipa pipa bear small pits on its back and they carry eggs in these pits. The number of eggs are about hundred. Each egg is placed in the groove made up on the back of the mother toad. Each groove or chamber is covered by a jelly like substance. After one or two weeks a young pipa toad hatches from egg. Now all young *Pipa* leave the chamber made on the back of mother. The mother cast off warty and dull skin and aquire smooth one (Fig. 17.5 D).

(e) *On exposed belly* : Female *Rhacophoras reticulata* of Sri Lanka carry their eggs on their belly. On removal of eggs by human hand the belly bear small grooves (Fig. 7.15 E).

(f) *In one pouch* : *Gastrotheca marsupial* bear a common pouch present inside dorsal surface of body wall. The eggs are placed in this pouch (Fig. 7.15 F).

2. Carrying Tadpoles

South American *Phyllobates* and *Dendrobates* carry their tadpoles on their back. Tadpoles remain attached on the back of parents with the help of sucker like lips. Tadpoles are carried by their parents to another ponds, if the pond becomes dry.

IV. DEVELOPMENT OF BROOD POUCH

Parents carry their eggs and tadpoles in their special natural brood pouches. These are of various types.

1. In small cell like pouches on back

Small cutaneous pouches are formed on the back of females of *Pipa cryptobranches* and *Desmognathus gastrotheca* species of frog. Eggs are surrounded by these cutaneous pouches. Each pouch is covered by a lid. These pouches are formed by the secretion of cutaneous glands. Each pouch consists of more than 100 eggs. Development of eggs and metamorphosis of larva occurs in this pouch. Fully developed young frogs come out from these pouches (Fig. 7.15 G) and lead free life.

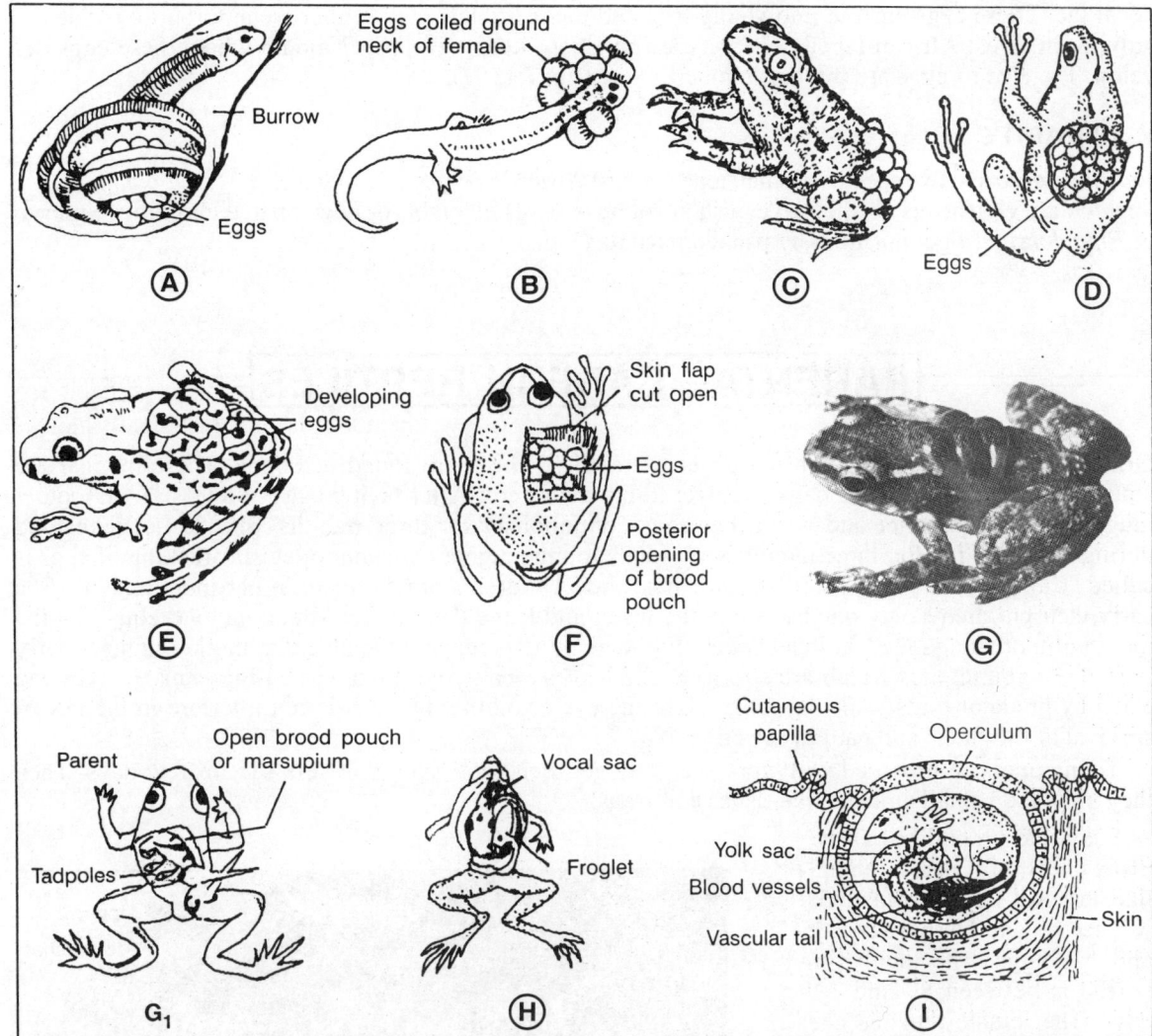

Fig. 7.15. Carrying of eggs and Tadpoles by Parent Amphibians. (A) Eggs around the body of Icthyophis. (B) Eggs on head and neck of Desmognathus. (C) eggs carried by male *Alytes* around their hind legs and pelvic region. (D) *Hyla goeldie* carry eggs on the back. (E) Female *Rhacophorus* carry eggs on back. (F) *Gastrothea* carry eggs on back in a common pouch (G & H) *Pipa* and *Desmognathus* females carrying their tadpoles in a cutaneous pouch made on the back (I) Development of pseudoplacenta in *Pipa dorsigera*.

2. Common pouch

Eggs are placed in a common pouch in *Notorima* and female marsupial frog *Gastrotheca marsupium*. This common dorsal pouch is formed only in breeding season. The pouch bear a small hole. The method of transfer of eggs in these pouches is still not known (Fig. 7.15 G_1).

3. In the mouth or gull pouch

South American male frog *Rhinoderma darwini* take eggs in their gull pouch. The gull pouch is modified vocal sac. These eggs emerge into young frog and these froglets may further metamorphose inside the gull pouch. West African female *Hylambates breviceps* keep eggs in her mouth where these eggs develop. The size of eggs are big but number is few (Fig.7.15 H).

V. VIVIPARITY

Pipa dorsigera and two species of small toads of East Africa *Psedophryne vivipara* and *Nectopharyenoides tortnieri* are viviparous i.e. they give birth to young ones. Their embryos develop in their uterus. Embryo of *Pipa dorsigera* get nutrition by pseudoplacenta (Fig. 7.15 I).

PARENTAL CARE IN REPTILES

Orinoko muggar is a rare parental species of reptiles. These are found in Logos. These muggar are aquatic but they come to the banks of river to lay their eggs. After laying eggs in mud or soil, mother muggar returns to water and watch her eggs continuously for three months. She do not take food during this period. After three months very small young muggar come out of eggs. Cracking of eggs is called "Calling of mother". Mohter come near their children and take them in her mouth cavity. She carry their children safely one by one in the water and leave them there. Young muggar come out the mouth of mother and lead an independent life. One thing is remarkable here that mother muggar carry only those young ones which are stronger. She leaves weak young muggar on the bank of river and eaten by predator birds. This happens before the eye of mother but she do not interfere in the law of survival of the fittest and natural selection.

Young ones are provided with york sac, they get their food from this yolk sac for few days. Then they prey upon small animals like fishes and frogs.

Estuarine crocodile (*Crocodylus porosus*) makes a mound-like nest on a sloping bank in the wet season and lay between 25 and 120 eggs. The incubation period is between 80 and 100 days. The female remains near the nest and defends it most carefully. She assists the hatchings to leave the nest, carries them to water and remains near them for a considerable period.

Female Muggar (*Crocodylus palustris*) starts digging trial nest pits atleast a fortnight before the actual egg-laying. The nest is made inside a burrow. The nest chamber is a wide mouthed pitcher-shaped structure, dug quite away from the edge of the water in a high sloping bank. The

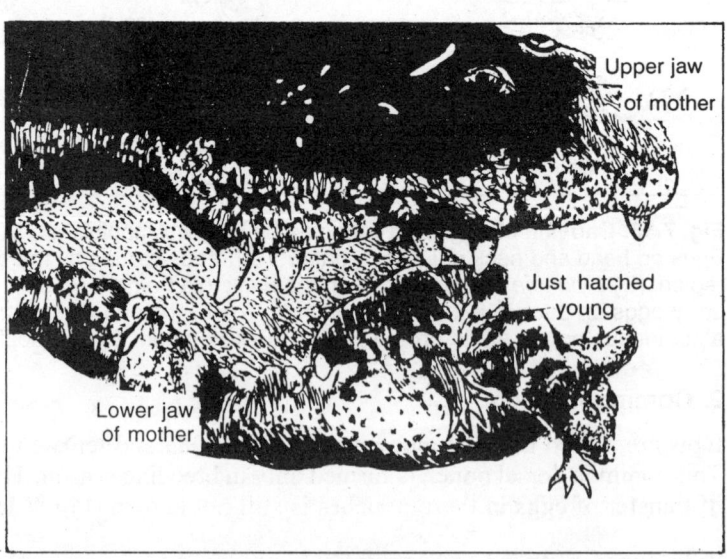

Fig. 7.16. A crocodile mother transporting her babies from sand to water just after they have hatched from her nest.

egg laying takes place between late February and first week of April. 10–35 eggs are laid in a clutch. The incubation period varies from 50-60 days. Hatching which are ready to emerge make grunting noise (calling mother) from within the nest, stimulating the mother crocodile to excavate the nest and carry them to water. Hatchings are from 25 to 30 cm. in length and weight about 60–100 g. Mother carry hatchings in her mouth from nest to water habitat.

Gharial (*Gavialis gangetics*) is amphibious crocodile. Nesting takes place from late march to mid April on sand bank of the river edge or mid-river islands. Between 18 and 40 eggs are laid is deep nests. Incubation period range from 83 to 94 days. The female guards the nest-site and also closely attends the hatchings for several months.

Female alligators demonstrate a delicate touch when the time comes for their eggs to hatch. After laying about three dozen, a female covers her clutch with mud and leaves, then protects them. As the embryos incubate in the sun, they exhale carbon dioxide, which seeps into the nest, forming a weak acid that coats the shell. Slowly the shell thins. After nine weeks, some hatchings can poke their snouts through the shell and emerge, while others emit grunts that elicit help from the mother. Gently grasping an egg in her mouth, she rolls it on her tongue, feeling for signs of life. After tongue-testing she eat up infertile eggs. It she senses something stirring, she gently cracks the shell open, and tilts her head forward to let her baby emerge.

With their (baby alligator) stomachs still heavy with egg yolk, newborn alligators are not strong swimmers and, lacking agility, are vulnerable to predators. So when venturing into water, they often hitch a ride with mother, who can keep a close eye.

PARENTAL CARE IN BIRDS

NESTING BEHAVIOUR : • Introduction • Origin of nesting behaviour • Steps in nesting • Season, selection of suitable places, establishment of territory • Eggs and Nests • Pairing • Types of nests • Birds which do not make nest but lay their eggs in safe places • Birds which do not make nest but incubate eggs on their body • Nest materials • Social nesting • Nest parasitism.

BROODING BEHAVIOUR : • Eggs and Ovulation in birds • Incubation • Brooding property • Types of young birds • Defending and feeding the young ones • Sanitation of nest • Guarding the nest.

NESTING BEHAVIOUR

INTRODUCTION

Birds are amongst the liveliest of creatures that constantly draw our attention to them with their marvelous nest construction. Before breeding, birds usually build a nest where the eggs are layed and incubated. After hatching, nestlings (young ones) are reared safely. Need of nest for offspring among birds is more important because birds have to face maximum struggle with the environment and predators as they are oviparous and usually without defensive organ. Incubation of eggs and taking care of young ones by parents is called brooding. Nesting and brooding are two important acts of parental care found in many species of birds. Parental care in birds is more complex than in fishes, amphibians and reptiles because parent birds take longer duration and provide food for the young.

ORIGIN OF NESTING BEHAVIOUR IN BIRDS

Birds are glorified reptiles and have developed many characteristic behaviours in course of evolution of nesting behaviour. The most striking feature is its adaptations for aerial mode of life and nesting behaviour. Reptiles have precocial offspring (young lead independent life after hatching). This pattern of development is the most primitive one and that altricial condition (young depend on parents for food and protection) represents a more recent stage of evolution. After hatching, altricial birds exhibit many instinctive behaviour which is required for growth and survival. They open their gapes wide to incite their parents to provide with a continuous supply of food. Because of their initial lack of feathers, they have to remain in the warm nest for the first few weeks of their life. Adult birds which produce altricial young must construct an appropriate nest and then feed their offsprings necessary for hatching to independence. Precocial birds, by contrast, emerge from the egg at a more advanced stage of development. Their eggs open and young have thick coat of down feathers. Many of them are able to find food unaided, almost from the moment of hatching. As a rule, their parents construct only a rudimentary nest, if they construct a nest at all. *Altricial offspring* require more protection and defence from predator than do *precocial offspring*, which are able to escape and pick up food. The first bird probably followed their reptilian ancestors in laying their eggs in crevices in the ground or in tree hollows and covering them with sand, earth or leaves. As the birds evolved, those species which became adapted for life in wetland and swamps developed the behaviour of seeking out small patches of dry land among the reeds. Subsequently, nest building above ground-level could have emerged as a response to folding and rising water level.

Territory : Selection of a suitable place is the first step of nesting behaviour. The main function of a territorial system is to ensure that the birds of one species are spaced out in such a manner that each can obtain enough food for itself and for bringing up its young.

Pairing : Some species such as *Ostrich, Swans* (*Cygnus*), *Geese* and *Indian robin* are monogamous and pair for life. Many birds i.e. house sparrow, parakeet, blue rock pigeon etc. pair for one breeding season only.

NEST MATERIALS

Birds use various kinds of materials for nest building, brought from far and near. Some birds use her own droppings to construct nest. Swallow of china supplies its own cement in the form of a glutinous saliva and uses this cement and its own feathers to construct a basin shaped cradle on the face of a cliff.

TYPES OF NEST

Before egg laying the birds build nest. Birds build their nests in the surroundings in which they are accustomed to live. However, exceptions are there. Nest construction is performed usually by the male, sometimes by the female or even both. The modes of making nest and materials used for it differ in different species of birds. The nests show great diversity in shape and size of the nest, materials used for nest constructions etc. Smallest bird is Humming bird and the diameter of nest of this bird is only about 1.8 cm. On the basis of site, shape and size, materials used nests have been classified as below:

Ground nest : Some ground birds simply scrape a little earth to one side and lay their eggs in depression. Indian stone curlew (*Burhinus oedicnemus*), Indian pratincole (*Glareola lactea*), make ground nest. Simple scrapes in the ground sparsely lined with grass and leaves e.g. Quail or with no lining as in lapwings (*Vanellus*) and ducks (*Anas*). Pheasants, partridges and curlews are arboreal birds but they lay their eggs on ground, at lonely places. Cormorants, Herons and Ducks are aquatic birds but they make their nest in bushes near the water reservoir.

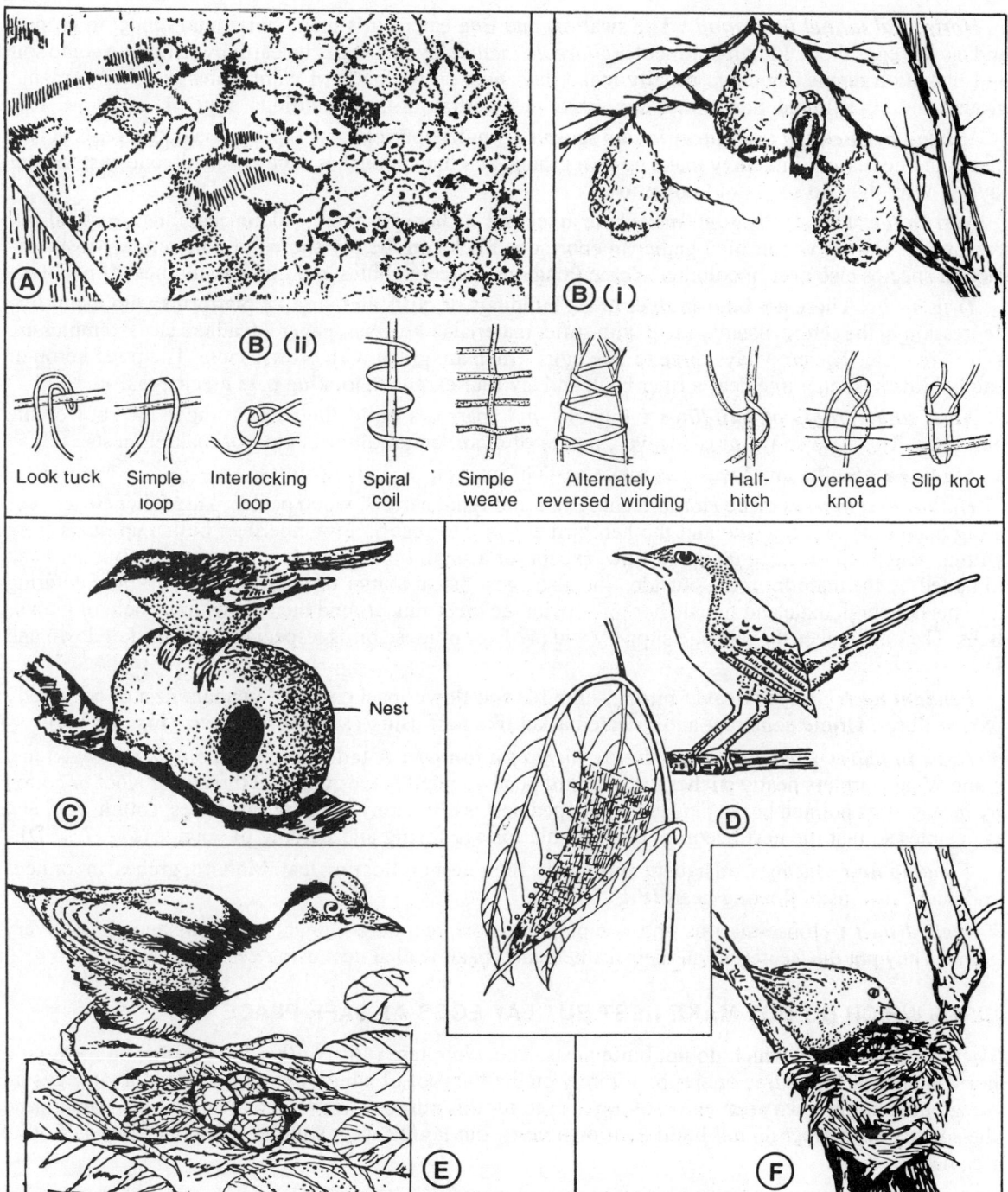

Look tuck | Simple loop | Interlocking loop | Spiral coil | Simple weave | Alternately reversed winding | Half-hitch | Overhead knot | Slip knot

Fig. 7.17. Different Types of Nests. (A) Tunnel nest made on ground by bee-eater birds. (Bi) Suspended nest of Baya. (*Ploceus cuscuttatus*). (Bii) Different types of stiches used by baya while making nest. (C) Oven nest of Rufous. (D) Pendent leaf nest of tailor bird. (E) Jakana make nest on leaves of floating plant on water. F. Nest of a bird made in between two branches of tree.

Horizontal tunnel in ground : The swallow and Bee-eater birds make horizontal tunnel in ground and lay her eggs there. Indian pratincole (*Glareola lactea*) lay their eggs on earth by removing some soil and making a ditch. Lapwings usually make their nest on the bank of calm water reservoir, grazing ground and big gardens. Sometimes they make nest on flat roofs of buildings (Fig. 7.17 A).

Making two nests at two places in one season : Singler sparrow and Towhee make two nests at two places in one season. First they make nest on ground and then in bushes. They use only one nest for egg laying. Why they do so is not known to us.

Nest on Ice : Female Penguins make hole in Ice and lay her eggs there. Adelie penguins are social and gregarious. During winter they gather in enormous flocks on the Icy shores of Antarctica. Most Cormorant species also nest in colonies. Some Penguins collect pebbles and make round nest of pebbles.

Twig nests : These are built in trees or on buildings or cliffs and are like platforms with a cup like depression in the centre, usually lined with softer materials like grass, papers, feathers etc. Examples are Kite, Crow etc. The crow lays three to five eggs which are green with brown spots. The pond heron or paddy birds nest on a tree near a river bank and lay four exquisite looking pale green eggs.

Nests under roofs of buildings : Pigeons and sparrows build their nests under the roof of the buildings. They use straw, grass, leaves, pieces of cloth, cotton threads etc. for making nests.

Mud nest : Swifts and Swallows make nests of mud on the side of cliffs.

Hollow nest in trees : The Hornbills of Africa and Asia, parrots, wood pecker, kingfisher etc. choose a big open hole in a big tree and the hen bird enters into that hollow. She then builds up walls from within, which would close up the hollow, except for a small hole through which she puts out her beak to be fed by the male from the outside. She also egest faecal matter through this hole. Before entering into the hole both male and female hornbills paint the tree trunk around the nest with the help of gum of trees. The gum makes the passage slippery and predator of these birds, especially snakes, fall down and fail to reach the nest.

Pendant nests : Baya (weaver birds), sun birds and flower packers build pendant nest of compactly woven fibres. Oriole construct an intricate basket like nest using twigs, threads etc. (Fig. 7.17 B).

Nests in leaves stiched together in the form of a tunnel : A tailor bird (*Orthotomus sutonus*) and some Wren warblers neatly stiches the edges of pendent plant leaves with the threads of wool or cotton by means of its pointed beak. This tunnel-shaped nest is ultimately lined by soft fibres, cotton wool and vegetables so that the nest becomes comfortable for egg laying and nursing of youngs (Fig. 7.17 D).

Floating nest : Jacanas, an aquatic bird, make their nest on floating leaf. Mallard, grebes, moor hens and coots also make floating nests (Fig. 7.17 E).

Walled nest : House-martins and common swallow secrete a cement like substance by salivary gland. They put this secretion on their feathers and make walled nest using cemented feather.

BIRDS WHICH DO NOT MAKE NEST BUT LAY EGGS AT SAFE PLACE

There are some birds which do not build nests. The white tern (*Gygis alba*) lay its eggs on rock, on a horizontal branch of a tree or shrub, or rarely on the flat roof of a building. Night hawk lay its eggs on the ground, but in town area, and roof top is used for this purpose. Birds like the green sand pipers and the solitary sand piper do not build their own nests, but lay their eggs in the abandoned nests of other tree nesting birds.

BIRDS WHICH DO NOT MAKE NEST BUT INCUBATE EGGS IN ITS BODY

Penguins generally lay their eggs in burrows or caves. King penguins incubate their eggs keeping them on their legs. The Emperor penguins pushes single egg beneath fold of its belly. The groove on belly

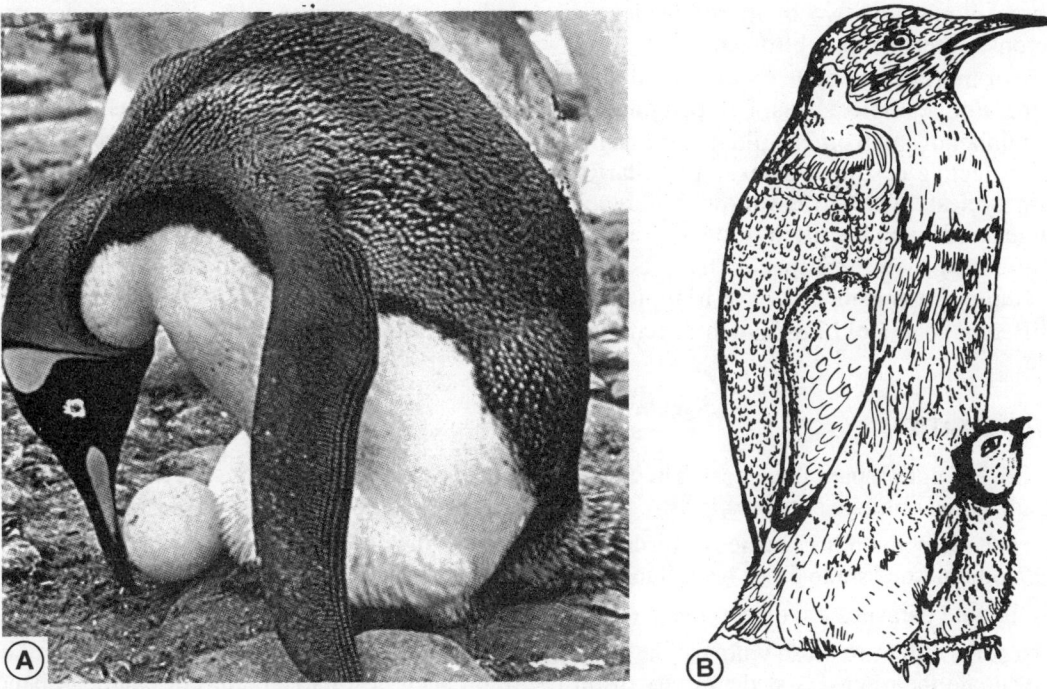

Fig. 7.18. (A) King Penguin trying to push egg inside the abdomen. (B) King Penguin keeping young on legs.

performs the function of a nest. It is a novel method of incubating egg in unfavourable condition where there is ice only. They also keep their young on her feet for some days (Fig. 7.18 A & B).

SOCIAL NESTING

Van Tyne and Berger stated that social nesting may involve :-

1. The members of a single species making uniform colony.
2. Members of two or more species making mixed colonies.

1. Members of a single species may exhibit two specialized types of social nesting

(i) *Communal nesting* : In this type, one to four pairs of birds build a common communal nest in which all females lay eggs. Incubation and feeding of the young are undertaken by all adults. Eg. Swamp hen, Guira cuckoo, Acorn woodpecker, Groove-billed anis.

(ii) *Co-operative nesting* : Flocks of numerous pairs of birds build the nest and each pair has its own nesting chamber. The size of such co-oprative nests may be enormous. For example, Weaver-bird (*Philatairus socius*), Buffalo weaver (*Bubalornis albirostris*) and monk parakeet of South America (*Myiopsitta monachus*).

2. Mixed Colonies

Birds of different species make mixed colonies. These may be of four types:

(i) Large number of two or more species nest together in a common area. For example, terns, herons, egrets, frigate birds etc.

(ii) One or more pairs of one species build their nest in the midst of a large colony of other species of birds. For example, skuas with penguins; gulls and tufted ducks in colonies of terns.

(iii) A number of small birds build their nests in close association with larger birds. This may be termed as protective nesting. For example, Starlings, House sparrows and Grackles build nests besides Osprey nests. The Cliff swallows build their nests near the nest of Prairie falcon. In such cases the larger birds who are often birds of prey tolerate the smaller birds.

(iv) Different genera and species have been observed to build their nests in close proximity. For example, Coppersmith, Myna, Magpie, King crow, etc.

(v) Different genera of birds live in different holes of same tree. For example, Pigeons, Myna, Parrot etc.

NEST PARASITISM

A few birds do not prepare their nest. They lay their eggs in the nests of other species. Such parasitic species are called obligate parasites.

There are still some other species of birds which incubate their eggs and take care of the nesting but lay eggs in the nest of some other bird. Such birds are called non-obligate parasites.

Non-obligate parasites are of two types (i) nest parasites and (ii) egg parasites.

(i) Nest Parasites are those who use the nests of other species in which they lay their eggs and host incubate their eggs. A wide variety of birds exhibit such nest parasitism. For example, banded finch, Jinete fly catcher, yellow tailed hornbill, pardalote etc.

(ii) The egg parasites are those which sometimes lay their eggs in the nests of other species, e.g. certain species of ducks, red head etc.

According to Van Tyne, obligate parasitism is found in five different families. These are :

(i) Cuculidae,

(ii) Indicatridae,

(iii) Anatidae,

(iv) Ploceidae, and

(v) Icteridae.

(i) Cuculidae

All members of this family do not exhibit nest parasitism. The cuckoos which are obligatory parasites are *Cuculus, Clamator, Eudynamis* (Koel), *Cacomantis, Cercococcyx, Chrysococcyx, Dromococcyx, Tapera* etc.

Crows guard their nest jealously and with pride. Still Koel (*Eudynamis scolopaceus*) manages to cheat the crow. At first, the cock koel flies to a tree where a crow is sitting on its eggs (taking utmost care to select a nest in which eggs have been newly laid) and starts cooing.

The angry crow at once attacks the koel, who flies away with the crow in hot pursuit. The clever koel can fly much faster than the crow and can easily get away if it tries, but it only flies fast enough to be just ahead of the crow, because it wishes to entice the crow to a safe distance from the nest.

While the chase is on, the hen koel quickly flies to the nest that the crow has left and deposits its egg in it. If it has time, the hen koel carries away one of the crow's eggs, but it flies quickly away before the crow returns after having abandoned the senseless pursuite of the crafty cock koel.

The returning crow does not seem to notice the strange eggs in its nest and sits on it quite happily along with its own. When the young koel hatches out of the egg, the crows feed it long after it leaves the nest.

The cuckoo is another bird, who lays its eggs in other's nests. They lay their eggs usually in that of the babbler bird also called 'the seven sisters'. Before laying eggs cuckoo make friendship with babbler and becomes frequent visitor in the nest of babbler. In an opportune moment cuckoo simply flies over the babbler bird's nest and drops its egg delicately into it. Babbler's eggs are blue and the cuckoo's egg is also blue. But the baby cuckoo, it hatched out of its egg, is so much larger than its foster parent and it is quite amusing to see it fed by its very small babbler parent, who often has to climb on to the large baby's back to feed him. It has been found that the parasitic young forcibly push out other nestlings from the nest so that only one cuckoo receives all attention from foster parents.

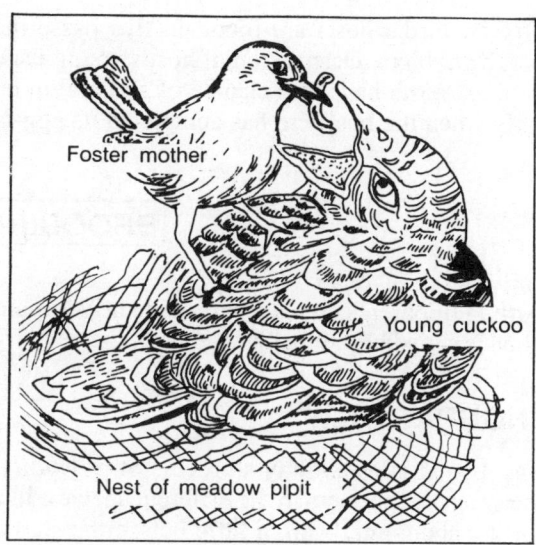

Fig. 7.19. A small foster mother (Babbler) feeding very large baby of other species (Cuckoo).

(ii) Indicatridae

Members of this family are commonly known as 'honey-guides'. Eggs are usually laid in nests of kingfisher.

(iii) Anatidae

This family includes the ducks. Only one species of this family *Heteronetta atricapilla* or black-headed duck of South America lays eggs in the nests of coot, rosybill, white-faced ibis and such other birds inhabiting marshes. The young rear themselves after only a short period of parental care and are least damaging to the host egg or nestlings.

(iv) Ploceidae

This family includes weaver-birds. Four genera of this family *Hypochera*, *Stegamura*, *Vidua* and *Anomalospiza* are nest parasites. First of three genera parasitize the nests of related estrildine species. *Anomalospiza* or the cuckoo finch exclusively parasitize nest of grass warblers like *Cisticola* and *Prinia* as reported by Fredmann (1980).

(iv) Icterodae

Only some cow-birds belonging to this family are nest parasitic. Bay-winged cow bird usually occupy nests of other species for egg-laying and incubation. The screaming cow-bird exclusively parasitizes the nest of bay-winged cow-bird. The giant cow-bird is reported to be parasitic in the nests of other member of the family. Eggs of bronzed cow-bird and brown-headed cow--bird have been found in the nests of nearly 60 and 200 other species of birds respectively.

Cow bird's hosts are found in five passerine families–thrushes, vireos, fly catchers, finches, and wood warblers. Destruction of host's young is mainly due to the rapid growth of cow birds. The young of most hosts have less chance of survival unless they hatch before the cow-bird and this is possible only when the host bird has completed its egg-laying before the nest is parasitized by the cow-bird.

BROODING BEHAVIOUR

Sitting of parents on eggs to provide heat to hatch them and taking care of young ones produced at one time is called brooding behaviour.

INCUBATION

Incubation is essentially a process of providing heat to the eggs. It is divided in different proportions between the partners in the different species. In most birds there develop incubation patches on the skin of the abdominal wall, a little before the start of incubation. These patches are also known as brood patches, and are formed in the apteria (tracts without feathers) by the loss of some abdominal feathers and by an increased vascularization of the skin or there may be only increase in the vascularization to provide necessary heat. On the basis of the contribution of the sexes to the process of incubation, Skutch (1975) has classified birds into three main groups : (A) Incubation by one sex only (B) Incubation by both sexes (C) More than two birds incubating eggs in single nest.

(A) **Incubation by one sex only :** This may be of three types :

    1. *Incubation by Female only* : Again this may be of three types :

        (a) The female sits continuously for many days. She may be fed by the male during this period, e.g. hornbill; or she goes without food, e.g., blue goose, golden pheasant etc.

        (b) The female may take long recess each day during which she does not incubate, e.g., some quail and guan.

        (c) The female may take more than one recess each day and sometimes by night also, e.g., most humming birds, mannakins, most song birds etc.

    2. *Incubation by male only* : This may also be of three types :

        (a) Continuous incubation by male who goes without food during the period, e.g., kiwi, emu, emperor penguin and weaver birds.

        (b) The male takes on long recess each day, e.g., some tinamou.

        (c) The male takes more than one recess each day, e.g., Ornate tinamou and Jacana.

(B) **Incubation by both the sexes :** Both the sexes take part simultaneously, e.g., red-legged partridge, sparrow, blue rock pigeons.

In herring gulls, the incubation duties are shared equally. This is essential because the eggs are quickly eaten up by other gulls, if left unguarded. Both the sexes participate alternately.

    1. Any one sex incubates by night having change-over at different intervals, e.g., Herring gull, Plover, Royal albatross, Sooty tern, Diving petrel etc.

    2. Female incubates by night, and during day. Both the sexes participate at different intervals, e.g., many Warblers, Pigeons, Doves, Amazon kingfisher, etc.

    3. Male incubates by night, and during day both the sexes share the duty, e.g., many Woodpecker, Ostrich, Anis etc.

(C) **More than two birds incubating in a single nest :** In this category the eggs may be laid by one female and several adults help in the task of incubation e.g., Bush tit. Or, *the eggs may be laid by two or more females* and incubation is done by several birds of both the sexes e.g., Acorn woodpecker. In some cases eggs which are laid on the ground get the necessary heat from surroundings, e.g., tree duck, Egyptian plover, Megapodes, Red heads etc.

Many birds start incubating after the last egg has been laid as in ducks. Some species as owls begin incubating as soon as the first egg is laid.

INCUBATION PERIOD

The incubation period (the time when the birds sit on the eggs until they hatch) varies in different birds. The average period of incubation for the smaller passerine birds is about 12-14 days. The eggs of the ostrich hatch in about 45 days. Those of the royal albatross, a sea-bird, have the longest period of incubation–about 80 days. The optimal incubation temperature is body temperature of the incubating bird.

There are some birds which raise their chicks in specially protected tubes. The chicks grow slowly and do not need to be fed much. For example, Baya.

PARENTAL CARE

A new-born is almost helpless in respect of food and protection and, therefore, it needs much attention from its parents. The process of the rearing of young birds (nestlings) follows a general pattern-the young hatch out, are fed by the parents and are protected from enemies, and finally become feathered and ready to live independently. This care or attention on the part of the parents is called the parental care. The parental care is behavioural aspect encountered among different groups of animals and is directly related to their survival.

The fully developed embryo cuts the egg-shell with an egg-tooth and during this activity the egg is said to be pipped. The hatching muscles help the chick in breaking out of the egg shell.

TYPES OF YOUNG ONES

There are two distinct types of newly hatched birds and they fit into the pattern in different ways.

1. PRECOCIAL YOUNG

The precocial young hatch out covered with down feathers, eyes open alert and are almost at once able to run or swim after their parents. They are also called 'nidifugae' (nidus-nest, fugere - to flee) or 'nest fugitives'.

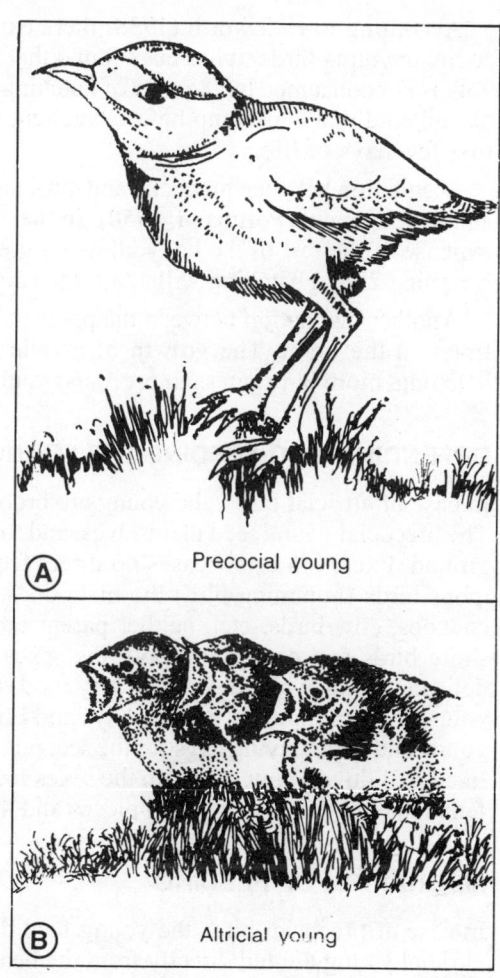

(A) Precocial young

(B) Altricial young

Fig. 7.20. Types of young ones : (A) Precocial young. (B) Altricial young.

There are different degrees of independence among the precocial young.

(i) Young quite independent of parents, e.g., megapodes.

(ii) Young follow parents but feed themselves, e.g., shore birds, ducks.

(iii) Young follow parents and Parents show them food, e.g., quail, fowl.

(iv) Young follow parents and are fed by them, e.g., grebes, hen.

(v) Young covered with down feathers and eyes open, but stay at nest and are fed by parents, e.g., terns, gulls.

2. ALTRICIAL YOUNG

Such young are naked, blind, weak and helpless when hatched and thus require greater parental care in getting food and protection. They remain confined to their nests for variable periods of time. They are also termed as 'nidicolous' or nest-dwellers. Examples : Pelicans, hawk, swift, kingfisher, cuckoo, passerine birds etc.

According to Heinworth (1938) there exists an interesting relationship between egg types and precocity in young birds. It has been found that eggs of precocial birds have greater amount of yolk and all yolk is not consumed by the time of hatching. On the other hand, eggs of altricial birds have less amount of yolk and that is used up before hatching and so there is less reserve food for sustenance during the first few days of life.

Distinction between precocial and altricial young has also been made on the basis of organ proportion and development (Portmann, 1950). In the altricial young the organs of metabolism are enlarged at the expense of the rest of the body allowing great metabolic efficiency and consequent growth. A cuckoo weighing 2 g. at hatching will attain the adult weight of 100 g. in only three weeks' time.

Another distinction between the precocial and altricial young is related to the development of nerve fibres in the brain. The growth of myelin sheaths which is regarded as a sign of maturation is, at hatching, more in progress in precocial young than in altricial young.

DEFENDING AND FEEDING THE YOUNG ONES

In case of altricial birds, the young are brooded by their parents as soon as the young are hatched out. The precocial young feed themselves, and the parents, particularly females, guide and locate the feeding ground. Except in a few cases no direct feeding takes place in precocial species. Among the polygamous birds (humming bird) the male does not help in brooding. In case of brood parasites, such as cuckoos, cow-birds, etc., neither parent ordinarily shows any concern for its offspring. In precocial shore birds and passerines, both the sexes participate in brooding. In general, the females feed the delicate young, while the males carry food. The red-eyed vireo perform about 75% of the feeding of the young. In some species, such as baya and English robin (*Erithacus rubecula*), the female may desert her young and begin laying eggs for the second brood, leaving the male alone to perform the duty of feeding. In case of doves, cow, etc. both the sexes feed their young in regular shifts. Male kestrel bring food and female break the food in small pieces and then feeds to young.

MECHANISM OF FEEDING

In case of precocial birds the young feed themselves by picking the food directed by parents, but the altricial young are fed directly from the beak by either parent. Opening of mouth of young depends on many stimuli. Side of mouth bear *Herbst corpuscles* touching tactile nerves. The beak of young opens like spring when mother touches her beak.

Directive marks in oral cavity of the young assist in co-ordinating the gaping of the young with feeding response of adults. The light-coloured, swollen corners of the mouth called 'oral flanges' serve as the simplest type of directive mark. More striking directive marks are on the palate that contrast sharply with the background colour.

Many birds swallow the food as they find, and later regurgitate it at the nest. In this method more food is carried in a single trip and the food is partly digestive juices of the parent. Egrets feed their nestlings by this method.

All pigeons and doves regurgitate *"pigeon's milk"* for their young, a substance rich in fat, protein and ash content.

FEEDING INSTINCT

In most birds the instinct to feed the young is brought into play when triggered by the reaction of the reproductive cycle at the proper time. In fact, the instinct appears even in the young birds so much so that the young of the first brood may assist in feeding their younger brothers and sisters of the second brood, e.g., swallows, blue birds, coots, etc. In some cases, anticipatory feeding is observed, that is, food is brought by the males before the young are hatched, e.g., wood warblers, tanagers, etc.

In case of altricial species the gaping response most probably depends both on the hunger and on the external releasing stimuli. The pattern and colour to the beak are remarkably effective releasers of the gaping response. It has been found that even imitations of the parents 'beak-form and colour', may elicit gaping response. It is interesting to note that it is possible to produce a model (imitation) which is super normal, i.e., it evokes a stronger response than does the natural object. Herring-gull chicks will peck at models of the parents' bill from which they are normally fed. The actual bill is clear yellow with a red circular patch on the lower jaw. The artificial bill is thinner and coloured red with three white bars at the tip. This model attracts more pecks from chicks that does a realistic copy of the natural bill.

FREQUENCY OF FEEDING THE YOUNG BY PARENTS

The frequency and amount of food vary according to species and depend on a number of factors such as the number of the young, the age of the young, the time of day, the method of carrying food, the season and the weather. Parent of owls (*Tyto alba*) bring prey about ten times a night. The young of the golden eagle (*Aquila chrysactos*) are fed twice daily. Small insectivorous birds, such as the great tit (*Parus major*), make as many as 900 feeding visits to the nest per day. On the other hand, during cold and wet weather, when insects are not flying, the European swift may not feed its young for days. The amount of energy expended by the parent in the performance of the feeding duty is remarkable. It has been observed that the parents, especially the females, lose about 17%–30% of their body weight in the act of feeding their young.

The nest is the home of a bird family providing shelter to the nestlings. Nests are kept dry and warm and are generally free from insects and predators.

Many precocial species leave the egg shells in the nest and lead their young away. Some (shore birds) remove the shells from the nest. A few altricial species leave the shells in the nest, but the majority of them carry the shells away or eat them up.

Many altricial species (passerines) remove the faecal sacs of the young immediately upon their discharge. The sacs are often eaten during the first few days of nestling's life, but later they are carried away. In disposing the faecal sacs, the swallows and martins pick up the droppings and toss them out. Wrens deposit them on branches away from the nest. The older young of some kingfisher turn their bodies around and discharge the faecal matter out of the nest opening. Probably babies have leant this hygienic habit from their parents. Many species of weaver-birds remove a decreasing number of faecal sacs as the young grow older, so that the rim of the nest becomes covered with them by the time they leave the nest. Some African and Australian ploceids do not remove the faeces at all.

Most altricial birds have a strong urge to keep their nests clean. Any foreign material kept in the nest is invariably removed, and when unable to do so they may as well leave the nest. Rings have sometimes been attached to the legs of the nestlings, and it has been observed that the parent pick up the nestling by the leg,

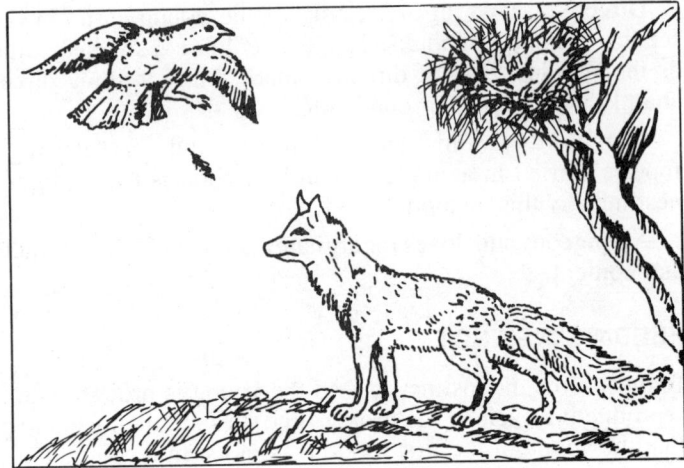

Fig. 7.21. Defence of Young by distraction method. A ringed plover lures a fox away from her chicks with the broken wing distraction display.

flies some distance away and drops it. The adult, in its effort to remove the ring, has been observed to even break the leg of the young.

The parent defends its young in precocial birds at the time of hatching or shortly after, and in altricial birds short!y before the young leave the nest. When parents are not present in the nest, the only defence the young has against emenies is to crouch in the nest or, if it can do so, to flee from the nest and hide in the surroundings.

Some species have been observed to perform distraction display to lure away the predator from the nest or from the young birds. In distraction action the parent bird flutters on the ground as if crippled and utters piteous cries. When the predator tries to catch the apparently crippled bird, the latter leads the former farther and farther away from the nest and then suddenly the bird flies away. In order to lure cats, dogs or foxes away from its nests on the ground, the ringed plover limp's along and clumsily flaps on wing as if it were broken. This is another example of distraction action (Fig. 7.21).

In case of need, parents carry their young by beak (*Grebes, Scoter*), leg (*red-tailed hawk*) or both by beak & leg (*American woodcock*). Nidifugous young instinctively respond to the warning calls of their parents. Different calls elicit different responses. At one call they freeze, at a second they scatter and freeze while the third call renders them immobile and the final call brings the young back to the parent.

NESTLING PERIOD

Nestling period varies with different species. In general, larger species have long nestling period. The nestling periods of small altricial birds–except of hole nesters and long-winged species like swallows and swifts–are about the same length as their incubation periods (Skutch, 1945). Nestling periods shorter than the incubation periods are characteristic of some genera of passerine birds, e.g., larks, some wood-warbler, ant-birds, etc. American robin, that nest in the open and whose eggs and young ones are exposed to environmental hazards, have shorter nestling periods than the cavity nesters. Some barbets, woodpeckers and toucans have nestling periods two or three times long than the incubation period.

HATCHING

The young peck their way out of the egg with the aid of the so called egg tooth (a projection or the upper mandible). It is used to cut the egg shell. The tooth disappears after hatching.

POST-BREEDING PHASE

The parental care does not end with the care of the nestling. For success in the struggle for existence, young birds need to be educated by their parents in various behavioural aspects, such as skill in finding and eating suitable food, skill in flight, learning to sing, social relationship etc. Some of these skills are developed as a result of instincts. The adults look after the young till the skills are perfected. The young of some birds of prey, like the hawk and kingfisher, are trained by their parents who place a prey before them and guide them to catch it. The singing ability comes from imitation, though it is an innate behaviour.

NESTING AND BROODING BEHAVIOUR AMONG FLIGHTLESS BIRDS BELONGING TO SUPER ORDER RATITAE OR PALAEOGNATHAE (OLD JAW)

- **Ostrich :** African ostrich (*Struthia*) are *polygamous* as one male attends several females. The male has a single solid retractile penis and the female has a clitoris. The nest is a simple hollow space in

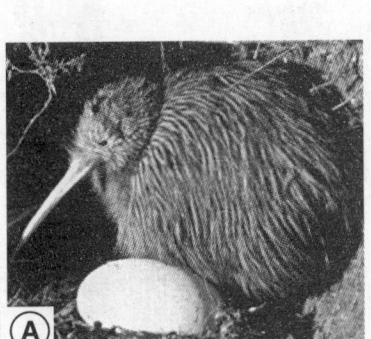 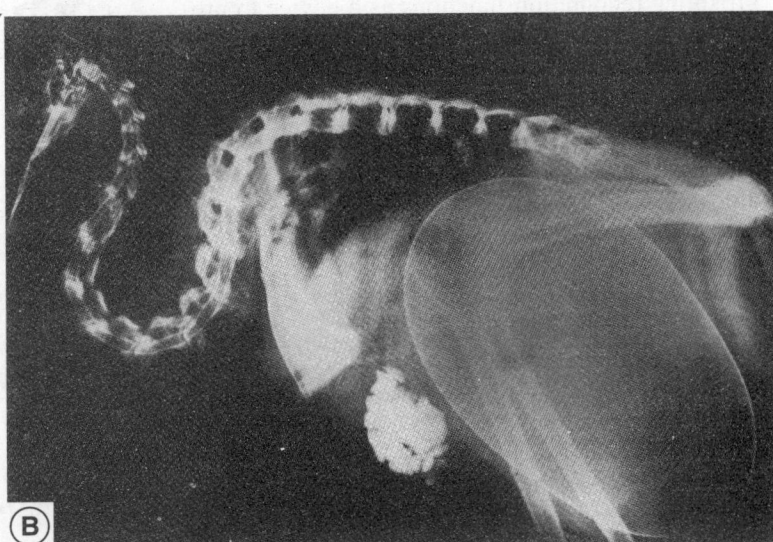

Fig. 7.22. (A) Male kiwi incubating egg. (B) A female kiwi weighing about 2.5 kg only but carry about ½ kg egg (X-ray, light) – one of the largest egg-to-body ratios of the bird.

Whopper of an egg is the Kiwi's burden :

Any mother-to-be stressed out by the ordeal or pregnancy should consider the kiwi's plight. This 2.5 kg female brown kiwi must carry a ½ kg egg (X-ray, rigth) – one of the largest egg-to-body ratios of any bird.

Studying brown kiwis in North Island's Waitangi Forest, researchers Barbara and Michael Taborsky found that an egg develops for 34 days before being laid – a record for birds. Greatest relief to mother kiwi is that only male incubates eggs. He sits across them and even then he is unable to cover egg completely.

The male is tied to the nest for about 90 days–another superlative–until the chicks hatch. The eggs have 60 percent yolk, which sustains the huge chicks.

the sand and several females lay their eggs in a single nest. Each egg is about 15 cm. in diameter and weights nearly 1.5 kg. The male incubates the eggs at night while the females sit during the day time.

- **Rhea** : (*Rhea americana*) is inhabitant of South America. The male is polygamous. Male incubates the numerous eggs of his flock of females and even broods the young for a time. During breeding season, the males become most savage and dangerous to approach.

- **Emu** : (*Dromais*) is represented by two species confined to Australia. Emu is invariably monogamous though seen in small parties after breeding. The nest is a shallow pit scraped in the ground. Each female has her own nest, but the male does the incubating and brooding.

- **Cassowary** : It lives in the jungle of Australia. The male cassowary is a devoted husband, for not only does he sit upon and incubate the eggs but also looks after the young ones.

- **Kiwi** : *Apteryx* of New Zealand is called as Kiwi by Maori (Tribal of New Zealand). This is the smallest living flightless bird. The female is larger than male and lays one or two eggs in a pile of soft grass placed at the end of her underground burrow. In proportion to the size of the body, the kiwi lays the largest eggs of any known animal.

OFFSPRING RECOGNITION

Offspring recognition functions as a device to prevent misdirected parental care. Offspring recognition is found more often in colonial species, where the risk of misdirected parental care is relatively high, than in solitary species.

Two swallows that nest in burrows in clay banks are the bank swallow, a colonial species (with a high risk of misdirected parental care), and the rough winged swallow, a solitary species (with a low risk of misdirected parental care). The two swallows belong to two separate genus but they are members of the same family of birds. They differ in various finer ways related to offspring recognition. For example, young Bank swallows produce far more distinctive vocalization than do young-Rough-wing swallows. Two other swallows–Colonial cliff swallow and Solitary barn swallow–also differ in their vocalization frequency.

Ground-nesting herring gull and cliff-nesting kittiwake are closely related and both are colonial species but even so, they also differ in the extent to which they risk misdirecting parental care to the offspring of others. Because herrings gulls nest on the ground and their young become mobile after they are a fews days old, parents may encounter juveniles that are not their offspring. To test the offspring recognition in herring gull, chicks older than

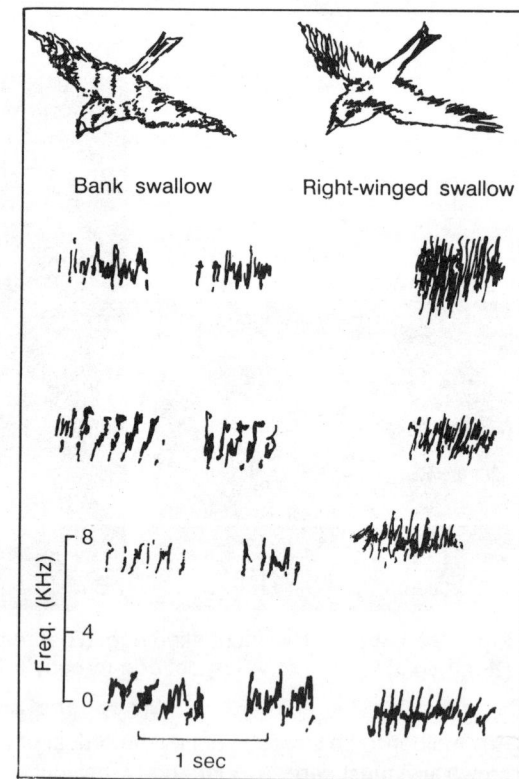

Fig. 7.23. Parental recognition of young in Bank swallows and Rough-winged swallows. Each sonogram represents a different chick's vocalization. Bank swallow produces a more distinct call rough-winged swallows.

4 or 5 days are transferred between nests, the adult gulls refuse to accept the substitutes and indeed may attack them vigorously.

In contrast, cliff nesting kittiwak's adults calmly accept strange chicks much older and larger or much younger and smaller than their own. In fact, one can replace a cormorant chick (very contrast to kittiwak's chick–Black and ugly) in kittiwake's nest and the adult kittiwakes will feed the cormorant's chick and will adopt them as their own offspring. The reason behind adoption of other chicks as their own by kittiwakes is that the adult birds do not recognize their young as individuals but instead rely on the location and behaviour of offspring as a guide to making feeding decision.

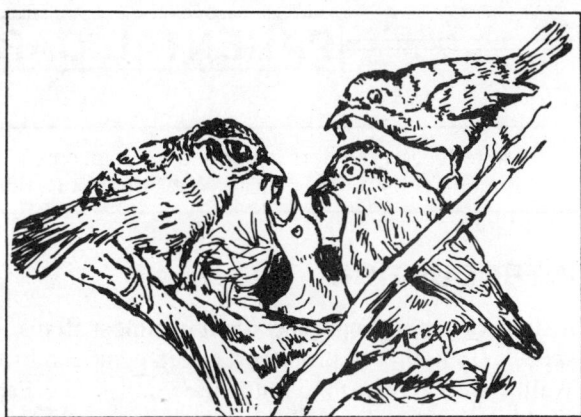

Fig. 7.24. Helpers at the nest in the Florida scrub jay provide food for the young, defense for the territory, and protection against predator.

HELPERS AT THE NEST

Some species of birds are now known to have helpers at the nest. The pied kingfisher is one of the species having helpers at the nest. A breeding pair of Florida scrub jays may have as many as six other individuals living with them in their territory. These non-breeding individuals may be 2 or 3 years old, or even older. They are physiologically capable of producing offspring of their own but instead defend the breeding pair's territory and feed the nestlings while detecting and repelling predators.

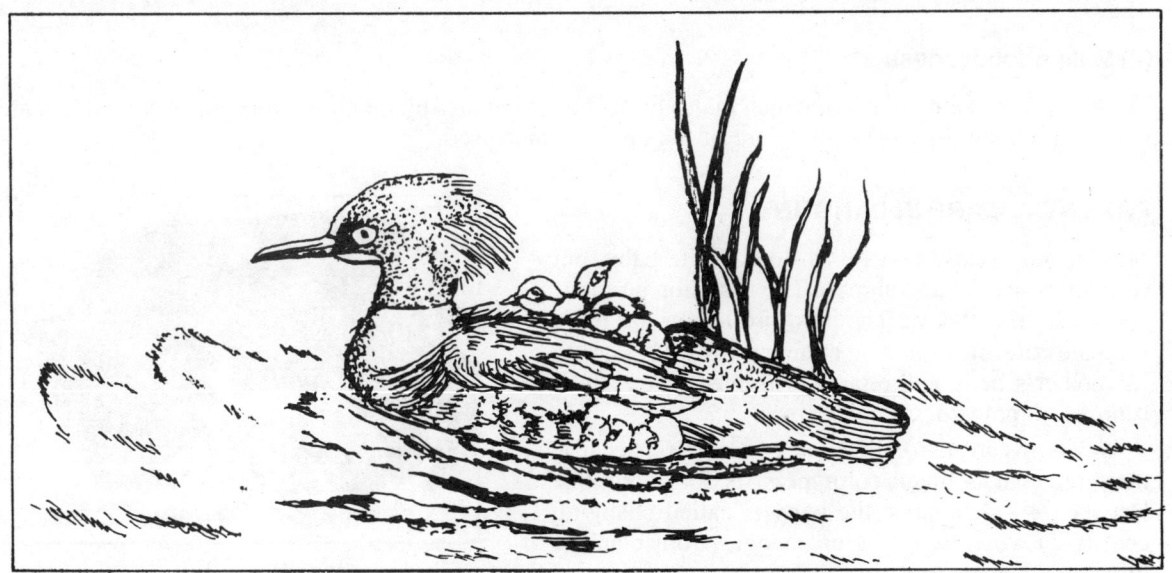

Fig. 7.25. Some duck carry her children on her back.

PARENTAL CARE IN MAMMALS

● Introduction : Factors governing parental care in mammals ● Categories of young ones ● Carriage of young ones ● Playing with young ones ● Duration of parental care in different species of mammal.

INTRODUCTION

Instinct of parental care is evident in almost all mammals. *Prototherians* are egg laying mammals. A few species (Echidna) of prototheria keep eggs in a brood chamber till hatching. *Metatherians* (Kangaroo, Wallby etc.) give birth to immature young ones. Female keep the young ones till they become matured. *Eutherians* give birth to fully matured child. Instinct of parental care is very high among eutherians and can be observed in even very ferocious animals such as lions, tigers, hyena etc. Female eutherians provide milk to the young and the males provide protection. Since males are not intimately associated with the brood male desertion is common. Even in species in which male are intimately associated with upbringing of brood (some primates and carnivores) do not show development of lactation.

FACTORS GOVERNING PARENTAL CARE IN MAMMALS

Maynard Smith (1978) discusses factors that govern parental care in mammal

(i) Female-effectiveness

The number of brood and care taken by the female vary. For smaller number of broods the female is more effective in providing parental care. For greater number of broods she is unable because she exhausts her energy in brood production.

(ii) Male-effectiveness

Those species of eutherians in which males protect their females by maintaining a territory tend to mate with less number of females but care of the brood is increased.

PARENTAL CARE IN LANGURS

The female usually gives birth to a single baby, but twin births are not uncommon. The gestation period is about 190 to 220 days. The newbord langur has more intimate co-ordination than a human baby. It clings to its mother's belly and retains grip even when she is running, jumping or climbing trees.

Newborns are also called black coats (BC) because their fur coat is black color persists for 3 months. Between 3 – 4 months, the baby is called changing coat (CC) when its fur color changes from black to brown and thence to white. Those above 4 months of age are called white coats (WC) and this lasts upto 7 months. Hanuman langurs upto the age of 7 months

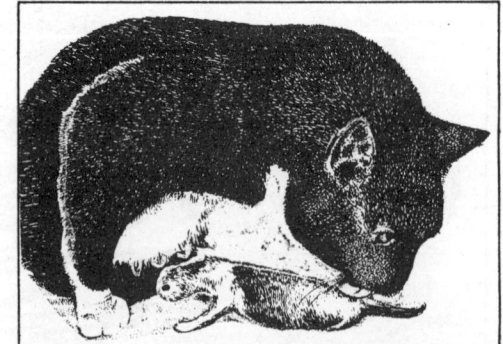

Fig. 7.26. A mother cat licking newborn young to remove the foetal membran and label it as its offspring recognition.

are designated "infant–I: Infants between 7 months to 1 year are considered" infant–II. This phase continues till the infants are weaned. Weaning is usually complete by 12 to 16 months. Weaned infants aged above 16 months and up to 3 years are considered juveniles. Females remain in cycle till they deliver their first infant around the age of 4 years are considered young adults. Females beyond 4 years of age are called as adults.

PARENTAL CARE IN RHESUS MONKEY

Monkeys are physical climbers. And, it seems, they are social climbers. Primatologist Frans B. M. de Waal found an unusual pattern of behaviour in rhesus monkey. A mother monkey holding her infant would pick up and also hold wandring second infant for periods ranging from a few seconds to ten minutes in lenth.

De Waal began to compile statistics on the frequency of what he calls "double-holds" and now belives that the mother was trying to choose her baby's friends. In more than 90 percent of the cases the mother would pick up infant from a family that ranked higher than hers in the monkey group's social structure.

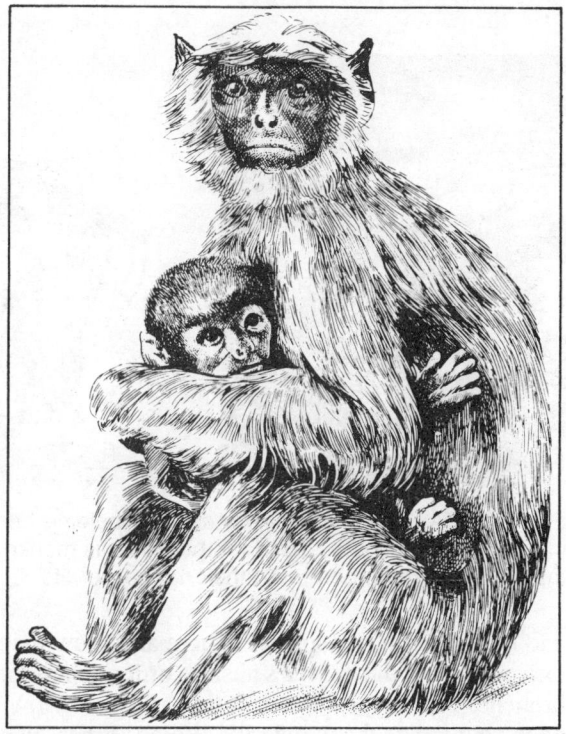

Fig. 7.27. Mother Hanuman Langur carrying her baby.

"He also believes that the purpose is to see their offspring play with peers from high-ranking families rather than low-ranking ones". And the sense of purpose is strong : in several cases, de Waal and his researchers saw a mother spot an infant from a higher-ranking family, rush off to pick up her own infant, then dash back to pick up the other for a double-hold. "It is an interesting human parallel".

CATEGORIES OF YOUNG ONES

It is possible to distinguish two categories of mammal young. In the first category are *entirely dependent* on their mothers for the early part of their lives. Examples are young rabbits and kittens which are born blind and without hair. In the second category are *sufficiently well-developed at birth* to move around independently. This is the case with many ungulates such as the roe-deer and the chamois (*Rupicapra rupicapra* - goatlike mammal).

Roe-deer and hares give birth on the ground, whereas the female rabbit digs a special burrow which she carefully closes off after each visit to the pups to suckle them.

Mammals make numerous kinds of house to protect their young ones. Some mammals, for example, most bats, make use of natural hollows such as rock fissures, tree hollows and caves. Mongoose (a small tropical animal with fur and that kills snakes) very intelligently occupy the termitarium of termites. Other dig burrows of varying depth and comlexity (mole, rabbit, vole) or take over and enlarge burrows which have already been dig by another mammal (fox). In certain cases nests are constructed above ground level and they may look rather like bird's nests, as in the case with those of the harvest mouse

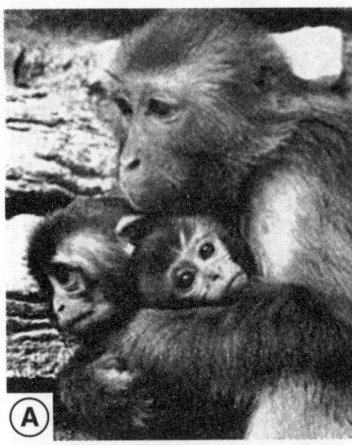
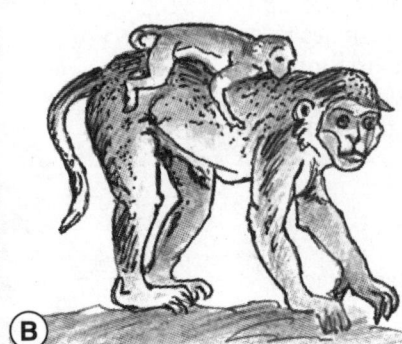
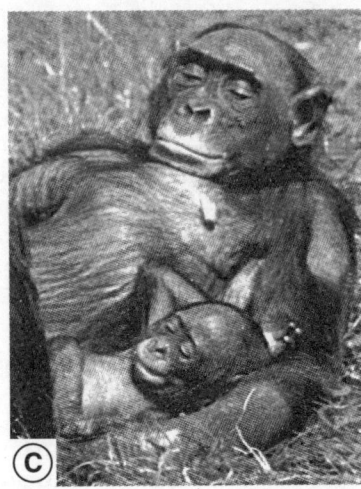

Fig. 7.28. (A) A mother Rhesus monkey holding her infant would pick up and also hold wandering second infant for some minutes. (B) A mother Rhesus monkey carrying her child on her back. (C) Unlike Chimpanzee male bonobo (son) bond with their mother for life.

and of some squirrel species. There are a few mammals which build their own nest. The most striking example being the beaver's nest. In order to build its den, the beaver will begin by accumulating a pile of branches close to the water. It then digs a burrow into the bank below the water level. This eventually opens out inside the wood pile. Which is then gnawed into appropriate shape in addition to the family den which houses a pair and their offspring. There are other dens which are temporarily occupied notably that which the male uses when he is separated from the female while she is in family way and giving birth.

The male may sometimes play an active role in the rearing of the young in mammals. In both wolves and foxes, the male provides a great deals of the food for the family while the young are being reared. The male roe-deer defend his offspring against intruders. Tigers and lions have no further relationship with the female after mating, even then the males sometimes show a certain degree of interest in their offspring.

CARRIAGE OF YOUNG ONES

Domestic cat, lion and the female leopard carries her cubs by the scruff of the neck when she feels they are threatened. A large number of mammal species exhibit this kind of infant transport.

Although true maternal behaviour starts with the birth of the infant, preparation for it occurs during the later stages of pregnancy in many animals. The female may move away from her fellows and begin to build a nest. The chest fur of female rabbits become loosened at this time so that it can be more easily plucked out to line the nest.

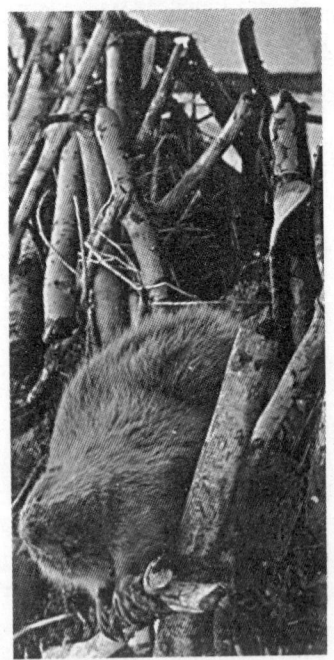

Fig. 7.29. Beaver's nest.

In the monogamous primate species a much greater degree of male parental care is evident (Passingham, 1982). For example, male marmosets (*Callithrix*) and tamarins (*Leontidues'*) carry young and returns them to the mother only for nursing. Similarly, male titi monkeys spend more time with the infants than does the mother.

COMMUNAL NURSING IN HOUSE MICE

House mice live in social units consisting of a single male and more females. The male mates with each female in his unit but provides no parental care to the pups. When there is more than one female in a reproductive unit, the females have ample opportunities for co-operation and conflict, especially since they all litter at about the same time and rear their pups in a commnal nest. The main reason for the better performance of mother rearing their pups in communal nests is that a given female suckles not only her own offspring but also those of her breeding partner-may be considered as *aunt behaviour*. Perhaps even more striking to the ethologist in the apparent inability of the

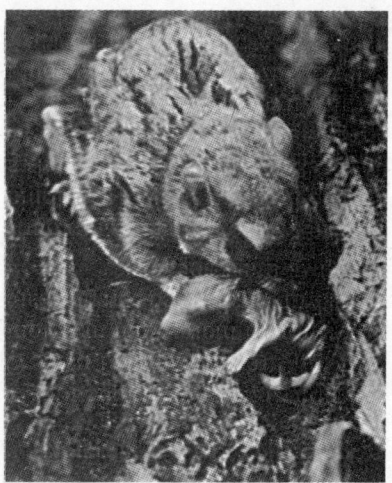

Fig. 7.30. Flying squirrel use hole on tree as nest. Here mother is carrying her young.

females in a communal nest to discriminate between their own offspring and those of their partners, even when there is considerable age difference between their own and alien pups.

PLAYING WITH YOUNG ONES

For many mammal species, play is at least as important as the mother's behaviour for determining the future social behaviour of the developing young. Play behaviour in the young can, in fact, depend quite heavily on maternal behaviour.

Harry F. Harlow showed that a young rhesus monkey deprived of its mother from birth onwards was unable to engage in play with other young monkeys provided as companions. The deprived youngster always proved to be indifferent, or even aggressive towards its companions, and on attaining sexual maturity it was unable to perform normal copulation. In physical terms play favours better motor co-ordination, improves respiratory functions and develops the musculature, thus preparing the growing animal more effectively for adult life. For this reason, play behaviour is particularly developed in predatory mammals. The cubs of lions, tigers, wolves and foxes, which are all rather clumsy and ungainly in their initial scuffles, rapidly acquire greater ability in both attack and avoidance. Chasing play also enables young gazelles monkeys to develop a capacity for high-speed running which improves their chances of escaping the jaws of their many predators. Many of these observations concerning the importance of maternal behaviour and of play also apply to human infants, to the extent that we depend in similar ways on the effects of experience.

DURATION OF PARENTAL CARE

The duration of parental care varies species to species. Period of parental care lasts for more than a year in grizzly bear. Human being take care of their children and grand children life long.

PARENTAL TOLERANCE OF SIBLICIDE

A kind of parental puzzle is the tolerance of some parent birds and mammals of lethal aggression among their offspring, or siblicide.

BIRDS

In the great egret, brothers and sisters fight for possession of the fish their parents bring to the nest. The dominant individuals in a brood may kill their sibling rivals by forcing them out of the nest.

A larger, first-born chick pushes its smaller sibling outside the nest and away from the shade provided by the brooding parent. Parents leave the ejected offspring to die of exposure before its very eyes. Parents do not interfear in nature's selection for survival of the fittest.

MAMMALS

Female spotted hyena give birth to their newborns (one to three are born at a time) at the entrance to a small undergroung burrow. Inside the burrow, the newborn hyenas can employ their fully functional canines and incisors in slashing attacks on one another. Some youngsters are able to kill their sibling by wounding them and by preventing them from leaving the burrow to nurse by mother.

Incidence of killing to sibling takes place in presence of nonintervening parents. Now the question arises how mother tolerate killing of her child? One hypothesis is that parents do

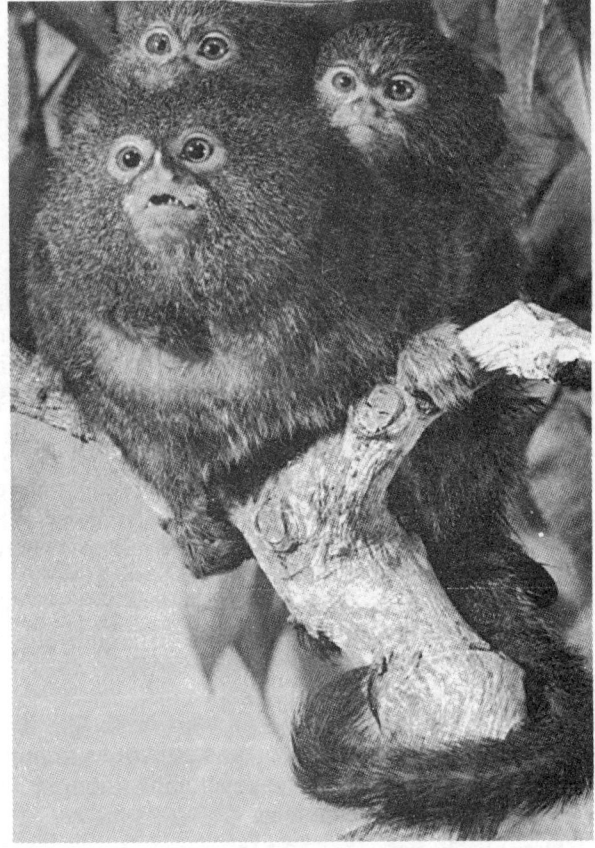

Fig. 7.31. A Marmoset father carrying his twin sons.

not gain from these actions, which have evolved because of advantages enjoyed by winning siblings, not because of selection on parental behaviour. There are situation in which we expect the fitness interests of parents and offspring to conflict with each other.

The significant feature of siblicidal attack is that they occur primarily when two sibs are of the same sex. Then, let us assume that fitness benefits to an offspring are derived from the removal of a competitor of the same sex but not one of the opposite sex. From a parent's standpoint, its fitness may well be reduced when siblicide occurs, particularly since the weak offspring could have survived, had its mother been permitted to care for it. Sibling rivalry and siblicide actually help parents deliver their care

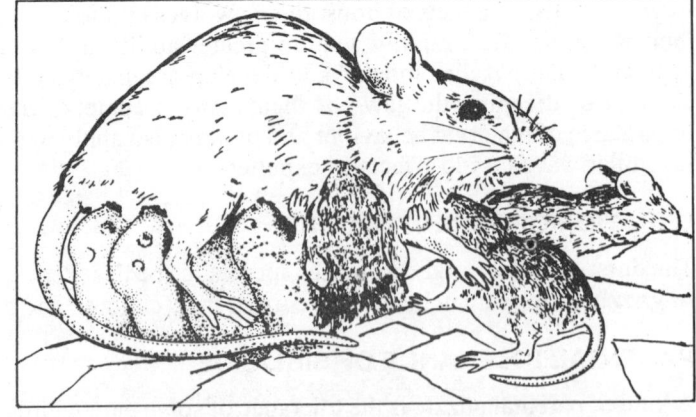

Fig. 7.32. Communal Breast feeding in rat.

only to those children that have a good chance of surviving to reproduce, while enabling parents to keep their food delivery costs to a minimum. Siblicide may be considered as indirect method of family planning and keeping the equal ratio of both sexes in population.

OFFSPRING RECOGNITION IN BATS

Pregnant females of Mexican free-tailed bat migrate to certain caves in the American Southwest, where they form vast colonies of millions of individuals. After giving birth to a single pup, the mother bat leaves her offspring clinging to the roof of the cave in an extraordinarily dense clusture that may contain about 4000 pups per sq. meter. When a mother returns to nurse her infant she should be confused due to shoulder-to-shoulder packing of pups. Early observers believed that females could not possibly relocate their own offspring and they nurse communally. Recent direct observation indicate that females and their pups are almost always able to recognize each other through vocal and olfactory communication.

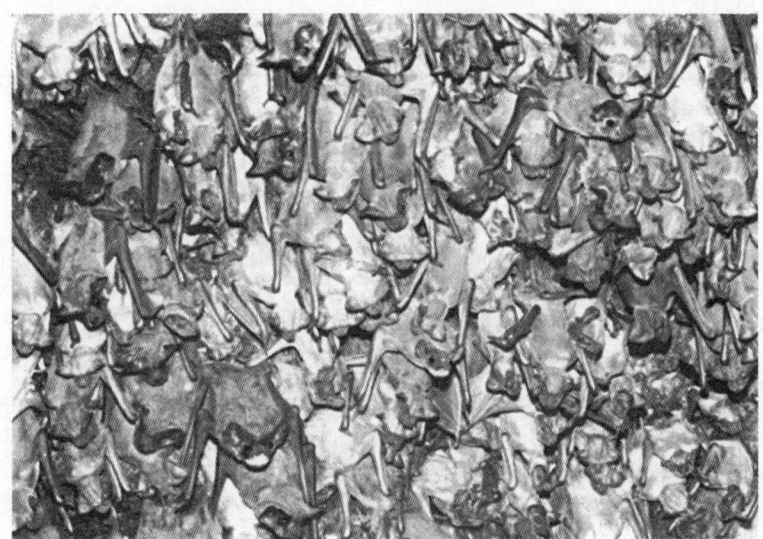

Fig. 7.33. Creche of Maxican Free-tailed Bat pups left together by their mothers, while they forage outside the creche.

WHY MOTHERS ARE SO MUCH MORE LIKELY THAN FATHERS TO PROVIDE CARE FOR THEIR OFFSPRING

In fact, females are considerably more likely than males to be the care providers throughout the animal kingdom as a whole in species in which only one sex provides parental care. One hypothesis to account for this fact is that because the female has already invested so much energy in contributing a large egg to the zygote, she is therefore predisposed to additional parental care to her offspring.

"*Low reliability of paternity*" links female parental care to the fact that female are more likely to be the parent of an offspring they assist than are males. If a female lays a fertilized egg or gives birth to an offspring, this progeny will definitely have 50% of her genes. A male has no such assurance, especially if his partner practices internal fertilization, in which case she may have already mated with another male and have used his sperm to fertilize her eggs. Therefore, to the extent that a male runs the risk of caring for progeny other than his own, the benefit of parental care falls for a male.

"Gamete order hypothesis paternity" is that the sex that provides care is determined by the order in which eggs and sperms are released. Whichever sex can leave first after mating is predicted to do so, leaving the other to care for the offspring, if parental care is to be given. By this theoretical argument, internal fertilization should be linked with female parental care, because after donating his sperm internally a male is free to desert his mate, leaving her with the decision to make about whether or not to provide parental care. But when fertilization is external, females often deposit their eggs before males shed their sperm, giving the females a brief moment in which to flee, leaving males holding the eggs.

EXERCISE

1. Define parental care and mention different aspects of parental care. Describe parental care in animals without backbones.
2. Give an account of parental care in fishes giving suitable diagrams.
3. Write an essay on parental care in amphibians. Give suitable diagrams to support your statement.
4. Write an account of brooding and nesting behaviour of birds.
5. Describe parental care behaviour of mammals.
6. Write short notes on nest parasitism, nest sanitation, and nesting period.
7. Describe different methods of carriage of young ones in mammals.
8. Describe nesting and brooding behaviour of flightless birds.
9. Write about Precocial and Altricial young.
10. What is incubation? Describe incubation of eggs in birds.
11. Write short notes on playing with young ones in mammals.
12. How parents tolerate killing of their children by stronger offspring?
13. Why mothers are so much more likely than fathers to provide care for their children?
14. Describe in brief "Offspring recognition in Bat".
15. Write a short note on "Parental care of Crocodile.

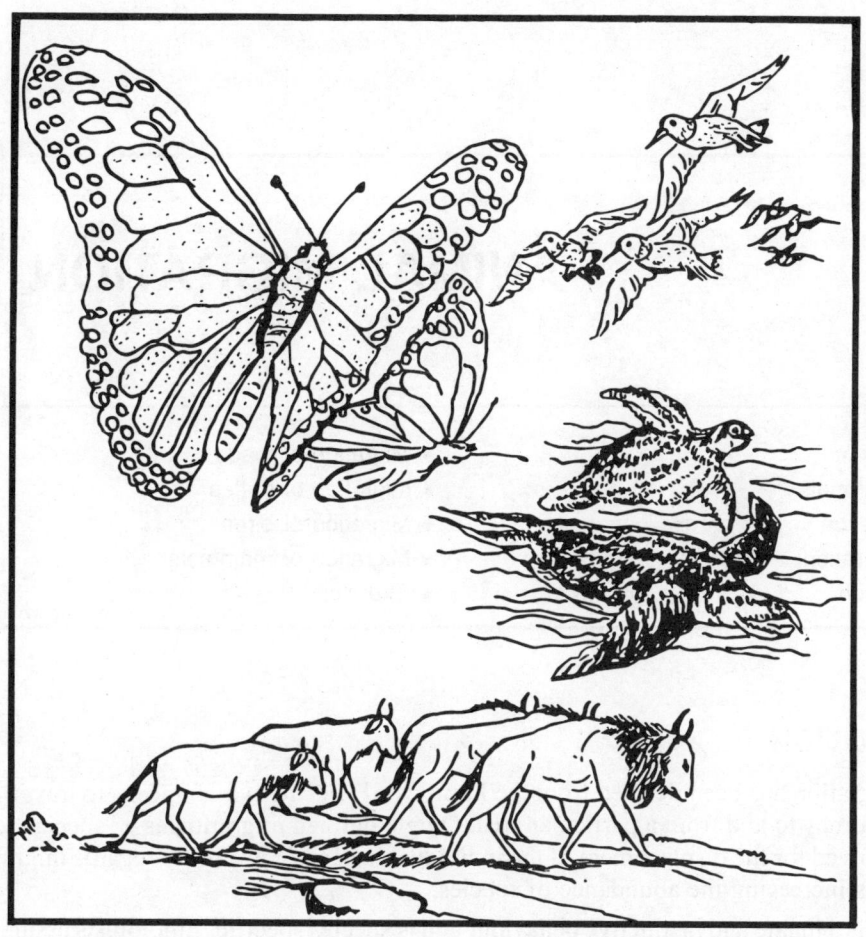

Environmental conditions on earth vary from place to place and also at the same place depending on the season. The seasonal changes in some parts of the earth are very adverse and threaten the survival of the animal population. Some species adapt and hibernate to meet the adverse conditions of the place they live. But many species escape from such adverse climate by moving to more favourable climate. On return of the favourable climate they return to their homeland. Journey of animals to and from a particular area is called migration. Migratory species take these journeys periodically.

If someone mentions migration, people generally think of birds. That is not surprising because bird migration is easy to watch and has fascinated many people for centuries. But birds are not the only creatures that migrate. Many other animal species make these seasonal journeys. They may not cover the same great distances, but they are still spectacular in their own way. Here is an interesting account of what it is all about.

ANIMAL MIGRATION 8

- Introduction
- Migratory animals
- Insect migration
- Lobster migration
- Fish migration
- Migration of toads
- Migration of turtles
- Migration of birds
- Migration of mammals
- Exercise

INTRODUCTION

The word migration has been derived from the Latin word *migrare* which means to travel. Migration is the regular journey to and from a particular area. Dingle defined migration as a "specialized behaviour specially involved for the displacement of the individual in space". Niekolky regards migration as adaptation towards increasing the abundance of species.

Migration is a innate and instinctive behaviour and is species specific. Ethologists assume that migration in some animal species was initiated as a means of survival but later on by virtue of Natural Selection, it became genetically determined fixed pattern of behaviour but differed from species to species.

Migration is different from unidirectional movement and those in which animals are helplessly carried by some other agency. In fact migration is a two way journey including *emigration* and *immigration*. *Emigration* is the outward journey from the feeding place to the breeding ground and *immigration* is the inward or return journey from the breeding place to the homeland. Migratory species take these journeys periodically. Thus migration appears to be a dynamic process and many animal species use this behaviour for their survival.

Migration creates many puzzles for persons interested in various aspects of phenomenon. What tells an animal where to go? What are causes of migration? How do migratory species (especially fishes – eels) know it is the same stream their parents left months ago. These are interesting questions regarding migration of animals and this chapter deals with these critical questions.

MIGRATORY ANIMALS

Following seven groups of animals may be considered as prominent migrants.

1. *Arthropods* : Crabs, Locusts and Monarch butterfly.
2. *Agnathans* : Petromyzon
3. *Fishes* : Slamon, Eel, Indian shad (Hilsa).
4. *Amphibians* : Frogs, Newts.
5. *Reptiles* : Green sea turtles.
6. *Birds* : Swifts, Sparrow, Robin, Oriole, Golden plover, Humming birds, Paradise flycatcher, Grey-lag goose, Cranes, Flamingo, Arctic tern, Black necked grebes etc.
7. *Mammals* : Caribou, Seals, Sea lions, Whales, Dolphins, Lemmings, Bison, Zebra, Wildebeest etc.

ARTHROPOD MIGRATION

Many insects travel long distances to find new sources of food and to colonize new places. Most insects make their journey through the air and rely on air currents and wind direction. However, such travel is not true migration. The insects do not return to where they started and their journeys tend to be accidental rather than deliberate.

Some butterflies such as Red Admirals, Painted Ladies and Clouded Yellows really migrate. They migrate northwards through Europe in spring. They cannot usually survive a British winter, but each spring they make their way north and reach the British Isles in varying numbers. Some will stay here to breed and there are a few reports of these butterflies flying south again in the autumn.

MIGRATION OF MONARCH BUTTERFLY

Another well-known butterfly migrant is the Monarch butterfly (*Danaus plexippus*). This butterfly is common over most of the Eastern United States and Southern Canada. It skims and dips in summer over fields and gardens from texas to New England, from Florida to Minnesota. But in winter the monarch vanishes from the colder regions. Where does it go? Canadian Zoologist Dr. Fred A. Urguahart with the tireless help of his wife, Norah, has spent much of his time since 1937 studying the migration of the monarch butterfly.

Millions of monarch butterfly move from Eastern United States and Canada to spend the winter in Mexico. A few Eastern monarch fly down the Florida peninsula and eventually reach Yucatan and Central America.

Migration occurs only in monarch population confronted with seasonal changes in the availability of the milkweed plants upon which females lay their eggs. In the Eastern United States milkweeds die off in late autumn and grow again in spring. Thus, there is a strong seasonal fluctuation in the resource base needed by monarch if they are to reproduce, and the butteflies living there migrate. In some areas of the Western United States milkweeds are present year-round, and here the movement of monarchs is much reduced.

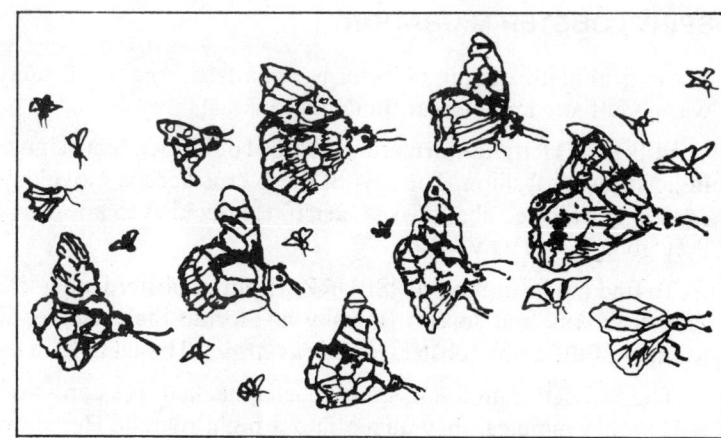

Fig. 8.1. Monarch butterfly – *Danaus plexippus*.

Monarch butterflies have evolved a migratory pattern that enables them to wait out the non-reproductive months with reduced risk of death from freezing. Inspite of exhaustion and desiccation during long distance travel the new land provide them suitable space for better life and therefore they prefer to travel long distance inspite of several adversities.

Monarch butterfly travel long distance from Canada and Eastern United States to Mexico. Once they are in Mexico, they hang together in masses on fir trees high in the mountains of central Mexico where they spend the winter. Monarch butterfly stream from winter roosts in fir trees in central Mexico to summer in northern latitudes, copulating and laying their eggs atop milkweeds to foster new generations along the way. Several generations are born, breed and die before the final generation reaches Eastern United States and Canada.

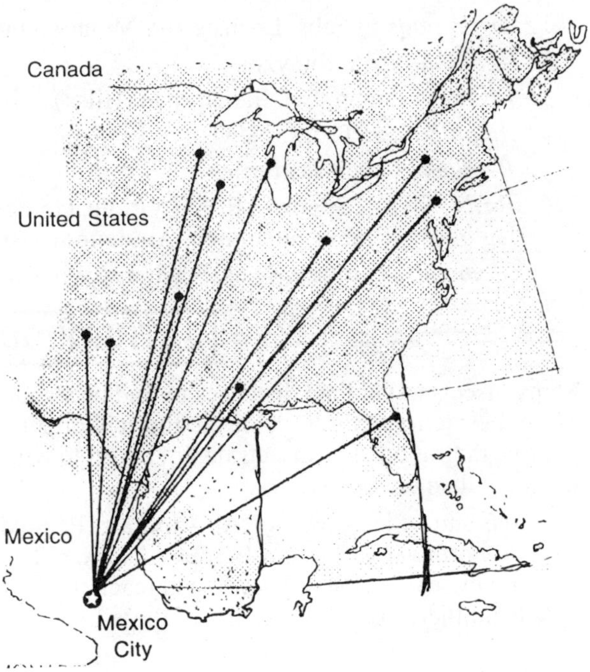

Fig. 8.2. Migrating route of monarch butterfly.

With the old monarchs died and all ties to the ancestral site apparently cut, an incredible thing happens to monarch butterflies that they have never been to Mexico, travel and roost there the next winter.

Dr. Urguahart also collected some other facts in context of monarch migration. He learned that almost all males die on the way north from the wintering grounds. He also confirmed that the insects would not fly at night. One tagged butterfly - captured, released and captured again - flew about 128 kilometers in one day.

SPINY LOBSTER MIGRATION

Zoological name of spiny lobster is *Panulirus argus*. It is a crustacean and found 25 feet down in the warm Gulf stream of Great Bahama Bank.

William F. Herrnkind, a marine biologist of Florida State University observed a row of lobsters marching in head-to-tail fashion. The row of these crustaceans move day and night several kilometers along the sandy, unprotected shallow sea beach. He decided to know : Where did they come from? Where were they going? And why?

To find out he organized "SLURP" (Spiny Lobster Undersea Research Project) in 1969 with scientist Paul Kanciruk and Joseph Halusky at Florida State University. They began probing the mysterious journey of the spiny lobster, *Panulirus argus*. The team focused on the Bimini area.

The SLURP team found spiny lobster stacked like cord-wood under a shelf off Bimini at dusk (Fig. 8.3) within minutes, they queue into a night march. The animals make initial contact with their long antennae; they keep aligned by touching their shorter inner antennules to the tail ahead - often hooking their front legs around it. Gluing a transmitting "saddle" to these migrants they tracked the creature with a directional receiver.

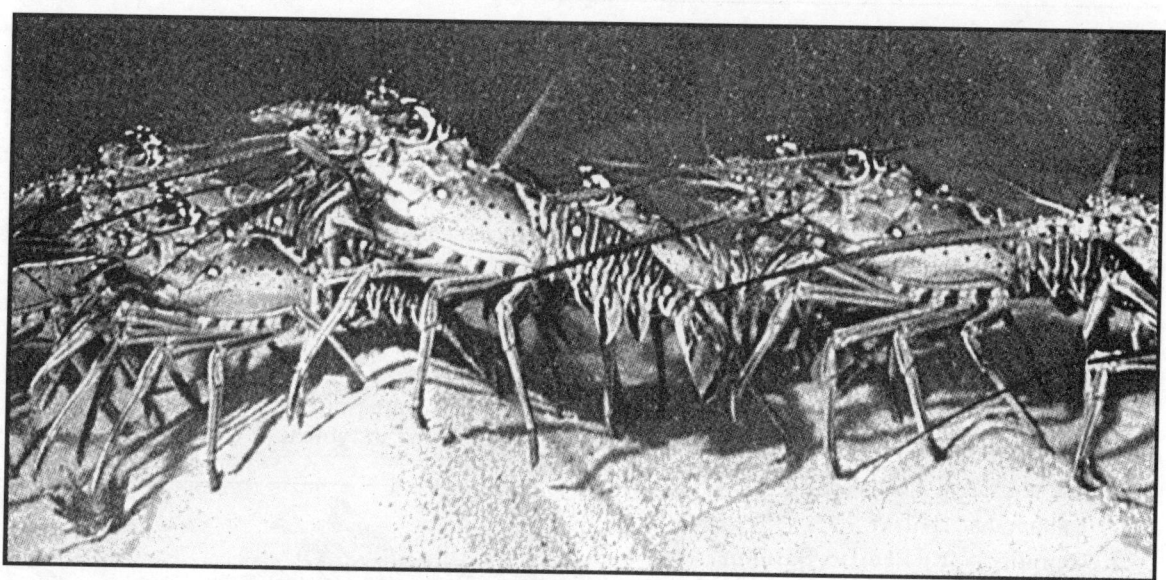

Fig. 8.3. Numerous spiny lobsters queue into a night march.

In one week Bimini lobster can move as far as 80 kilometers, heading almost south across 1.25 kilometer wide plateau formed by the islands and the western edge of the Great Bahama Bank (map). This lobster is nocturnal but unstoppable while migrating. When they transferred one group of migrating lobster to a vinyl pool at Bimini's Learner Marine Laboratory, these lobsters marched around it day and night for two weeks.

In the wake of these lobster caravans, a trail of mysteries remains. As yet, SLURP, team is not certain of the animals' precise origin and destination. However, autumn's waning daylight appears to be a factor that catalyzes the migrations.

They gave one result : population redistribution to new feeding grounds and possibly new breeding grounds too, since all the migrants they saw were sexually mature or about to mature.

But the instinctive behaviour may well be an evolutionary holdover, a living echo from glacial periods, the last some ten thousand years ago. To survive the much colder waters, perhaps the lobster had to find a warmer seasonal habitat—or perish. By retaining the inner drive today, in an interglacial period, it may thus be prepared for the next ice age. But this theory needs further study.

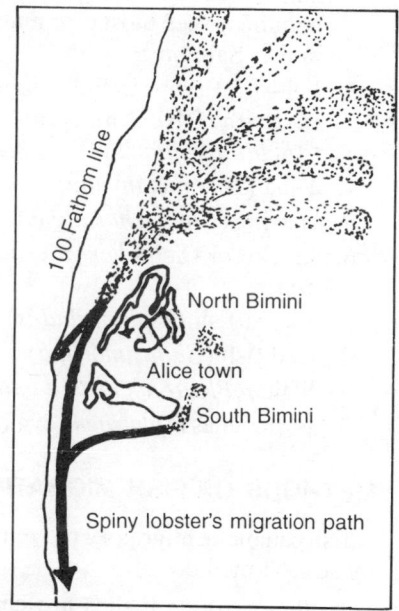

Fig. 8.4. Dr. Herrnkind and his team discovered the migration path of spiny lobster.

FISH MIGRATION

• Introduction • Migratory fishes • Types of fish migration • Diadromous, Potamodromous, Oceanodromous • Fish navigation • Causes of fish migration • Speed and distance covered during migration • Advantages and disadvantages of fish migration.

INTRODUCTION

Usually fishes live in a constant habitat and restrict their movement within a particular territorial limits. But there are a few fish species which migrate from fresh water to sea water or vice-versa. In mature adult fish, migration is mainly for spawning and feeding.

MIGRATORY FISHES

According to Cohen (1970) about 8000 fresh water species, 12000 marine and a few estuary species of fish are migratory. Approximately 70% of total migrants are found in typical (warm) waters.

A few migratory fishes are :
1. Indian Shad (Hilsa)
2. Salmon – (a) Pacific Salmon (*Onchorhynchus nerka*). It is threatened species (b) Atlantic Salmon (*Salmo salar*). Instinct of homing is seen most prominently in the 'Salmon'.
3. Eel – (a) European Eel (*Anguilla rostrata*) (b) American Eel (*Anguilla vulgaris*)
4. Tuna (*Thunnus thynnus*)
5. Herring (*Clupea harangus*)
6. Mackerel (*Seomber microlepidotus*)
7. Sword fish (*Xiphia gladus*)
8. Cod fish (*Gadus morhua*)
9. Plaice (*Pleuronectis platessa*)
10. Barracudas (*Sphyraena zygaena*)

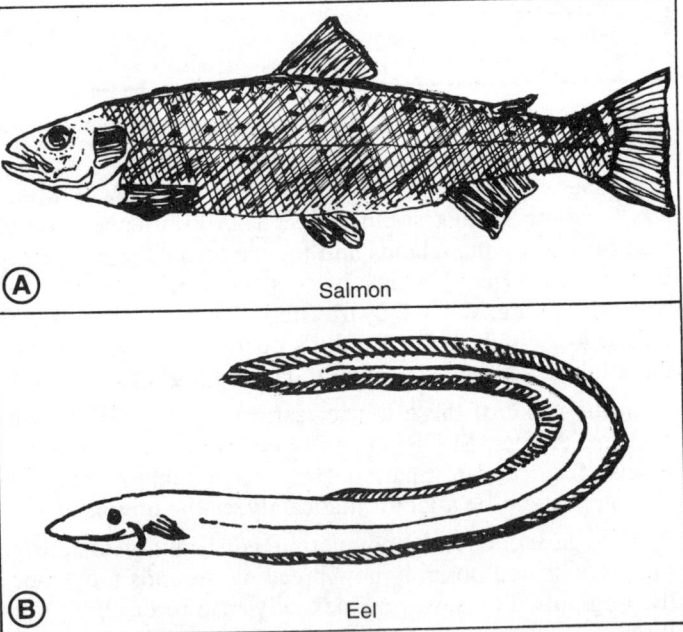

Fig. 8.5. Salmon and Eels are true migratory fishes. Eels breed in the sea and the young of some species migrate to freshwater viz., rivers where they grow into adults. Those that live in European rivers, return to the sargasso sea near the West Indies to breed and their young then travel to the same traditional rivers in Europe. Salmon behave quite differently. They breed in rivers but spend part of their lives at sea. They only come back when they are ready to breed.

METHODS OF FISH MIGRATION

A fish can make migratory movements by several methods :
1. *By drifting* : Fishes are carried passively by water currents.
2. *Random locomotory movements*: Locomotory movements that is

random in direction. Fishes released from a point in a uniform environment and spreading out in all directions; the process is called dispersal and lead to uniform distribution of the species.

3. *Oriental swimming movements* : Fishes move in particular direction.
   (a) Either towards or away from one habitat.
   (b) At some angle to an imaginary line running between them and the source of stimulation.

TYPES OF FISH MIGRATION

On the basis of procurement of food, spawning, climate, osmoregulation, water current etc. fish migration is recognized of following types.

1. *Alimental migration* : Migration in search of food and water. Examples are Salmon, Cods, Herrings, Tunna (marine fishes), Grass-carp, Chinese roach, Gudgeons (fresh water fishes) etc.

2. *Spawning or gametic migration* : Migration for the purpose of spawning is migration in true sense and is also called gametic migration.

3. *Climatic or wintering migration* : Migration to secure more suitable climatic conditions. It is initiated due to low BMR (Basic Metabolic Rate) either after feeding or before spawning. Examples are Salmon, Sturgeons.

4. *Osmoregulatory migration* : Migration, for the propose of spawning, feeding and wintering can all be regarded as protective or osmoregulatory migration.

5. *Detanatant/Contranatant* : During migration fishes move either in the direction of the water current or against it (i) The swimming of fishes in the direction of water current is known as detanatant. (ii) Movement of migrating fishes against the water current is called contranatant. Movement of adult salmon from sea to river is an example of contranatant migration.

On the basis of direction Myers (1949) recognised three patterns of fish migration :

1. Diadromous
2. Potamodromous, and
3. Oceanodromous.

1. DIADROMOUS MIGRATION

Fish migration between fresh water and sea is known as diadromous migration. Diadromous migration is further classified into the following three categories :

(i) *Anadromous migration or Anadromy* : Journey of marine fishes from sea to fresh water (river) for spawning (breeding) is called Anadromous Migration. Many marine fishes like Salmon, Salmo (trout), Shad (Hilsa), Striped bass, Lampreys travel long distances in the sea and run up to the river to spawn in fresh water.

Salmon and Hilsa travel several thousand Km. in the sea, and then several hundred Km. into the fresh water rivers to reach the spawning grounds. They migrate in pairs. Black spots develop on the body of female Salmon and red spots on the body of male Salmon during the journey. The reproductive organs ripen and the alimentary canal shrinks. Female makes a saucer shaped nest in the river bed. Females lay the eggs in this saucer shaped nest. Then the male releases the sperm and the eggs are fertilized. After egg laying, the spent fishes return to their home i.e. feeding place in the sea. This upstream and downstream journey takes about one year.

Young Salmon do not immigrate immediately. They grow in full size and then return to sea. Salmon attain sexual maturity in about seven years. After attaining full sexual maturity they return to fresh water rivers for breeding purpose. As they proceed up the rivers, they come to many path and turns, water falls etc. but they return to their exact place of origin where they took birth seven years ago.

Both the Atlantic (*Salmo*) and Pacific (*Oncorhynchus*) forms have this practice, but there are some differences between the two. After spending three to four years at their feeding grounds at sea, the Salmon return and ascend the fresh water streams. Both sexes make the journey together. After spawning the Pacific species die. But some of the Atlantic species survive and return to sea again. They are able to spawn a second or third time. From the time they return to fresh water until they spawn, the Salmons stop feeding and depend on the fat present in body for energy. After hatching, the larval fish live for some time in the streams before immigrating to sea. Some species stay here only for a few weeks, but others may remain for months. Young Salmon do not return to the sea until their salt-secreting cells had developed. Experimental evidence show that strong olfactory sense of Salmon determines its homing into the original birth place for different odours.

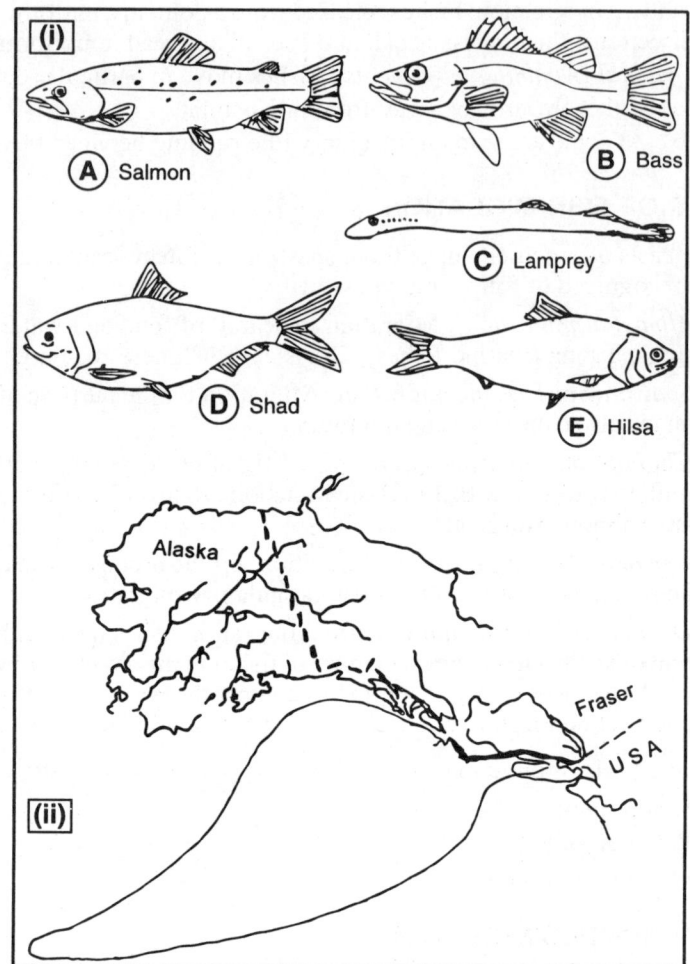

Fig. 8.6. (i) Anadromous fishes. (ii) Anadromous migration by salmon. Salmon live in northeastern Pacific Ocean (Black dot area) and migrate to British Columbia's Fraser River to breed.

Hilsa also show Anadromous migration. These fishes travel from Estuary to fresh water rivers during the breeding season. They travel from Bay of Bengal to Ganges and have been reported upto Allahabad during breeding season. Farraka dam is disturbing its migration and breeding and therefore, Hilsa fish is on the verge of extinction.

Some fishes travel from sea to estuaries. These are called semi-migratory-fish. Roaches and white fishes are known examples of semi-migratory fishes. The three-spined stickleback (*Gasterosteus aculeatus*) live in sea but enters fresh water to breed.

(ii) *Catadromous migration or Catadromy* : Fish which spend most of their life in fresh water, but travel to the ocean for spawning are called Catadromous. Fresh water eel (*Anguilla*) is the best example of this types. There are 16 species of fresh water eels. *Anguilla japonica* spawns in the North pacific sea. *A. australis* spawn in the South Pacific sea. *A. rostratta* (American eel) and

A. anguilla (European eel) spawn in the western North Atlantic (Sargasso) sea.

European eel (*Anguilla anguilla*) is yellow in colour which represent their feeding and growing phase. 8–10 years old male eel and 10–18 years old female eel prepare for migration. This changes from yellow to silvery eels which represent their breeding phase with the approach of autumn. Their digestive tract compresses and become functionless and they stop feeding. Gonads cover the entire coelomic cavity. Eyes become large, lips thinner, the pectoral fins more pointed.

The silvery eel migrate down the rivers reaching the sea in late summer. These eels travel 3 to 4 thousand km, reaching their spawning grounds in the Western Atlantic Ocean, South of Bermuda. It is believed that the eels spawn at a depth of about 400–500 meters below the surface at 16–17^{0}C. The parents die after spawning. Eggs hatched into a larva known as leptocephalus. The larva is flat leaf-like transparent, tiny creature, provided with long needle like teeth. These possess large

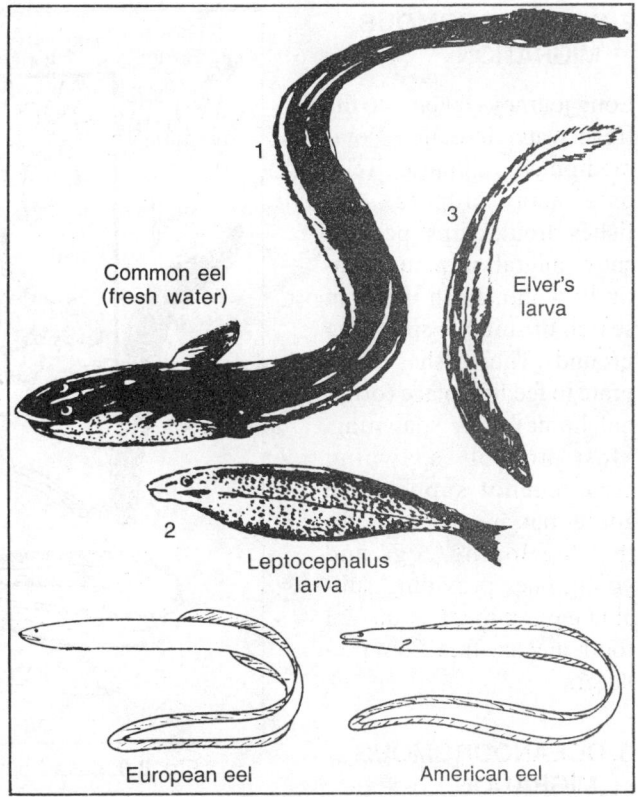

Fig. 8.7. Catadromous fishes. Fresh water Eel is catadromous. Two types of larva (leptocephalus and elver) are found in life cycle of fresh water common eel.

eyes and lead pelagic life. The larvae swim and begin their long homeward journey and move in the easterly direction. They take 3 years in reaching their home in the river. During journey leptocephalus metamorphose and attain a length of about 8 mm and now called *Elver's larva*.

For the first lap elver's larva rely on drift. They are swept by the current up towards the North American and European coastline. Once at the coast, it is time for the elver to show its mettle. When the ebb tide turns away the shore, the elvers lie close to the sea floor, letting the tide wash over them. But when the current turns towards the shore, they rise to the top and are carried closer to the estuary. From then on, the passive life is over and they kick actively against the current to get into the right river. How do they know, it is the same stream their parents left months ago? Behaviourists think it is the odour of the water that elvers identify–*Bulce Domum*, the sweet smell of home.

(iii) *Amphidromous migration* : Migration of fishes from sea to rivers and vice-versa but not for breeding purpose is called amphidromous migration. This is mainly for food and change of environment. This travel may occur regularly at some definite stage of their life cycle. The only example is **Gobies** (Fig. 8.9).

2. POTAMODROMOUS MIGRATION

Long journeys taken into the fresh water is called Pota-modromous migration. Tele-osts, many clupeids, cat fishes, trout, carps, perches show migration pattern en-tirely within fresh water in search of suitable spawning grounds. These fishes immi-grate to feeding place (origi-nal home) after spawning. Most probably spawning areas cannot support the adults but are essential for the developing eggs and young ones providing suit-able environment, abundant food, and are free from pre-dators.

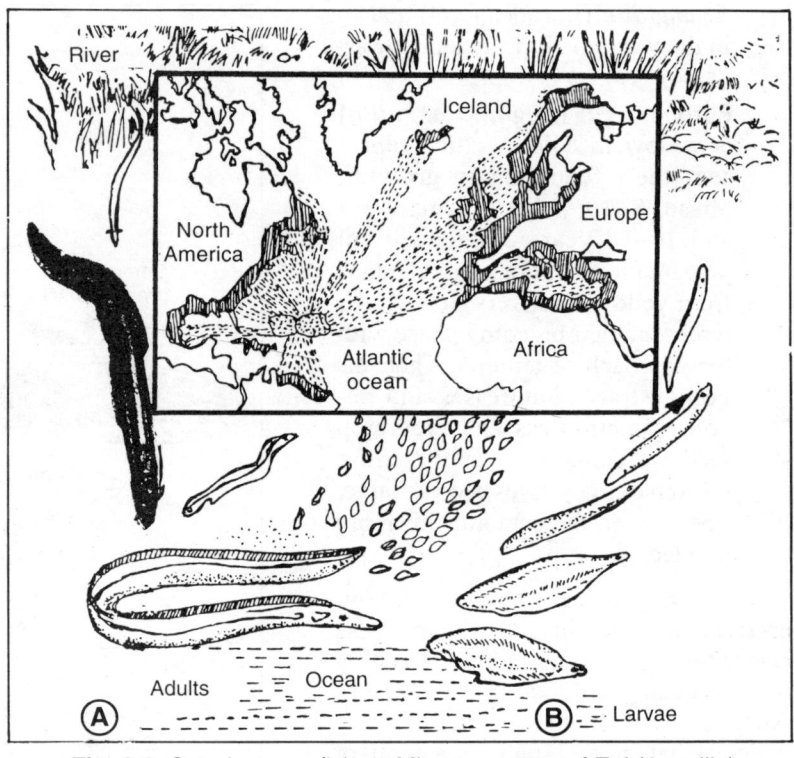

Fig. 8.8. Catadromous fishes. Migratory route of Eel (Anguilla).

3. OCEANODROMOUS MIGRATION

Long to and from journey confined to the sea is called oceanodromous migration. Cod, Mackerels (Scomber), and Atlantic herrings (Clupea) take long journey in the sea from deeper hotter ocean water to the shallow colder shores for the purpose of spawning. This is during breeding season. After spawning they return to their original home.

OTHER KINDS OF MIGRATORY FISHES

(i) *Swordfish and Barracudas* : Swordfish (*Xiphias gladus*) and Barracudas (*Sphyraena*) living in warm tropical sea perform latitudinal migration moving towards the north in spring and south in autumn. These fishes migrate only for suitable climatic conditions and cannot be considered migratories, in strict sense.

(ii) *Herring* : Herrings live in North Pacific and N. Atlantic Oceans. The Atlantic herrings show annual spawning migration, to the spawning ground close to the coast. Eggs do not float but sink (dem-ersal type of eggs). Larvae are pelagic and these larvae are carried by the currents from the spawning ground to the wintering area near the coast, where they feed and grow. The young fish live for two years in coastal

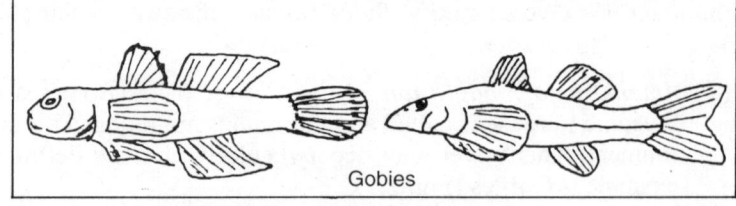

Fig. 8.9. Amphidromous fishes : Gobies.

water and then move along with the older fish in the migration cycle. After spawning parent herrings move towards their summer feeding place (between warm Atlantic and cold Arctic waters). In autumn they move in south-westerly direction along the

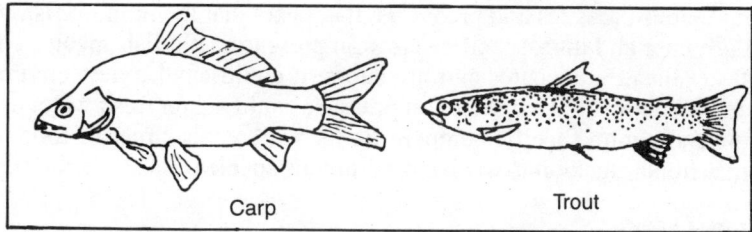

Fig. 8.10. Potamodromous fishes : Carp and Trout.

western coast the Norwegian sea. Then they move to a south-easterly direction in the East Icelandic current. In winter, the ripe herring concentrate in the north of Faroel and then to Norwegian sea. Thus they complete their annual migration. They cover about 3000 kms during this migration.

(iii) *The Arcto Norwegian Cod (Gadus morhua)* : Several distinct population of this species live in the N. Atlantic ocean, Banks island, New Foundland, Labrador, W. Greenlands, E. Greenlands, Island, The North Sea, Baltic Sea, Barent's Sea and Foeroerne. The summer feeding place of cod is Barent's sea.

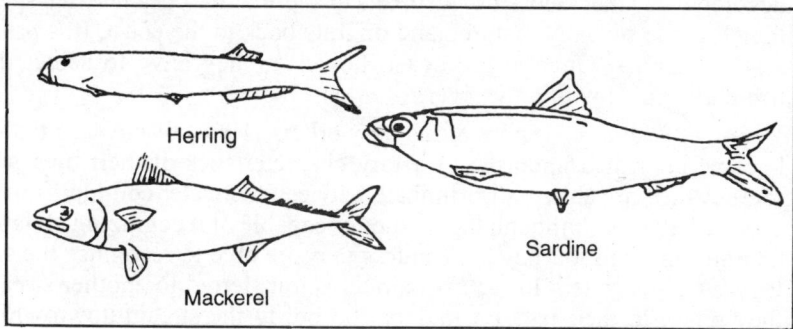

Fig. 8.11. Oceanodromous fishes : Herring, Sardine and Mackerel.

Distribution of cod recedes in autumn but during winter dense concentrations are noted in Bear island. Later, the mature fish leave Bear Island for the Norwegian coast. They reach spawning grounds within the Lofoten Island and spawns from February to June here. Fertilized ova hatch in about 15 days. Larva feed on zooplankton for 6 months. Later they move to the bottom and feed on crustaceans and pelagic fish. On becoming older they join mature fish of the same population and return to their home ground. They cover about 1000 kms during migration.

(iv) *Flat fish (Pleuronectes platessa)* : This fish live in coastal water of N. Europe. Adult fish is bottom dweller but eggs and larva are pelagic. They are carried by current from the spawning to the nursery areas. In about 8 weeks larva metamorphose into young ones. Young ones become bottom dweller and sexually mature at about 3–4 years of age and return to the same spawning grounds. This fish live for 20 years and repeat migration cycle several times.

(v) *The Tuna* : Tuna is the only fish known to be warm blooded. These live in Atlantic and Pacific oceans. This species is known to cover a distance of 10,000 kms. One race of Tuna spawn in Mediterranean in the month of May and June. After spawning the spent fish begin the migration cycle within the Mediterranean sea. Spawned fish migrate usually through the strait of Gibralter and northward as far as Norway. During winter, they travel southward and finally enter the Mediterranean sea to spawn.

Why fishes cross the barrier of salinity?

In context of fish migration question arises why some species move from fresh water to the sea, whereas others move from sea to rivers? Fish in both the environments have evolved along with their numerous parasites and predators. It appears that the migrant fish may have become diadromous due to both inter and intra-specific selection pressures. If a fish species could evolve into a euryhaline species faster than its parasites and predators, it could enter a new environment and escape specific diseases and predators. Such a selection pressure could act on fresh water as well as marine species. Besides this inter-and-intra specific competition for various resources of food in the fresh water or ocean, could act in a similar fashion to evolve diadromous species.

FISH NAVIGATION

The most complex form of fish migration is navigation. What tells a fish where to go? Ichthyologists and behaviourists have pondered this puzzle and come up with temporary answers. Navigation requires not only a directional sense, but also some kind of map. On their long distance migration, fishes use landmarks, particularly as the destination is approached. Migratory Pacific salmon (*Oncorhynchus*) hatch in marine streams of the western United States of America and Canada. After the long stage of development, they swim downstream to the Pacific ocean. After spending two or three years at sea, they become sexually matured and migrate back to the coast. It is probably accomplished by means of a sun compass. Once at the coast, however, they have to select the correct river and the correct tributary stream within the river.

Long research of Hasler & his co-workers (1960) discovered that during the development the fish become imprinted upon the olfactory characteristics of their own native stream. During their return journey they are able to discriminate between the water coming from their native stream and that from other tributaries. Although the Salmon is capable of recognizing all landmarks on their way, they cannot continue on their journey back unless they are able to recognise the scent associated with the tributary they were imprinted. In fact, if Salman is transferred to another stream after the period of imprinting, they return to their native tributary and not to the stream down which they passed on their outward migration. Thus fish navigation studied in Salmon appears to be a complex form of instinctive (innate) and imprinted (learnt) behaviour.

FACTORS CAUSING FISH MIGRATION

The migration of fish is caused by both *intrinsic* and *extrinsic* factors.

A. *Extrinsic factors are* :
1. Searching of food.
2. Photoperiod.
3. Environmental factors, such as salinity, P^H, water current, turbidity etc.
4. Imprinting

B. *Intrinsic factors are* :
1. Instinct.
2. The ripening of gonads, hormones, biological clock etc.

A. Extrinsic factors

1. Searching of food

Availability of food is one of the important factors that is responsible for large scale migration of many species of fishes going out in search of feeding areas. The water current influences considerably the direction of movement of fishes. Eggs and juveniles are transported passively along with the water current to their feeding grounds. After spawning spent Salmons are carried by the river currents towards the sea.

2. Photoperiod

The intensity of light and photoperiod also influences migration of fishes. Lampreys and Sturgeons migrate during the night and Herring migrate during full moon. Rise in temperature of fresh water rivers during summer provides a stimulus to influence upstream movement of Salmon for spawning. Higher temperature of sea water in summer provides a stimulus to Salmon for migration.

3. Environmental factors

Salinity, P^H value, smell and taste of water influence fish migration. Most of the fresh water fishes are stenohaline (almost intolerant to salinity changes). They restrict their activities to fresh water only and do not undertake long distance migration. A few species of fishes-Salmo, Anguilla, Hilsa, Onchorhynchus etc. are euryhaline (tolerant to salinity changes - sea water to fresh water). They travel from sea to river and vice versa.

4. Imprinting

Smell also appears to guide fishes during migration. Strong olfactory sense of Salmon determines its return to the original birth place where its hatching and early development had taken place.

B. Intrinsic factors

1. Instinct

Migration is an innate and instinctive behaviour and it is genetic make up that develop this instinct in the concerned species.

2. Physiological Factors

The ripening of gonads, hormones, biological clock, etc.

The ripening of gonads, hormones, food, biological clock, etc. are the biological factors influencing the fish migration. A number of hormones secreted by the pituitary gland such as Prolactin, Corticotropin, GH etc. are responsible for osmo and ion regulation in fishes during migration. The fresh water to sea water migration and vice-versa in diadromous fishes is associated with well marked endocrine changes.

METHODS OF STUDY OF FISH MIGRATION

Two methods are most commonly used for the study of fish migration :
- (I) Marking and tagging
- (II) Echo ranging technique.

I. MARKING AND TAGGING METHODS INCLUDES THE FOLLOWING TECHNIQUES

1. *Physical marking* : It is generally done by climpping the fins in an orderly fashion. These are commonly used for flat fishes.
2. *Internal marking* : Metallic markers are introduced within the body cavity by specialized marking guns. Internet markers can be detected by special electro magnetic detectors. This method is commonly employed for Herrings.
3. *Hydrostatics tagging* : It consists of a small celluloid cylinder. Within this cylinder printed instruction are kept for the finders, regarding information pertaining to the fish and address of

contact. The method is used for long distance migrants like cods. Other tags in use are the Gilbert tag and internal tags for clupeoids.

4. *Numbered bait hook tagging* : Fishes are marked by numbered bait hooks which the fishes seizes along with the bait. This method is used for Red fish and other deep sea forms.

5. *Plastic flag tagging* : Plastic flag like structures are attached to the back of the fish by nylon thread. This method is used for Cod, haddock and whiting.

II. ECHO RANGING TECHNIQUE INCLUDES TWO METHODS

1. *Acoustic transponding compass system* : A small radio transmitter is fitted inside the body of the fish which transmits a pulse. Special receivers pick up this pulse. This reference pulse is then read through a digital decoder. The position of transmitting fishes is found out and plotted on maps. This method is used for continuous monitoring of the position, depth and direction of movement of a fish.

2. *Ultrasonic transmitter system* : An ultrasonic transmitter is fitted in the body cavity of fish. The transmitter sends out ultrasonic sound waves with the help of which movements of the fish can be found out. This method is usually used to study the migration of Salmon.

Speed, Distance, Duration of the fishes during migration

The average speed of fish migration is 3 times the length of the fish per second (body length x 3/sec.). The distance covered by Salmon, Cod and Eel between feeding and spawning ground may be over 1100 kms. The duration of migration varies species to species.

Advantages of Migration to fishes

The greatest advantage derived from the migration is the better utilization of new habitates and their resources. In other words "migration is an adaptation towards abundance". The nursery of spawning grounds alone do not have sufficient food to maintain both mature and immature members of a large population. Hence, it would be advantageous to have separate feeding, breeding and nursery grounds. Migration provides suitable climatic conditions for breeding and survival of the young.

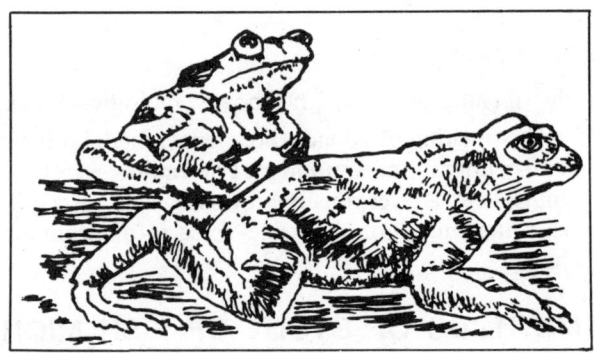

Fig. 8.12. Migratory Toads.

Disadvantages of Migration to fishes

Long journey is wasteful and many migrating fishes get lost while migrating. Numerous migrating fishes are eaten by predators. Construction of dams check migration and the concerned fish species become extinct. Due to Farakka dam constructed in Ganga river, Hilsa fish is facing the danger of extinction.

MIGRATION OF TOADS

Toads breed in water but for much of the year live away from water and at the first sign of spring they migrate to their breeding ponds - often in huge numbers.

MIGRATION OF REPTILES

Some turtles live out at sea, but need to come a shore to lay their eggs. They have favourite, traditional beaches where they bury their eggs. They visit these beaches year after year.

Green sea turtles nest on Ascension Island, a tiny speck of land (8 kilometers wide) in the centre of Atlantic Ocean between Africa and Brazil. The adult female turtles visit the island only to deposit their eggs in beach sands. They swim 1600 kilometers or so to warm shallow water of Brazil, where they feed on marine vegetation for several years before returning, usually to the same beach, to lay another clutch of eggs.

How could a round-trip journey of thousands of kilometer evolved? Perhape in some cases long distance migration have been derived from short-distance dispersal tendencies that took individuals from one region to another adjacent area. Subsequent changes in climate or geology may have gradually increased the distance between the regions with useful resources, favouring even more "ambitious" dispersers. Amazing Atlantic migration of green turtles have grown longer and longer as the continents of Africa and South America have slowly drifted apart. At first glance, this idea may seem a bit far-fetched. But sea turtles were swimming in the Earth's oceans and breeding on beaches millions of years before Africa and South America separated from the earlier continent of Gondwana land.

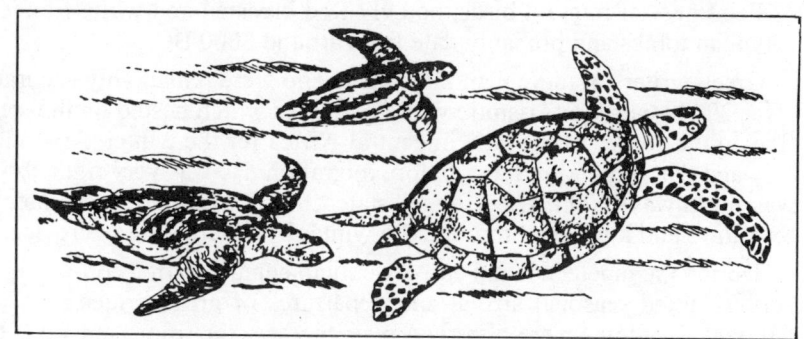

Fig. 8.13. Migration of green turtle.

Logger head turtle hatchings head for the Atlantic ocean near Florida when the sand cools at the dusk. Researchers have believed that the brighter area towards the sea attracts the hatchings.

MIGRATION OF BIRDS

● Introduction ● Discovering migration ● Pertinent questions about bird migration : Why birds migrate, evolution of birds migration, how many types of bird migrations are there, modes of bird migration, what are the factors stimulating migration, how birds find their way, homing ● Significance of bird migration ● Methods of studying migration. Bird sanctuaries of India.

INTRODUCTION

Bird migration is one of the marvels of the natural world. They travel from continent to continent without any passport, visa, and need not any aircraft. Bird migration is a regular *to and from* a particular area. The most common migrations are linked to the seasons of the year.

Birds have traveled from continent to continent for tens of thousands of years. Their behaviour can still surprise modern scientists. So, let us enter this fascinating and secret world and discover some of the wonders of birds migration.

DISCOVERING MIGRATION

Most of the discoveries of bird migration have been made during the last few centuries of twentieth century and first decade of twenty first century, but the arrival and departure of bird migrants has been observed for thousands of years. First explanations for the arrival and departure of migrant birds were often wide the mark, but sometimes they were accurate.

Paintings of migrant birds, notably Red breasted and white fronded geese, appear on the walls of Egyptian tombs and probably date from around 3000 BC.

Greek writers of more than 2000 years ago were remarkably accurate in some of their observations. Over 2000 years ago Aristotle wrote of cranes which nested on the steppes north of the Black sea and flew to the source of the Nile in central Africa for the winter. Aristotle also noted that cuckoos left in July and that birds were fatter before migration. He was very right about his observation. But Aristotle was not always right. He wrongly stated that Redstarts turned into Robins for the winter, and that Swallows and kites slept through the winter by hibernating in crevices.

During the nineteenth and early twentieth century various observers noted seasonal arrival and departures of great strides. Migrant Swallows were observed over the sea, far from land, and, as world travel and specimen collecting became more widespread, so the theory of migration became more accepted.

Bird watchers were fascinated with the subject. Records were gathered from light-house keepers because large numbers of night-time migrants were attracted to these large, powerful lights. In addition, many collectors shot and stuffed migrating birds, especially rare migrants.

There were several early attempts to mark birds in some way. Later on attaching a light-weight, numbered ring to the legs of individual birds became the basis of migration studies. Discoveries were made about where some birds spent the summer and winter, the routes they took and their life-span.

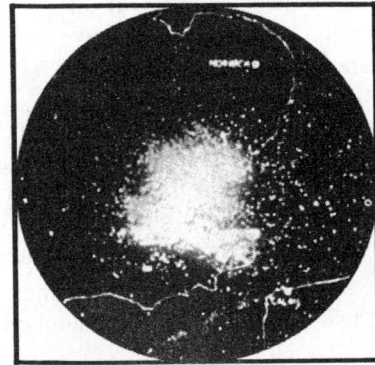

Fig. 8.14. Angel's seen on radar during world war II, were a mystery until people realized they were migrating birds.

The use of radar during world war II showed that flocks of migrating birds could be seen. Ornithologists used radar images as one of the methods of tracing migration routes.

PERTINENT QUESTIONS ABOUT BIRD MIGRATION

Bird migration is very interesting topic but many questions regarding bird migration arise in the mind of even a lay person. Such as,:

   I.   Why birds migrate?
   II. How evolution of Bird's Migration took place in the past?
   III. How many types of bird migration are there?
   IV. Modes of bird migration?
   V.   What are the factors stimulating migration?

Ornithologists and behaviourists along with scientists of physical sciences have pondered these puzzles and come up with temporary answers.

I. WHY BIRDS MIGRATE?

Birds face numerous adverse situations and risk their lives during long journeys. They may run into bad weather or they may be attacked by predators, and there may be food shortages or drought at their journey's end. Many birds that set out on migration do not survive, so why do they do it? The answer is that the species is greatly benefited by migrating. Individual birds may not survive, but the whole species does better by undertaking this annual or biannual journey.

Every year, millions of willow warblers leave Central and Southern Africa and fly to the forests of northern Europe and Asia to breed. Here they get abundant insect food which the warblers need to raise their young. In winter the forests of northern Europe and Asia become cold and dark and insects are hard to find. So, the warblers leave in the autumn and return to Africa which is their home area.

Another advantage of moving away from the equator to breed is that there is longer day length means more daylight. In summer in the Arctic there are almost 24 hours of daylight which means that birds, such as Bewick's swans (which nest on the tundra of Siberia) have much more time to feed.

Bewick's swans feed on the nutritious new plant growth of the Arctic and finish nesting and rear their young in a little over 1000 days. After summer they must leave the place before the snow and ice return.

Dotterels migrate from Africa to nest on the tops of the highest Scottish mountains. They wait on lowland fields for most of the snow and ice to melt and then return to the high tops to mark out and defend the best territories. Dotterels face no competition because other plovers (members of the same family) nest at lower levels.

Another reason for migrating is that certain places are ideal for nesting and, therefore, birds visit these places year after year. Seabird colonies, for example, are full of birds for a short, hectic breeding season, but are largely deserted at other times. Suitable cliffs for Gannet colonies are not very common, but, once established, they may be used for hundreds, even thousands of years.

Young Gannets swim and fly away from their colonies as soon as they are able to leave the cliffs. They make their way to wintering grounds off the west coast of Africa. Young Gannets attain sexual maturity in one or two years and return to the cliffs where they were hatched. They nest on the cliff and produce new generation.

Migration of Barnacle gees to Arctic fulfill dual purpose. It gives a supply of food and safe places (rugged cliff) to nest.

II. THE EVOLUTION OF MIGRATION

Bird migration has probably been taking place for millions of years. But question arises how did these migration journeys come about.

There are several theories to explain the causes of bird migration but none of which seems satisfactory in all respects.

1. Environmental effects

Seasonal change, food scarcity, varying day length, increase of cold etc. forced animals to migrate. In this context Northern ancestral home theory and Southern ancestral home theory are given.

(A) Northern ancestral home theory

This theory suggests that the original home of birds was northern hemisphere of earth and they were non-migratory. By the end of Pleistocene epoch (1 million years ago) there was sudden changes in climate. Northern hemisphere was covered with ice sheets due to glaciation. In this cold and adverse condition birds were forced to move towards Southern hemisphere. On return of normal climate in northern hemisphere (glaciers receded in northern hemisphere) they returned to their homeland. They lived in northern hemisphere (original homeland) until they were forced to move southwards due to climate change. By constant repetition of moving from northern hemisphere to southern hemisphere and vice-versa, birds developed the habit of migration.

The above explanation about origin of bird migration seems to be very logical but question arises as to how first migrant birds came to know that now favourable climate had returned in northern hemisphere when they were at least 4000 kms away from their original homeland?

(B) Southern ancestral home theory

This theory assumes that the ancestral homeland of birds was southern hemisphere of earth and they were non-migratory. Owing to over population they were driven to the northern hemisphere. But when climate to northern hemisphere became very cold due to seasonal climatic cycle, they returned to southern ancestral homeland. This *to and fro* journey was repeated for many years periodically. Gradually this habit became innate instinct.

The above theory also seems to be a matter of speculation only. Both the above theories do not have any scientific base and as such cannot be accepted unless there is a scientific proof.

2. Evolutionary theory

The most logical and convincing theory that explains the phenomenon of bird migration is the evolutionary one. In the end of Pleistocene epoch, tropical birds, probably spread out in colder northern latitudes, where food was abundant. They were however forced to move southward when winter arrived. The repetition of this *to and fro* movement became innate instinctive behaviour through long history of race. This may be cited as an example of Lamarck's theory of inheritance of acquired character.

The migrations that take place in Europe today began about 10,000 years ago when the ice sheet which covered much of Europe, Asia and North America started to melt at the end of the last Ice Age.

The vegetation of Europe would have been very different then, even Southern Europe would have had Arctic tundra. Gradually the climate warmed and the ice retreated, the forests of birch and pine spread north and the birds such as Bramblings, which lived in them, also spread northwards. Crested tits and other species which could find food all year round became residents but many, like the willow warbler which ate insects, spread into these new feeding areas to take advantage of the food and to rear young. When their food became scarce in autumn, and there was short day length in which to feed, willow warblers and many other insectivorous birds flew back to their original homes.

Most of the migrants that visit Europe in spring travel from Africa where they spend the winter. There are similar patterns in Asia where birds, such as Arctic Warblers (which breed in the Baltic Republics in summer) spend winter in south-east Asia. Also, in North America, many summer migrants

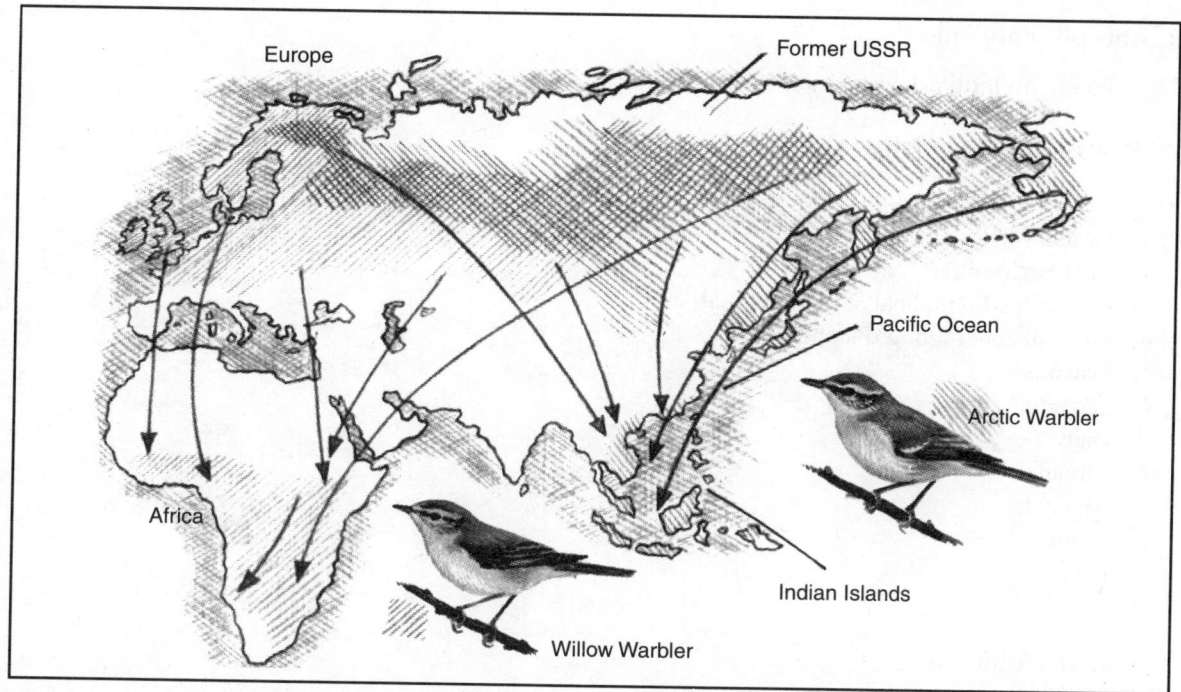

Fig. 8.15. The breeding and wintering areas of Willow and Arctic Warblers : two closely related species which breed in similar areas, but have quite separate migrations. This is because one species was split by glaciation into two – an eastern and a western species.

spend winter in Central or South America. Whereas, which visit northern North America and originate in Europe or Africa, continue to return to their original homeland.

During the evolution of migratory behaviour, some birds have changed their habits. The Barn Swallow of America is the same species as the Swallow of Europe and Africa. It, too, migrates, but it flies to South America. All Swallows once migrated to Africa, but presumably those in North America found that if they flew southwards, rather than following traditional routes, they reached very similar habitats and travelled only half the distance. As there was less competition and more chances of survival, they would be able to return to their nesting areas earlier and fitter the following spring.

3. Gonadal stimuli

Physiological changes in gonads i.e. hormonal change force birds to migrate to suitable place for breeding.

4. Thyroid hypothesis

Thyroid glands secretion regulates the metabolic activities of bird. The changes of metabolic activities lead the individual to migrate.

5. Metabolic aspect

Before migration, fat deposition takes place in the body due to metabolic changes, which stimulate the birds to migrate.

6. Anti pituitary role

The role of anti pituitary hormones also effect the migration.

III. KINDS OF BIRD MIGRATION

There are twelve types of bird migration :

1. Partial/Total,
2. Regular/Irregular,
3. Altitudinal/Latitudinal & Longitudinal,
4. Short distance/Long distance,
5. Seasonal,
6. Circadian,
7. Daily,
8. Climatic,
9. Alimental,
10. Gametic,
11. Local,
12. Cyclic.

1. Partial / Total

On the basis of number of migrants, two types of migration may be recognised :-

(i) Partial Migration

When only a few member of a species participate in migration, then the phenomenon is called partial migration. Sometimes the young will leave and the adults stay or one sex may leave and the other will stay behind.

Robins are partial migrants. In Britain, most stay there for whole year, but in continental Europe the northern robins are long haul migrants which spend winter around the Mediterranean.

(ii) Total Migration

When all members of a species participate in the migration, then this phenomenon is called total migration. Cranes, Flamingo, Greylag Goose, Swift, Barn Swallow, Paradise Flycatcher, Robin etc. are total migratory birds.

2. Regular / irregular (Depending on the routes)

Migration may be of two types :

(i) Regular Migration

Migratory birds follow the same route during emigration and immigration. Most of the migratory birds are regular migrant.

(ii) Irregular or Erratic Migration

Irregular or erratic migration is found among Great blue heron, Cuckoos, Thrushes and Warblers. In such birds, after breeding, both young and adult fly in all directions irregularly over many or a few hundred kilometers in search of food and suitable place.

3. Altitudinal / Latitudinal / Longitudinal (depending on direction)

Migration may be of three types :

(i) Altitudinal Migration

Birds that spend the summer in the higher reaches of mountains come down during the winter to low valleys in winter is known as altitudinal migration. This type is very common in India where the mighty Himalaya lie close to the Indo-Gangetic plain. Common examples are Wood cock, Bush Chat, *Scolopax rusticola etc.*

Some foreign mountaineer birds exhibiting altitudinal migration are Grebs and Coots of Argentina. Violet Green Swallows of England and Willow Ptarmings of Siberia. The brown Plumage of Willow Ptarminges becomes white in winter as their food habit changes. They become insectivorous to as against being herbivorous. They start taking buds and twigs of willow trees instead of insects.

(ii) Latitudinal Migration (N.......S)

Greylag goose, Pintail, Common teal, Shoveller, Mallard duck, Pochard etc. are latitudinal migrant. The movement of birds occurs to north temperate and sub-arctic region for feeding and resting during summer months and then retire to south for winter

(iii) Longitudinal Migration (E.......W)

The migration of birds from eastern region to western direction and western region to eastern direction is called longitudinal migration. Each bird species living in southern hemisphere religiously observes longitudinal migration. The starling travels from a breeding area in eastern Europe or Asia to Atlantic Coast, to avoid winter. The Potagonian plover migrate from southern Potagonia to Falkland island in summer and return to Potagonia in winter (Sep. and Oct.) for breeding.

4. Short Distance / Long Distance

(i) Short Distance Migrants

Some species are local migrant. They move out of one area into another, not very far away. This kind of movement is particularly noticeable in North India where the seasons are clearly marked. Birds that spend the summer in the higher regions of mountains come down during the winter to the lower foothills or even the plains. This type is very common in India where the mighty Himalaya lie close to the Indo Gangetic plain. Pedaki live in foothills of Himalaya in spring season and migrate to Nepal and Sikkim in summer for breeding. Tits may leave a wood in order to reach for food in gardens of England: this is local migration. Waxwings leave their breeding sites and wander in search for food : this is called *nomadism.* Cross bills leave an area if food runs out and move into a new area where they may stay and breed : this is an *irruption.*

(ii) Long distance Migrants

Long distance migrant cover long distances from feeding place (homeland) to breeding ground. White wagtails live in northern part of India and plains of China in winter season. On arrival of summer season they migrate to eastern part of Baikal lake of Siberia which is the breeding ground. They return to India and China in winter season.

Ruff breeds at Siberia and migrates to England and India, travelling a distance of 9,600 kms. Siberian white cranes travel from Baikal lake of Siberia to India every year in Winter. They cover more than 7000 km. to visit India. The American golden plover (*Pluvialis dominica*) live in North America in summer but migrate to South America in winter covering a distance of 1,000 km. They again return to their original lomeland on arrival of summer season. Thus they enjoy summer of two places each year and do not experience winter at all.

5. Seasonal (Depending on season)

Following types of seasonal migration have been recognised :

(i) Summer Migration

Migration of birds from the hot southern parts to comparatively cooler northern part in spring season for breeding and nesting and again back in the summer of autumn is called summer migration. Participants are called summer visitors. In Britain, swifts, swallow, nightingales and cuckoos are summer visitors. They arrive in north in spring from the south remain there and breed. They leave for the south in autumn. Swallows return to the migrants. In Finland, Robins are summer visitors.

(ii) Winter Migration

Migration of birds from cooler northern parts to the hotter southern parts in winter is called winter migration. Participants are called winter visitors. Some birds such as Fieldfares, Snow buntings and Redwings are winter visitors. They spend winter in southern part and return to northern part in spring. In parts of Spain Robins are winter visitors.

SOME SUMMER AND WINTER MIGRANTS OF EUROPE

SUMMER MIGRANTS

The summer migrants of Europe are Wheatear, Cuckoos, Sedge warblers, Swifts, Garganeys ducks, Swallows, Sand Martins, House Martins and Black caps etc.

Songbirds like cuckoos, swallows and many warblers sing sweet songs in countryside of England in summer season. After dark one can hear song of nightingales in Southern England.

The first summer visitor to England is wheatear. It comes from Africa on coasts of England in March. At about the same time chiffchaffs visits here from Mediterranean. Willow warblers, swifts and swallows are African birds and they come Europe in the month of April. Spotted Flycatchers and Reed warblers and many arrive in the month of may. All migrants breed there. These birds take advantage of a temporary supply of food and then return home again.

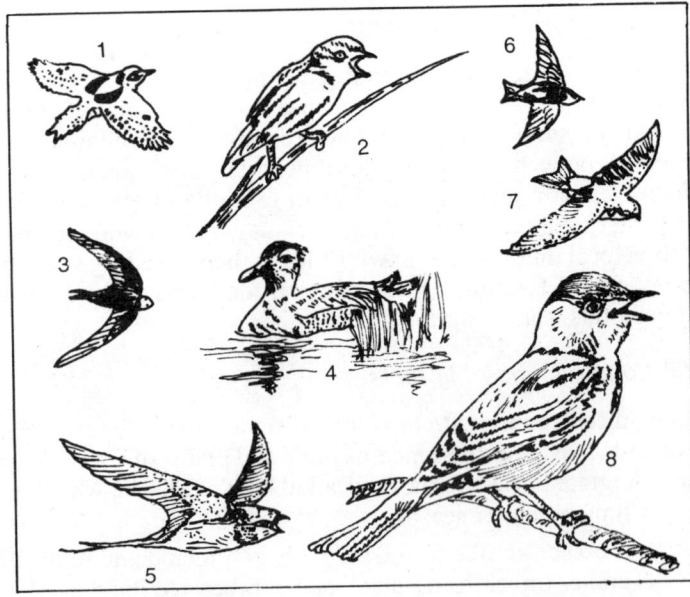

Fig. 8.16. Some summer visitors of Europe.

Cuckoos is the first migrants to leave the British Isles after breeding. They leave the place in July and go to south. Swifts leave the place in early August. Upto the end of October all migrants leave the Europe.

WINTER MIGRANTS

For birds that breed in the Arctic and in the northern and eastern Europe, the winter weather in the English isles seems mild. Most lakes are unfrozen. The soil is soft and there are sufficient food to cater the need of winter visitors.

The important winter visitors of Europe are wild Gees and Swan (Goldeneyes, whopper swans, shovelers), short-eared owls, Redwings, Fieldfares, Bramblings etc.

The first winter visitor to European region is wild geese and swans. They arrive here in October. Redwings and Fieldfares follow wild geese and swans. First they feed on berries and, when the berries run out, they feed on worms and other small animals which live in the soil. They nest here in winter and leave the place after breeding in the month of March/April.

SOME SUMMER AND WINTER MIGRANTS OF INDIAN CONTINENTS

Siberian crane, white wagtails, ducks, teals, pochard etc. visit Indian subcontinent viz. Keoladeo bird sanctuary, Bharatpur, Rajasthan from Baikal Jheel of Siberia in winter season. They return to Siberia in the beginning of summer.

The rufous turtle dove (*S. orientalis*) ("काला फाख्ता") breeds in central Siberia, Japan, North and Central China, Tibet and Nepal. In winter it migrates southwards all over Eastern India and as far South as Deccan.

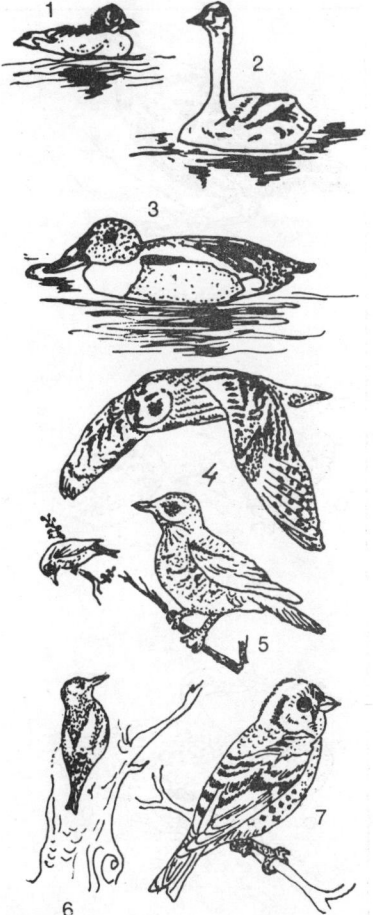

Fig. 8.17. Some winter visitors of Europe.

The central starling (*Strunnus vulgaris porphyronotus*) ("गोधुनी") is found in the North-western part of India in winter. In summer, it migrates to Turkistan and Tianshian mountains to breed.

The brown shrike (*Lanius cristatus*) ("लाहटोरा") breeds in Eastern Siberia in summer and migrates to India and ceylon in winter.

The white wagtail breeds in Eastern Siberia and migrates to India in winter.

Migratory birds come across the Himalaya from northern parts of Asia and Europe to India to escape from the severe winter prevailing there and enjoy the much warmer and longer day length with abundant food in Central and Southern India. Teminx stint (पनलब्बा), Common Teal (अधंगा), Ruff and Rib (बगवद), Spotted sand piper (चुपका), Pintail (लालसर), and Fantail swipe (चाहा), White eye pochard, Cranes, Wild ducks, Geese, Flycatchers and Wagtails (खंजन) are important visitors. They arrive in September/October and return in March/April.

MIGRATORY INDIAN BIRDS

There are 1200 species of Indian birds but only 300 species are migrants. Koel (*Eudynamys scolopacea*) emigrate from southern part to northern part in spring season and immigrate to southern India and Sri

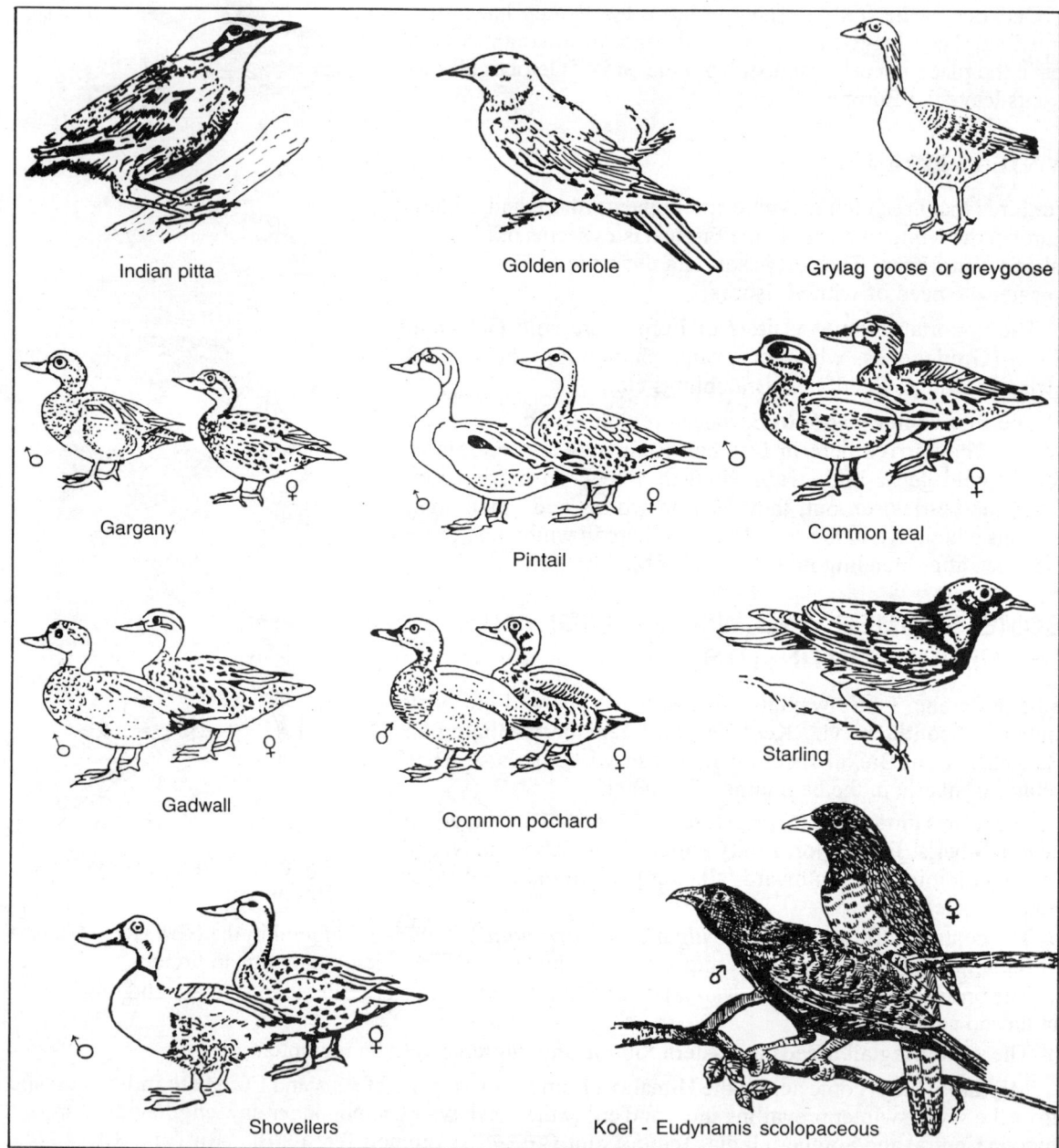

Fig. 8.18. Indian migratory birds.

Lanka in winter season. *Neelkants* emigrate from Himalayan range to plains of India in spring season (March/April) and return after breeding. Shoveller, Teal and Red Crested Pochard etc. remain present in spring season (March/April) in plains. On return of summer they return to their homeland (feeding ground.)

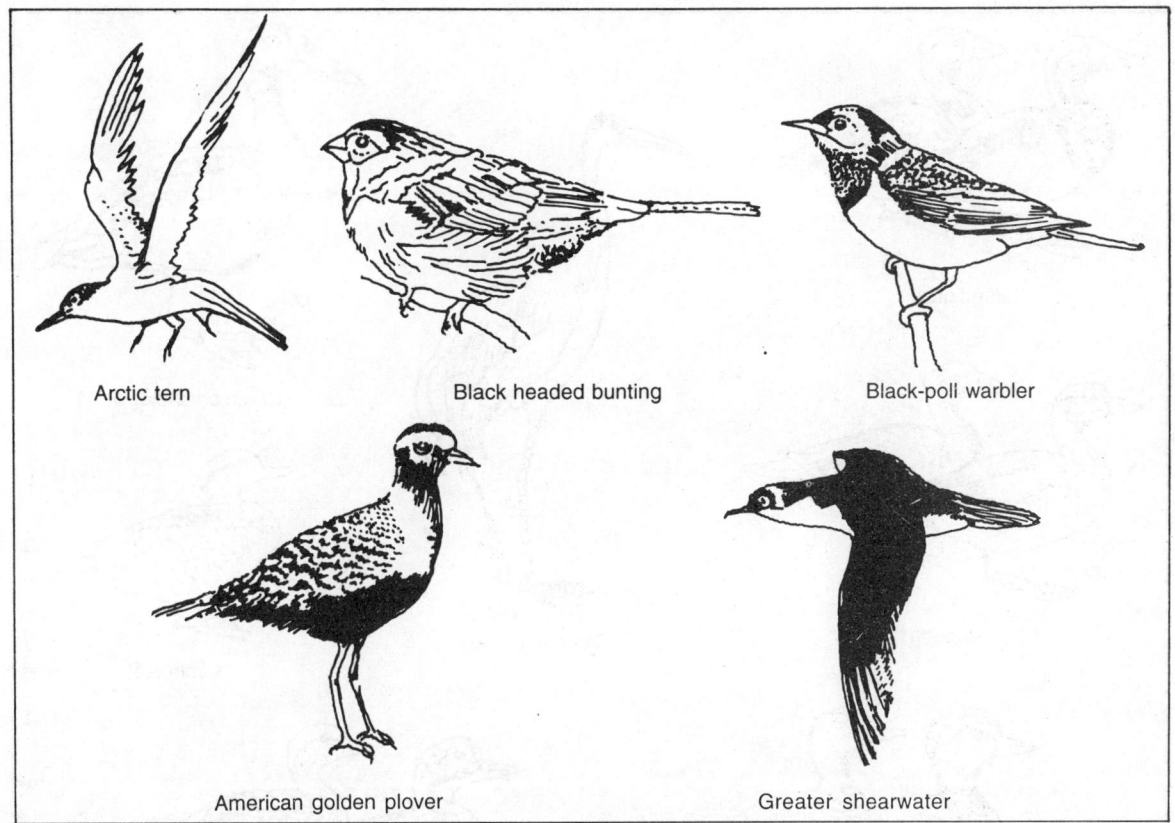

Fig. 8.19. Long distance migrants.

(iii) Cyclic migration

Migration of some bird species depends on season but not at regular intervals. They migrate at 3 to 5 years interval. One proper example is Snowy owl found in USA.

(iv) Birds of passage

Certain birds such as Great snipes and Sandpipers while migrating drop in their way for a few days. They are called birds of passage. They are seen twice a year in the middle of their route as they stay in both *to and fro* journeys. Sand pipers and Great snipes are birds of passage.

6. Circadian (Depending on day and night)

Two types of migration are there :

(i) Diurnal Migration

The migration of birds during day time is called diurnal migration. Many birds such as Swallows, Ducks, Robins, Pelicans, Geese, Crows etc. travel in day time. Diurnal migrants have tendency to travel in well organized (Ducks. Geese and Swans) or loose (swallows) groups.

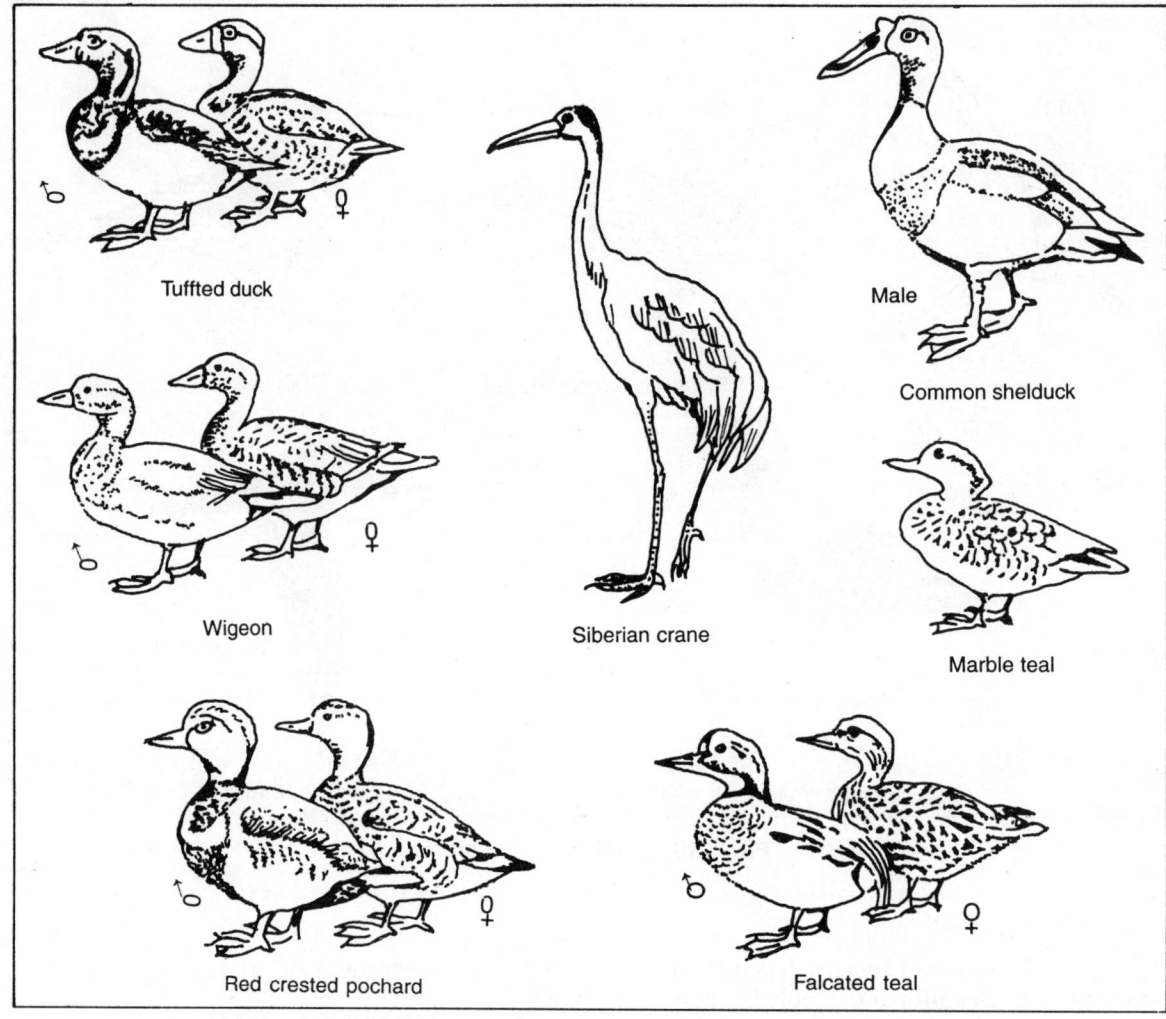

Fig. 8.20. Migratory birds visiting Keoladeo National Park (Rajasthan).

(ii) Nocturnal Migration

The migration of birds during night is called nocturnal migration. These include mostly small sized birds, such as Sparrows, Thrushes, Warblers etc. Indigo bunting is also a nocturnal migrant. Nocturnal migrants escape their enemies under the cover of darkness.

(iii) Both Diurnal and Nocturnal Migrants

Some migratory birds such as Ducks, Gulls Shore birds travel both by day and night time.

7. Daily or Local Migrant

Certain birds, like house-sparrow (*Passer domesticus*), parrot or parakeet (*Psittacula krameri*), crows and gulls, fly away from their hideout in the early morning in groups and return to the same place in the evening. This is an example of daily migration.

8. Climatic Migration

It occurs as a result of seasonal changes in the climate of the environment. The well known North - South migration of many Ducks and Geese is a good example of climatic migration.

9. Alimental Migration

This type of migration occur as a result of food or water shortage and may take place any time in a year.

10. Gametic Migration

Occurs as a result of need to occupy some special region for reproductive process. Most migratory birds perform gametic migration.

11. Local Migration

Few birds migrate short distance. Some Indian local migrants migrate from base of the Himalaya and forests to warmer states of India for breeding in spring season. Neelkanth or blue jay or Roller (*Coracias*) is a local migrant. They migrate from woodland area of the Himalaya to plains (warmer part) for breeding in spring season. They breed in plains and return to woodland area of mountains by the time their young ones become able to fly.

12. Moult Migration

Before moulting, some species go on a special moult migration to an area which is safe from predators and where there is sufficient food.

IV. MODES OF BIRD MIGRATION

The time, speed, duration, distance or range, altitude, regularity, routes, segregation, sustenance during migration etc. are important points to discuss while studying migration.

Time : Some birds fly by day e.g. Swallows, Robins, Hawks, Cranes, Geese, etc. Some fly both by day and by night. But most of them speed on their way through darkness after the sun has set e.g.. night Hawk, Warbler, Sparrow etc.

Speed : Migratory birds do not fly at their fastest. The migration speed is usually from 48–64 kmph. Most shorebirds fly between 64 kmph and 80 kmph. Cranes, Crows and Finches fly with a speed of 48 kmph. Maximum speed recorded so far

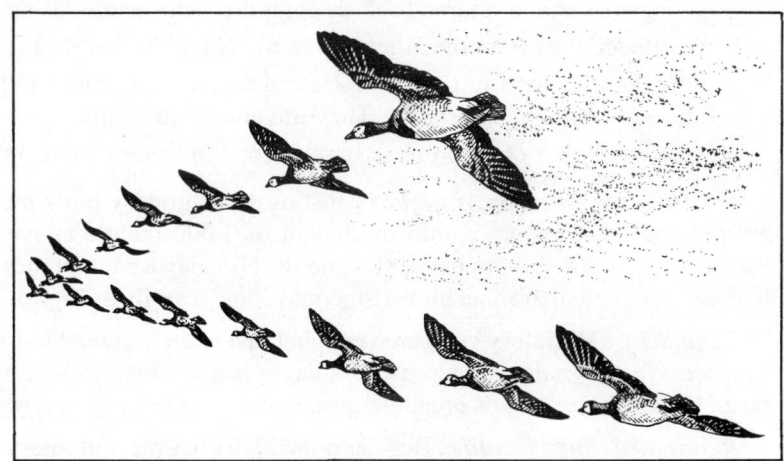

Fig. 8.21. Cranes and Geese fly by V-shaped formation. Flying in formation saves fuel for geese and cranes or other larger birds. The bird in front sets up turbulance which helps those that follow.

is 272 kmph by Indian Swifts. Ducks travel at 80–90 kmph. Migrating birds do not generally fly very high; they fly at under 900 meters, but some travelers have been found at greater heights.

Travel in flocks : Birds usually travel in flock (group of birds of the same kind). The V-shaped formation of Cranes and Geese draw our attention as they fly in the sky. Shallows, Flycatchers, Warblers, Shorebirds and Waterbirds begin to gather in flocks (each with its own kind) and after a great deal of excited fluttering, twittering and calling, they rise up into the air and away they go. Usually the male birds go first to their breeding grounds and the female birds follow them in a few days.

Duration : Some migratory birds fly great distances without pausing to rest and feed. The golden plover cover non stop flight by about 4,000 kms from Hudson Bay and Alaska to South America. Migratory birds usually travel not less than 5 to 6 hrs. per day. Some birds make the long journey in easy stages, stopping to rest on the way.

Range : The range of migration varies from few kilometers to thousand of kilometers but it is almost constant for a particular species of bird. Some migratory birds and distance covered by them is given below.

1. Himalayan snow parties—One or two km only.
2. Starlings of Berlin—2,000 kms.
3. Manx shear water (A sea bird)—4,940 kms. It crosses Atlantic ocean from Boston to west coast of England.
4. Storks and swallow—6,000 kms. Migrate from North Europe to South Africa.
5. Cranes—about 5,000 kms. From Baikal lake of Siberia to India (Bharatpur and Ghana of Rajasthan).
6. Golden Plovers, Sand pipers cover a distance of 9,600 kms. The American Golden Plover (*Pluvialis dominica*) travel 12,800 kms. south in the plains of Argentina. Thus enjoying two summers each year.
7. Bobolink and Bam swallows cover 14,400 kms. from the Arctic to the grassy plains of Argentina or the Potagonian beaches in South America.
8. Arctic Tern covers longest distance of 17,600 kms. from northern part of Canada to Antarctica during winter and returns back through the same route during summer.
9. Woodcock flies from the Himalaya to the Nilgiri without a pause, a distance of 2,400 km.
10. Wild ducks come from central Asia and Siberia to Kanwar and other lakes of Bihar state (India). They cover about 3,200 kms. They travel over the Himalaya.
11. The rosy Paster come from Eastern Europe to Central Asia a distance of more than 3,000 kms.

Velocity and Altitudes of flight : Most of the migratory birds prefer to fly close to the Earth while routine migration occurs within the height of 1,000 meters above the earth. Some species of birds (Siberian crane) even cross the Andes and the Himalaya at an altitude of 666 meters or even higher. It is interesting to note that some birds (Siberian Crane) can fly as high as a boeing jet (above 5,000 meters).

Regularity : Migratory birds are very punctual in their time of journey, unless they are delayed by bad weather. We may calculate almost to a day when we may expect birds to return. The Purple martins reach to their homeland or breeding ground on the same day every year.

Return to definite locality : Besides punctuality in time, migratory birds return in the selected locality every year. For example : Swallows (from their winter abode in South Africa to Europe) visit same village and even the same tree. Cranes migrate from Siberia to Bharatpur (Rajasthan, India) in the same area.

ROUTES OF MIGRATION

Every species of birds travel through a definite route :

(a) *Sea routes* : Marine birds adopt sea routes. Migratory birds can cross 650 kms. long sea at a stretch.

(b) *Coast routes* : Some travel through coast routes. Coast routes are East Atlantic coast line, West Atlantic coast line, etc.

(c) *River Valley routes* : Many birds migrate from mountains to plains and plains to mountain through river routes. Sometime they cross mountain ranges. The river valleys, mountain ranges and coastal routes provide good landmarks for migratory birds. White storks (*Ciconia ciconia*) that breed in western Europe fly to their wintering grounds in Africa by westerly route over Spain and Gibraltar, whereas those breeding in Eastern Europe take an easterly route.

The other route used by birds from Mongolia and Chinese Turkestan is over the passage in the north-eastern Himalayas. The main routes of entry into India are through the passage on the north-western and north-eastern sides of the Himalayas, but certain birds on the direct route fly straight across the main Himalayan range and do not detour.

Sparrow comes from the Himalayan region and Central Asia to the plains. Smallest of all, the willow warbler–half the size of a sparrow–covers as many as 3,200 km. to reach India every winter. Main migratory movement is generally north to south in autumn and vice-versa in spring. Thus the main travellers come to India from the north-west and start from between lake of Baikal and sea of Aral in Siberia. But some Storks come over from as far as West Germany.

SEGREGATION DURING MIGRATION

Night hawk, kingfishers, swifts etc. travel in separate companies. Turkeys, Bluebird, Swallows etc. travel in mixed companies of several species. This may be due to similarity in their size, food habit etc. In some cases male and female members of same species travel separately. Males travel ahead of females to reach first to build the nest for eggs and young. Female birds reach behind.

MIGRANTS OF OTHER PLACES

(i) Marine birds also make extensive migration. The great shear water (*Puffinus*) breeds on Tristan da cunha but comes to Greenland in may, returning again after months of wandering at sea, apparantly without a landfall.

(ii) The Arctic Terns (*Sterna paradocoe*) ("धुरी की नाई") breeds in the North Temperate zone (Canada, Northern Ireland and West Coast of Greenland) in summer and in winter migrates to Antarctic continents along both sides of Atlantic islands.

(iii) The broad-billed Rover, breeds in Madagascar from December to May and migrates northwards to the Congo Basin between June and November.

(iv) The Widens breeding in Iceland, migrate to Europe and cross over the Atlantic to reach North America.

(v) Some birds enjoy two summers in a year. They breed during summer in the Northern Hemisphere and cross the Equator at the approach of winter to live in the summer of Southern Hemisphere. The American Golden Plover (*Pluvialis domestions*) "chotta battan" breed in north of America in Arctic circle. In autumn it moves south until it arrives in the South America where it spends winter. It returns to the Arctic region in April, thus covering 20,000 kilometers and enjoying summers in one year.

MIGRATION OF BIRDS BY SWIMMING AND WALKING

Bird migration does not always take place by means of flight. Some birds migrate by swimming and even walking.

(i) Penguins (*Spheniscus*) : In summer these breed on the land of Antarctic continent. In the winter they move hundreds of kilometers on floating packs of Ice and return south in summer. They cover a greater distance by swimming in the sea and marching to their nest site.

(ii) Guillemots (*Uria*) mostly swim for many kilometres across the country.

(iii) Coot (*Fulica*) walks for several kilometers across the country.

FUEL IN MAKING THE JOURNEY

How birds, both large and small, can find the fuel to travel so far?

This fuel is fat which gives them the energy for prolonged journey. Before migration a bird defends a feeding territory and store quantities of extra fat. The amount of fat stored depends on the length of the journey to be flown.

Ruby-throated humming birds increase their body weight by a half before they make a 800 km. flight across the Gulf of Mexico. Waders, about to fly from Western Europe to their Arctic breeding grounds, put on similar amounts of weight. Sedge Warblers, which fly from Britain to Central Africa, double their normal body weight before leaving.

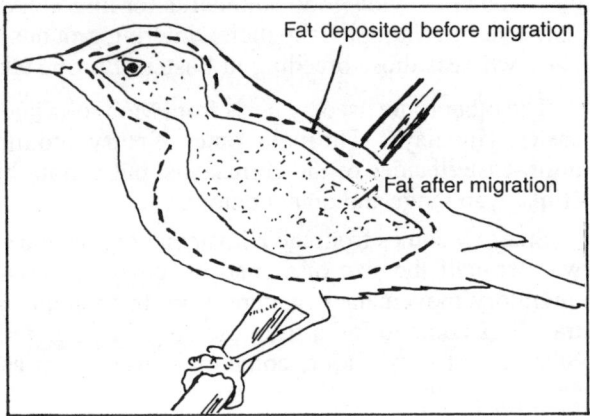

Fig. 8.22. Weight loss during migration : The area inside the dotted line is where a sedge warbler stores its fat; the dark area shows how much weight it can lose during migration.

THERMALS

Large migratory birds rise high to cross long distances. These large day flying birds such as Buzzards, Eagles, Storks, Cranes, Pelicans and Cormorants need thermals viz. upcurrents of warm air to rise high to cross long distances. Using thermals migratory birds hardly need to flap their wings, so they get to the greatest height with the minimum amount of energy.

Thermals form where the ground is heated more quickly than the surrounding area. This often happens on the side of a hill which is warmed by the sun. In Pennsylvania, USA one hill known as Howk Mountain is a famous point to watch migrating birds of prey. On average 17,000 birds of prey pass over it every year.

High flying migrants avoid sea crossings because there are no thermals. The mediterranean is a huge barrier to soaring birds when they leave Europe. The natural route from Western Europe is across the strait of Gibralter. The Eastern European birds fly around the eastern Mediterranean, crossing the Bosporus near Istanbul in Turkey and continuing around the eastern end of the Mediterranean and into Africa via the head of the Red sea.

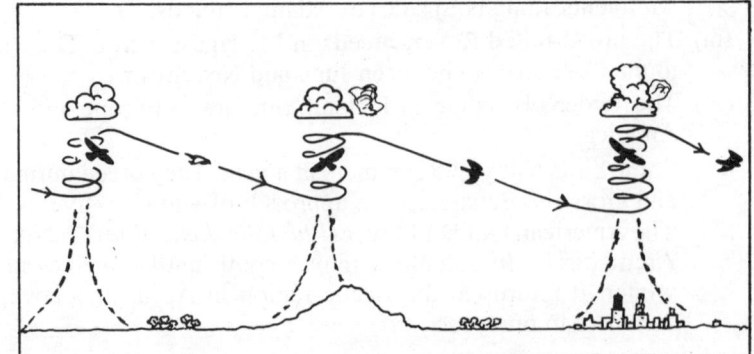

Fig. 8.23. Soaring birds using thermals.

SUSTENANCE DURING MIGRATION

Many birds cover several thousand of kilometers nonstop. Golden plover covers nonstop flight of 3,840 kms. without food and drink. Premigratory deposition of fat is used during travel. Besides energy, fat also provides water to cope with the high rates of metabolism and breathing. Swallows and Swifts capture insects as food while flying.

V. FACTOR STIMULATING MIGRATION

What stimulates birds to migrate periodically is an important question for ornithologists and etholo-gists. Is there any one or many factors stimulat-ing birds to migrate from one place to another at the same time through same route each year?

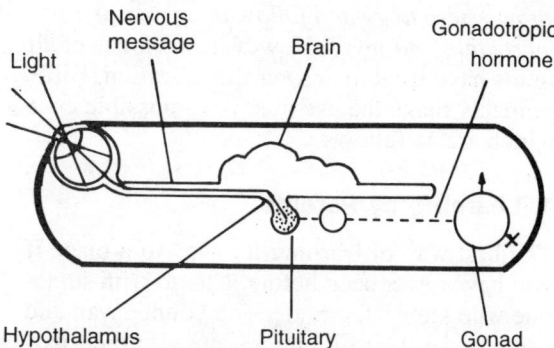

Fig. 8.24. A system in which light acts on the retina which sends nervous messages to the hypothalamus through nerves. Hypothalamus stimulates the pituitary gland to release gonadotropic hormone.

Ethologists agree that there are many factors stimulating and operating throughout bird migration. All factors may be grouped under two heads :

1. Exogenous factors

Environmental factors such as light, temperature, humidity, scarcity of food etc. may stimulate bird migration. The most regular and predictable seasonal changes of the environment is the fluctuations in the photoperiod i.e. day length and temperature.

2. Endogenous factors

The effect of light (day length) and fall in temperature on migratory behaviour is ultimately mediated by hormones, especially sex hormones. The increased and decreased photoperiod received by the eye is converted to electrochemical messages. The message stimulates hypothalamus. Hypothalamus secretes neurohormones to stimulate pituitary gland. Pituitary glands release gonadotropic hormones. Gonadot-ropic hormones bring physiological changes causing migration in birds. Thus one can say that fluctuation in photoperiod and temperature (Exogenous factors) ripening of gonads and instinct (Endogenous fac-tors) compose together migratory behaviour of birds. The exogenous factors can initiate bird migration only when urge of migration is within the bird. Thus environmental conditions and physiological condi-tions of birds are equally essential for bird migration. Before migrating birds start deposition of fat and their gonads start ripening. Thus migration is a part of sexual cycle. Birds move to migratory route as soon as their gonads begin to ripe and by the time they reach the breeding ground the gonads ripe completely.

Migration is an innate instinctive behaviour. Newly hatched migratory birds kept alone migrate without any previous learning. They show restlessness if kept in prison during migratory season.

Thus it seems that both exogenous and endogenous factors stimulate bird migration. But the endoge-nous factors may be considered as the dominating factor. Without urge or drive, external factors cannot force birds to migrate. The complete mechanism of bird migration still need further investigation.

VI. NAVIGATION

Many migratory birds travel amazing distances when migrating. Swallows fly from one continent to another and still are able to return to the same place that they nested in the previous year. Whitethroats migrate at night and may fly across the sea in the dark, but still they return to the same breeding sites year after year. One of the intricate questions before ethologists is that "*How do the migratory birds*

*know where to go and follow their way on their
incredible journeys?*' However, scientists of all
fields have tried to answer this question. Birds
probably make the use of several possible cues
which are as follows :

1. Learning by Parents

The best way of learning the way to a place if
you have never been before is to go with someone who knows the route. The young swan and
geese make their first migration with their parents as a family group, they get to know the
route and stopping points.

2. Instinctive behaviour

Migration may be instinctive. Birds do learn to
change their direction if they are blown off from
their fixed route.

Petrels breed on the tiny island of Tristan da
cunha and find their way across the Atlantic
ocean. Every year, starlings from the east of the
Baltic sea fly to England and Northern France.
Behaviourists discovered that young birds have
an innate tendency to fly in the southwesterly
direction. To study this tendency further, a young
flock of Starlings was interupted midjourney at
the Hague and transported south to Geneva.
When released they continued southwest to land
in unfamiliar Spain. When this experiment was
repeated with older birds, they flew north from
Geneva back on course. This suggests that
learned behaviour also help in navigation.

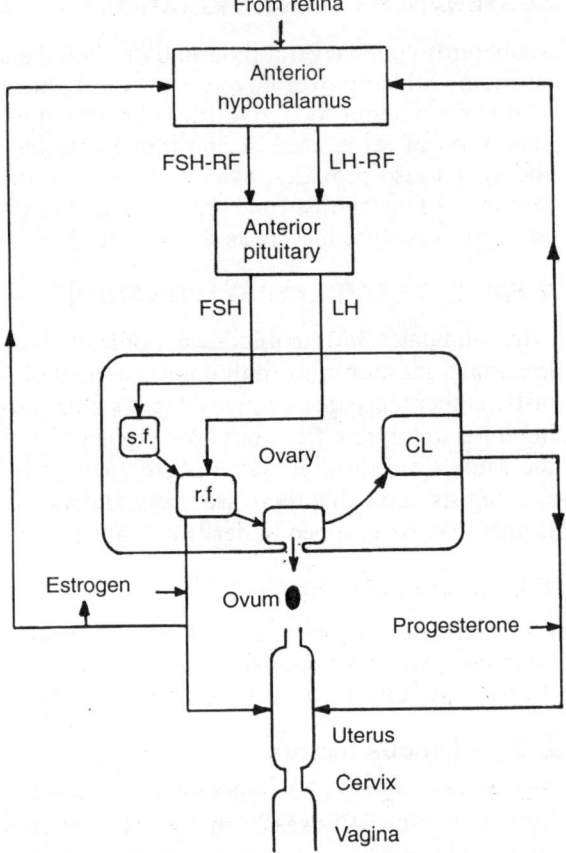

Fig. 8.25. Principal hormonal pathways involved in a
ovarian function in a typical vertebrate. FSH-RF,
Follicle stimulating hormone releasing factors; LH–
RF, luteininzing hormone releasing factor ; sf. small
follicle, rf. ripe follicle, CL corpus luteum

There are marked seasonal changes in body weight, gonad size, food preferences, restlessness etc. in
long distance migrants such as the Garden Warbler (*S.-robin*), the Sub alpine Warbler (*S. cantillans*),
and the willow Warbler (*P. trochilus*).

These species winter in Africa and migrate across the Sahara desert to Europe. When they are
maintained under constant laboratory conditions in Europe having been raised from a few days after
hatching, the events that are known to be seasonal in free living birds appear in caged members of the
same species as well.

When kept in cages, blackcaps (*Sylvia articapilla*) caught in Germany and Austria orient in a south
westerly direction during their migratory restlessness, consistent with their destination being the western mediteranean. Birds caught in England in the winter and returned to Germany oriented instead in a
northwesterly direction, consistent with England being their destination. When the offspring of birds
caught and bred in England in the winter were returned to Germany, they also oriented in a north
westerly direction, indicating that even the direction of migration is specified by instinct.

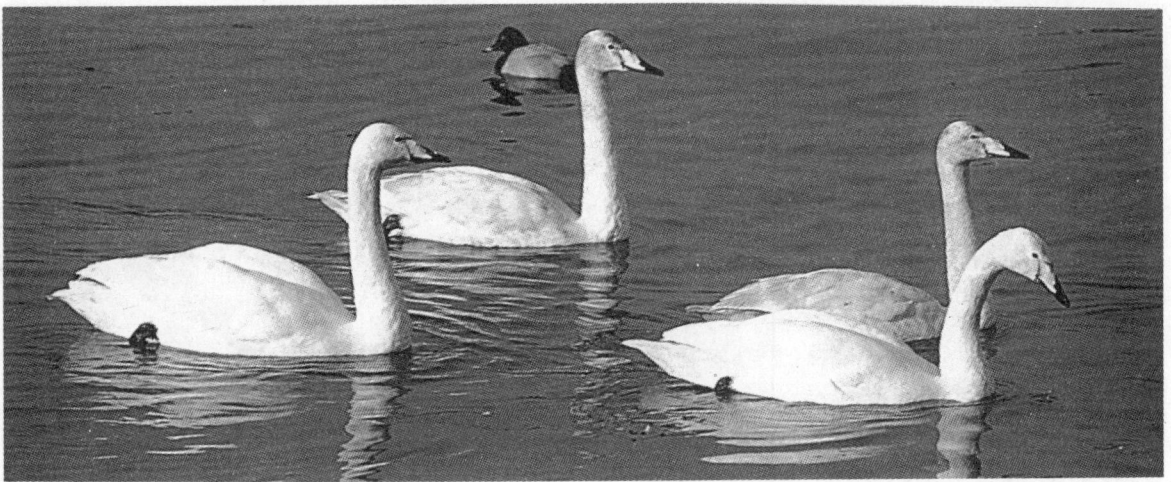

Fig. 8.26. This family of whooper swans travelled from their Arctic breeding grounds to winter in Western Europe. Adults and young birds travel and winter together.

Some migratory birds have to change their direction while migrating so that they can avoid major natural features such as a mountain range or wide sea crossing. Garden Warblers fly south-west through Europe but once they have crossed the Mediterranean, they head off due south to their wintering grounds in southern Africa.

It is surprising to know that migratory birds can also change their direction according to the time of the year. Experiments using Garden Warblers in captivity have shown this fact. Garden Warblers were kept in captivity in Europe. When set free, Garden warblers changed the direction they wished to fly at about the same time that wild birds would have been flying south through Africa.

VISUAL LANDMARKS

Birds in flight have a good view of landmarks such as lakes, hills, coastlines etc. The birds recognize and remember these landmarks. A returning young swallow remember the village, the meadow and even the perch it used the previous year. But one question arise that how nocturnal migrants see the visual landmarks?

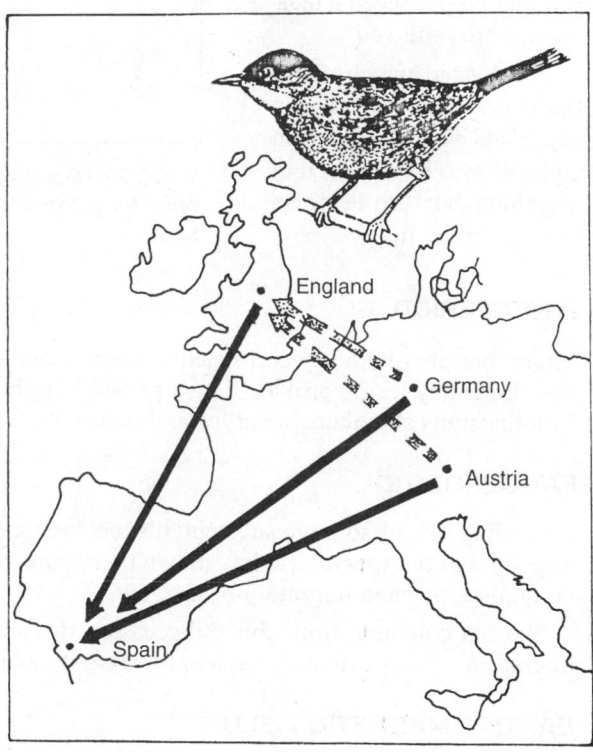

Fig 8.27. Old (Solid line) and new (broken line) migration route of blackcaps (*Sylvia articapilla*).

HORMONAL CONTROL

Some birds make outward journey to north in spring when their gonadal activity increases. Contrary to this their inward journey to south is associated with regression in gonadal activity. Bullough stated that prenuptial journey is stimulated by sex hormones and back home journey is allowed essentially by their absence. There are arguments both in favour and against this suggestion. For example, northward journey of European starling is associated with increased gonadal activity. European starlings migrate even if their gonads are removed.

The thyroid, which exhibits cyclical changes has been suggested by Hans, Oaklson and Lilley to be involved in migration, but its role is also not confirmed fully.

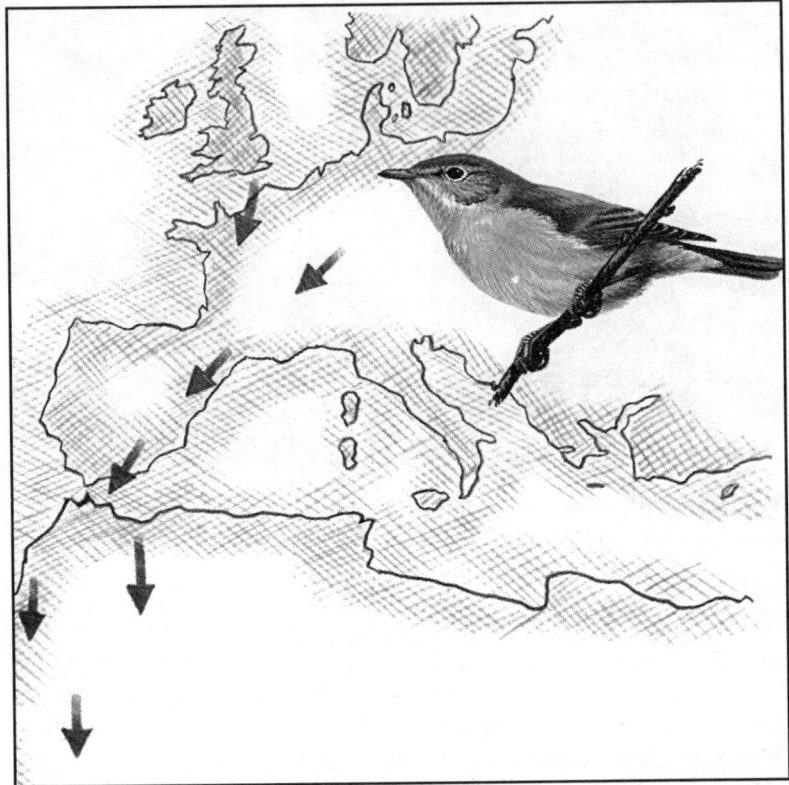

Fig. 8.28. Migratory route of Black poll - migrate south-west in Europe, but once they cross the Mediterranean they take a different course and fly south.

PHOTOPERIOD

Migrations are obviously correlated with the season and changes in the amount of daylight or photoperiod. Long day length provide longer period of light received by eye. This stimulate hypothalamus. The hypothalamus stimulate gonad through hormone. The hormone act on brain. Brain decide to migrate.

FAT DEPOSITION

According to Wolfson, the substantial subcutaneous and visceral fat deposits play an important role in migration of the species. He has shown that photo-stimulation leading to gonadal activation is followed by fat deposition in migratory birds.

We can conclude from above discussion that many external and internal factors stimulate birds to migrate and birds use many factors to navigate while migrating.

EARTH'S MAGNETIC FIELD

Gravity is a fix factor of environment and Van Middendroff and Henry L. Yeaglev gave the idea that some birds obtain information about direction from the Earth's magnetic field. A built in compass in animal's brain helps in finding ways. It is equivalent to our idea of north, south, east and west. These compasses use magnetic field of earth and position of sun. Griffin (1948) suggested that birds are guided by the earth's magnetic fields. Bird's internal ear reacts to the mechanical coriolis effect produced by the rotation of the earth. This theory got acceptance with the work of Eastwood (1965). Eastwood worked with Waterfowl and demonstrated that birds can migrate correctly under cloudy skies with the help of magnetic field of the earth as a source of directional information. Robins (*Erethaeus*) oriented their nocturnal activity in the migratory direction even without visual cues but not if they were equipped with small magnets released under cloudy skies. Other birds of same groups without instalation of the magnets were able to orient correctly in cloudy skies. This proves that earth's magnetic field helps in proper navigation.

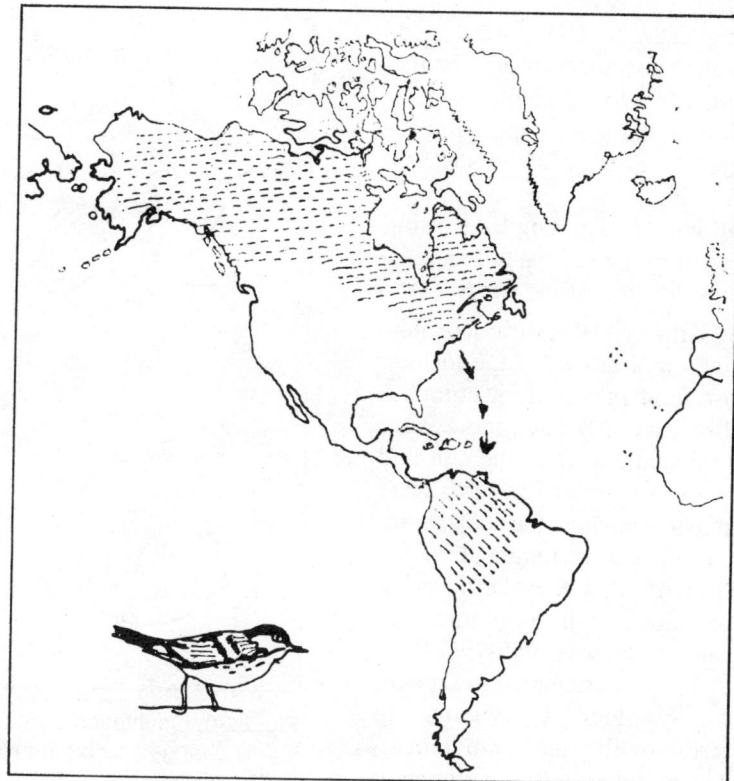

Fig. 8.29. Transatlantic migratory path of black poll.

How the magnetic field of the earth works is not fully understood, but a tiny magnetic crystal has been discovered inside sparrow and pigeon's skull. A sixth sense which allows birds to recognize direction to explain many of the mysteries of migration.

SENSE OF SMELL

Many of the 'tubenosed' seabirds, such as Shearwaters, Storm Petrels etc. have an extremely good sense of smell and are able to smell their way home from far out to sea.

INFRA SOUND OF EARTH

Sound with a frequency of 10 cycles/sec. is called infrasound. Humans cannot hear it but birds and many animals are able to hear infrasound. Infrasound may also help migrating birds to find their way. Infra-sound is the name given by scientists to the noises given off by the land. A flying bird is able to detect the differences in sound between sea and land, mountains and forests, open ocean and rocky coast. These sounds may be audible at a great distance and help in finding path of migration. Many migrating birds call as they fly. This keeps flocks together in the dark (Yodlowski et al. 1977, Kreitthen, 1978).

Sun Compass

Kramer (1951), Hoffman (1954), K.Schmidt-Konig (1958–51), Matthews (1965), Mc. Donald (1972–73), Whiten (1972) etc. demonstrated that many diurnal travellers use the sun as compass. They also suggested that migratory birds make allowances in their course according to the changing position of the sun as the day progresses. Some of them successfully altered the direction of flight of diurnal migrating birds using big mirrors to give a false apparent direction of the sun.

Kramer (1951) trained Starlings in a circular cage to look for food in a certain compass direction. All landmarks were excluded and only the sun and sky was visible. The birds were able to maintain a particular compass direction throughout the day showing that they could compensate for the movement of sun. Matthews (1955-1968) and Colin have attempted to account for the pigeon's navigation in terms of the sun's movement. The ability of a flying pigeon to determine the altitude of the sun has never been demonstrated, and this is an essential ingredient of sun navigation theory.

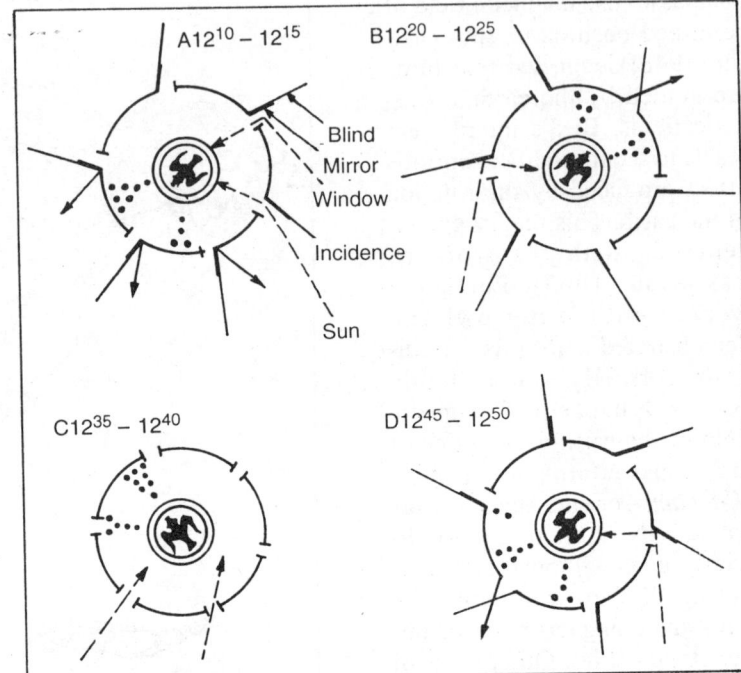

Fig. 8.30. Orientation of Starlings when the apparent direction of the sun is changed by big mirrors.

POSITION OF THE MOON AND STARS

Night migrants use the moon and stars in the night sky. The different phases of the moon are probably too complicated to be of help, but the patterns of the stars are used to navigate. This was discovered through experimenting with captive birds in a planetarium.

Navigation by the sun during the day and the stars at night is not possible in cloudy weather. Some birds get 'lost' in bad weather, but migration does not stop even when the sun and the stars are hidden by cloud. The position of sun and stars may help birds in navigation but there must be another aid to navigation used by birds.

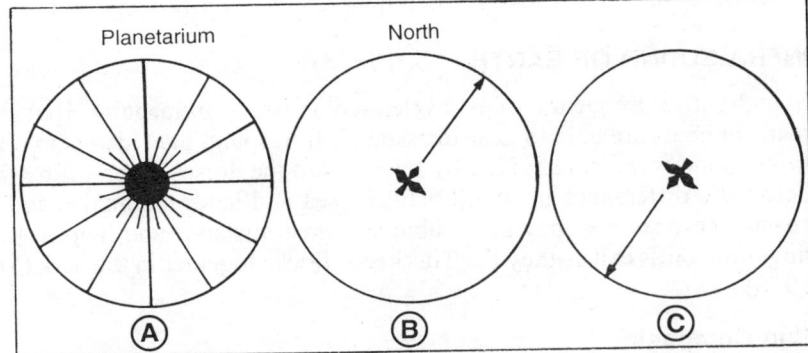

Fig. 8.31. Saucer's experiment with Warbler in a planetarium to show that night migrants use stars for guidance of routes.

Saucer and Saucer (1955) experimented with Songbirds and came to the conclusion that these birds use stars as guide for navigation. The work of Saucer was verified and later improved by Steve Emlen (1966-1972). Emlen performed this experiment on Indigo buntings (*Passerine cydnea*).

Emlen kept a few Buntings in a planetarium where the seasonal star patterns could be manipulated at will or shut off to stimulate a cloudy night. When these buntings in autumnal migratory condition were exposed to natural star filled sky, they could not orient themselves in a southward direction. This happens regardless of whether the planetarium sky pointed to true south or not. The Buntings lost the ability to orient themselves when the stars were not visible. He showed that hand raised Buntings without any sight of the sky were unable to orient properly during migration.

Radar observation of migratory birds suggests that the sun or stars (celestial bodies) are necessary for avian migration. But confirmation of this theory requires more investigations.

Ambient pressure

The birds can detect very minute difference in barometric pressure change (Kreitthen and Keeton, 1974: Delius and Emmerton, 1978). This sensory ability may provide birds with an accurate physiological altimeter.

Odour

Henton et al. (1966), Shumake et al. (1969) discovered by physiological methods that the olfactory sense in pigeons is sufficiently good to be used in navigation. Schmidt and Koenig (1979) confirmed the above finding in other bird species.

Polarized light

Normally the wave-like vibration occurs equally in all planes. In polarized light, the vibrations are greater in one plane. When unpolarized sunlight is scattered by atmospheric molecules, polarization occurs, greatest for the light scattered at an angle of 90 degrees to the rays of the sun, which means there is a pattern of polarization in the sky that changed according to the position of the sun.

Experiments show that pigeons are able to perceive rotations in the plane of polarization of light (Kreitthen and Keeton, 1974 : Delius et al. 1976). But it is not known how migratory birds interpret this information. The pattern of polarization of the sky can provide an indication of the sun's position even when the sky is overcast by clouds.

Biological clock

Mathew put forward the view that the birds are equipped to use a "biological clock" which enables them to make necessary adjustment in their course according to the changes in the position of the sun and stars.

Migration of birds is only possible when there is urge for migration within the bird. This urge is initiated in definite time of season by biological clock. Schmidt-Koenig (1985) have shown by experiment that the biological clock depends on the light dark cycle and can be upset by providing an artificial cycle out of phase with the natural one.

HOMING

The ability of birds to return to their exact native place, (in some cases they return to the same tree) is called homing. Scattered knowledge suggests that they return to their homes by instinct just like other animals (ants, bees, migratory fishes and mammals). Homing experiments with carrier pigeons have proved the importance of vision in navigation. Once a bird reaches in the general home vicinity they find their exact locality by recognising the familiar land marks.

SIGNIFICANCE OF MIGRATION

Advantages

1. Migration saves birds from extreme cold and heat. This provide suitable climate for living.
2. Birds emigrate from home ground in winter when there is extreme cold and no food. They reach to warmer region where suitable climate and sufficient food is available. They immigrate to original habitat when the condition is becoming suitable. Thus by alternatively utilizing two different habitats, birds are able to exist.
3. Breeding ground provide better and rich food which is essential for breeding.
4. In breeding ground birds get longer working hours to gather more food to feed young ones.
5. Migratory bird arrive in breeding ground in large numbers hence the pressure of predation is divided among a great number of eggs and young and this results in greater individual survival.
6. Migratory birds are subject to greater ecological diversity and therefore, have a greater range of adaptability than resident birds.

Disadvantages

Migratory birds face many dangers and hardships while travelling long distances over hills forests, and plains and over large stretches of water. Sometimes sudden storms arise and drive them far off their course. Often they are blown right out to sea and they are drawn in the wild waves. Then at night bright lights attract and confuse the birds. Small birds are eaten by predators during their travel. Many migratory birds die by electric and telephone wires. Hunters also kill migratory birds.

METHODS OF STUDYING BIRD MIGRATION

RINGING

Bird ringing is a technique which provides information on migration. Ringing is done by capturing young and adult birds. Birds are captured by light-sound, Mor-tatti, chargodi, teengodi, banana leaf method and with the help of Dhannijal and Mist Jal. Now numbered light band of metal or plastic is put on the leg of migratory bird. For ringing the birds, help of Mirshikar ("मीरशिकार") and Sahni (साहनी) type experts are taken. Birds are ringed on the upper portion of leg. The band bears a number, date, identification mark, and the address to which the finder is requested to return the ring. The bird is then set free. Sometimes tags made up of coloured plastic are attached on the bird's bill by a very thin nylon thread passing through the nostrils called nasal tags. Rings are of various shape and size - Z, A, AB, B, C, F, G, K and L. Z shaped ring is used for smaller birds like sparrow and L. shaped ring for bigger birds. Each ring is embossed with B.N.H.S. (Bombay Natural History Society). This is world wide Network for the study of ringed birds.

The bird ringing laboratory at Lawrel and Maryland in USA have maintained more than thirty million banding records and add a million new ones every year. In India, at Keoladeo National Park, Bharatpur, (Rajasthan) extensive research on migratory birds is going on. More than 1.5 lack birds have been ringed during past 30 years. By ringing method it has been possible to establish the migratory routes of birds. The ringing at Keoladeo National Park, Bharatpur has revealed that European swallows return not only to the same locality but even to the same tree for nesting year after year, covering a distance of

9,600 km. Dr. Salim Ali, the birdman of India observed that a ringed grey wagtail returned from Himalayan breeding place to a particular lawn in Bombay year after year on the exact date in September covering a distance of about 900 km.

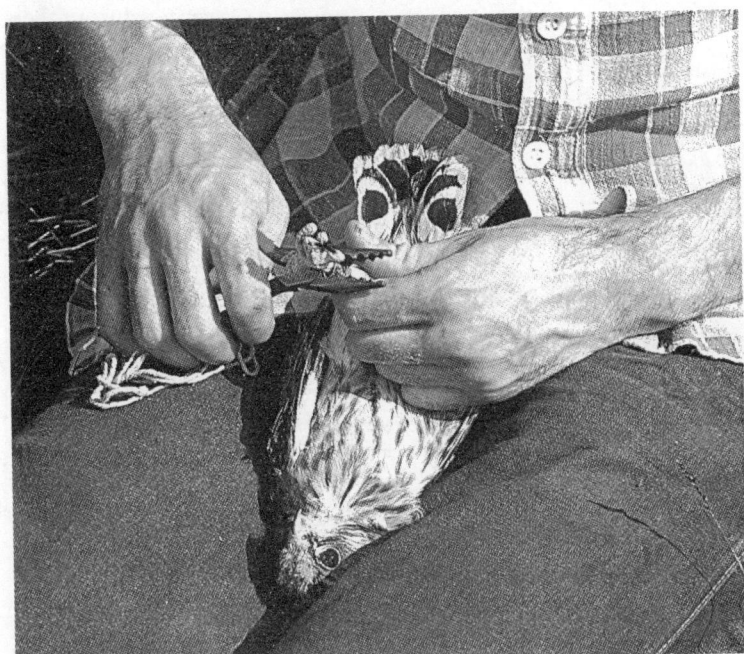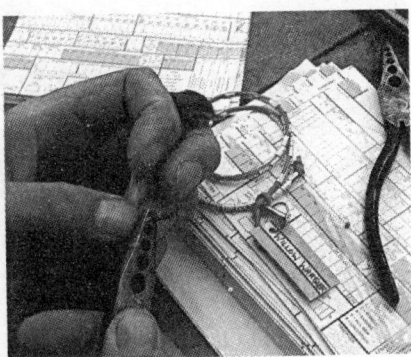

Fig. 8.32. Different rings and special pliers are used to tag birds ranging from Goldcrests to mute swans. People who ring birds are specially trained so that the birds can live a normal life, bearing a ring, after release.

By obseving movements across the face of the moon. The principal equipment needed, is a telescope. The birds crossing the face of the moon are counted.

A radio-transmitter and receiver is used for radio tracking when a bird cannot be followed visually.

By radar

Transmitter is implanted around the neck or stuck with a adhesive to the skin of the back between the wings and signals are received by radar.

By Tape recording or chip counting

The bird calls through a tape recorder, with the help of a parabolic receiver, microphone and amplifier. This is used to estimate the number of migrating birds by tabulating the call notes heard at night.

Birds Sanctuaries of India

1. Govind Sagar Bird Sanctuary   – Bilaspur, Himachal Pradesh
2. Ranganathittu Bird Sanctuary   – Mysore, Karnataka
3. Keoladeo Ghana Bird Sanctuary   – Bharatpur, Rajasthan
4. Kanwar Jheel Bird Sanctuary   – Begusarai, Bihar

MIGRATION OF MAMMALS

WILDEBEEST

Great herds of wildebeest live on the grassland of Africa but their food supply depends on the rains. They undergo long migrations to reach suitable feeding areas. They follow tradinal routes during their journeys which cross fast flowing rivers and through country side where there is no food.

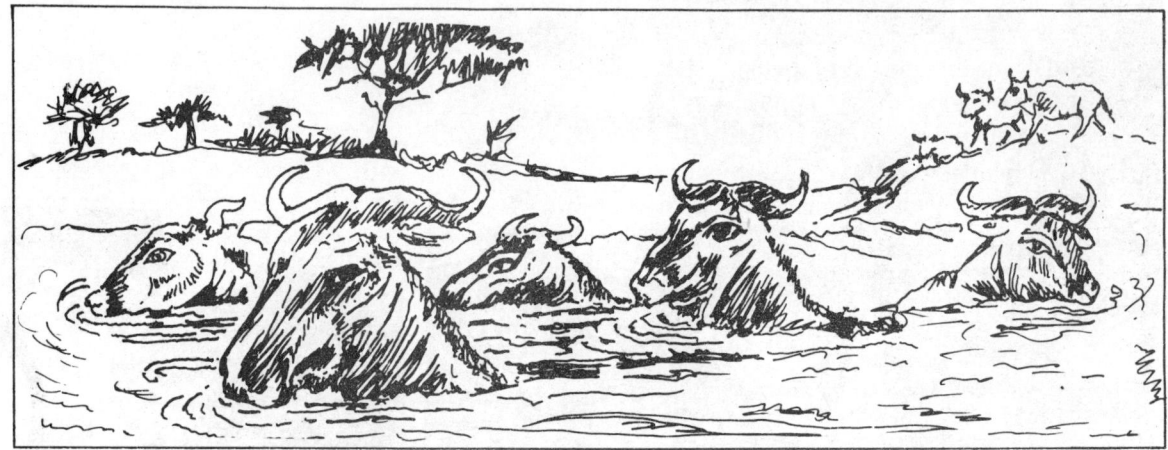

Fig. 8.33. Migrating wildebeest.

GREAT WHALES

Great whales are huge mammals. They are largest creature of the planet earth. They are found in all the oceans. Humpback whales give birth in warm sub-tropical seas. There is one population around Hawaii and another near the West Indies. In late summer, after breeding, these whales migrate northwards to reach feeding area on the edge of the Arctic. The Hawaiian whales swims to the waters off the coast of Alaska and the west Indian whales move north to feed on the Grand Banks off the east coast of America before proceeding further north to fishing grounds of Labrador.

EXERCISE

1. Define migration. Describe the migration of fishes. (Civil services, 1968)
2. Name at least 5 migratory fishes. What purpose migration serve to migratory species.
3. Mention factors causing fish migration.
4. Describe advantages and disadvantages of fish migration.
5. Give an account of the migration of fishes. Explain its significance and controlling factors. (Civil services, 1978)
6. Describe navigation of fishes. Support your answer with suitable example.
7. Describe migratory behaviour of Tunna, Herring, Sword fish, Arcto Norwegian cod and flatfish.
8. Describe different methods of study of fish migration.
9. With special reference to reptiles give an account of reptile migration.
10. With special reference of Indian birds give an account of bird migration. (Civil services, 1969)

11. Give a critical account of the migration of birds. What role is played by the endocrine glands during migration. (Civil services, 1975–1977)
12. Describe navigation of birds. Support you answer with suitable example.
13. In what way migration is the greatest mysteries of bird life? Mention methods of studying bird migration.
14. Describe Different methods of studying bird migration.
15. What is the difference between :
    (a) Diadromous and Potamodrormous fish.
    (b) Amphidromous and semi migratory fishes.
    (c) Detanatant and Contranatant fishes.
    (d) Resident and migratory birds.
    (e) Altitudinal and Latitudinal migration of birds.
    (f) Alimental migration and Gametic migration.
    (g) Leptocephalus larva and Elver's larva.
16. Describe migration of wildebeest and back hump whale.

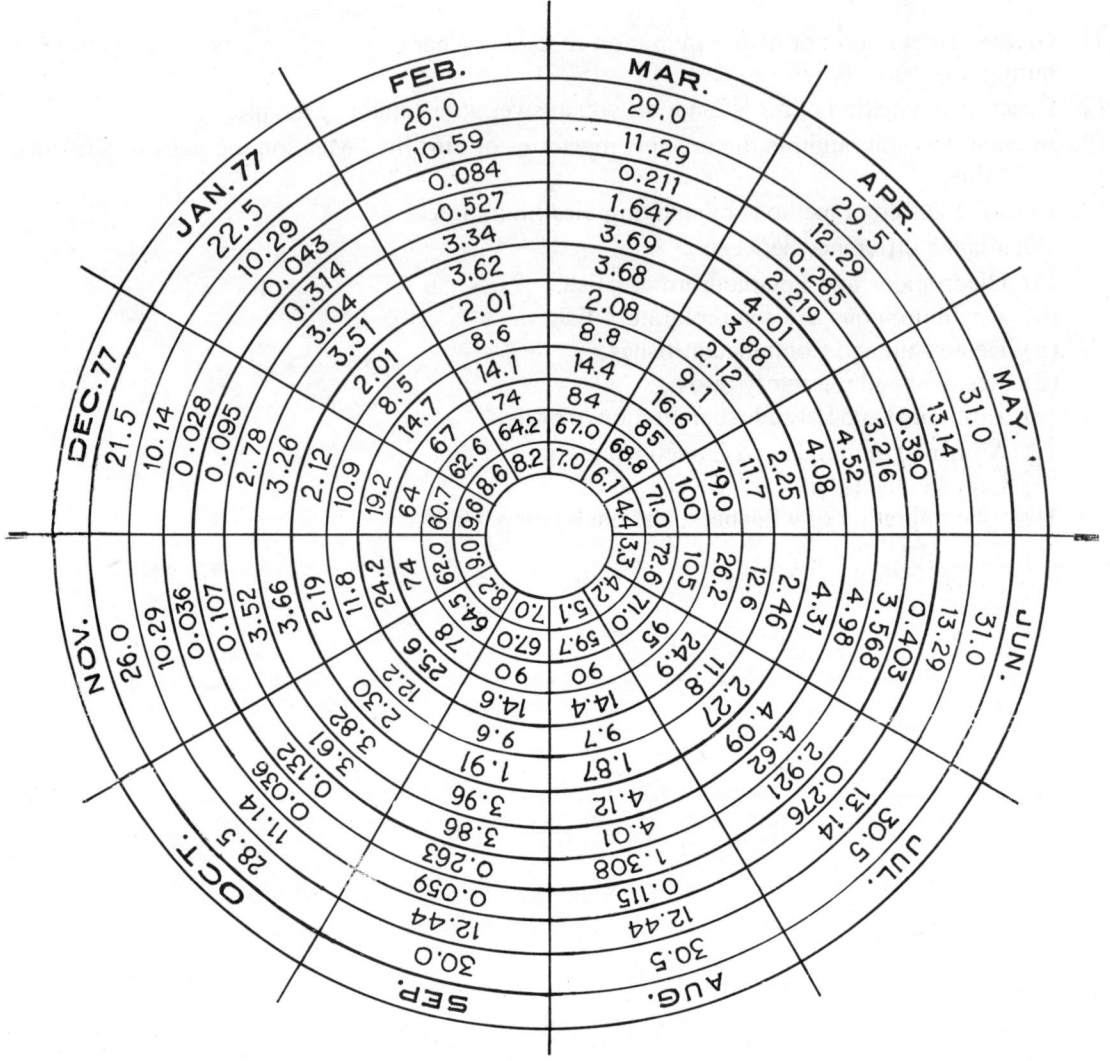

We use watch for knowing the time of day and night. Do plants and animals have time sense? The answer is yes, they have better time sense than us. The opening and closing of flower of lotus takes place in a definite time in morning and evening respectively. Sun flower faces to east as soon as sun rises in the morning and rotates its position during day time with the rotating angle of the sun. In the evening sunflower face to the west and lowers its head as soon as the sun sets. Mosquitoes attack us in the evening at twilight. Birds start foraging in the morning and return to their nest at a definite time in the evening even in cloudy or rainy weather. Again a question arises "how do plants and animals know about time of the day or night?" Plants and animals have a built in clock called biological clock. The biological clock help them to know the time of the day and night. This chapter deals with biological clock of organisms.

CHRONOBIOLOGY 9

- Introduction
- Historical perspective
- Exogenous rhythms and endogenous rhythms
- Biological clock
- Origin and evolution of biological clock
- Rhythm gene
- Various types of endogenous rhythms :
  - Circadian rhythm : Mechanism of circadian rhythm
  - Circannual rhythm
  - Breeding rhythm : Breeding cycle, hibernation, diapause, migration
  - Lunar rhythm : Swarming of Palolo worm, Grunion fish, ovulation in cattle, dictyota, diseases
  - Tidal rhythm : Influence of environmental cycles upon biological clock of organism
  - Main endogenous sources of biological clock
- Exercise

INTRODUCTION

Rhythmicity is a wonderful phenomenon of nature. Day night cycle, seasonal cycle, moon cycle, tide cycle etc. are examples of rhythm of nature. Organisms also exhibit rhythmicity in behavioural activities. Rhythmicity in behavioural activities of organisms are known as biological rhythms or biorhythms. There are numerous examples of biorhythms.

You must have experienced that you tend to wake up almost at the same time everyday in the morning and start feeling sleepy at certain time as the night falls. In other words man is diurnal but bat is nocturnal. These are examples of circadian rhythm of 24 hours, matching the cycles of day and night. Courtship displays and nesting behaviour of birds in the spring and the migration of certain bird species in autumn are examples of circannual rhythm. Circannual period of a year, matching the season.

The breeding of the palolo worm and grunion fish coincides with the rotation of moon, circular rhythm of 29 days, matching the moon cycle. Shore crab and Fiddler crabs have daily rhythm matching the tide cycle of 12.4 or 24.8 hours, called circatidal cycle. The time interval between activities can vary from minutes to years depending on the nature of the activity and species. For example, the polychaete *'Arenicola marina'* lives in U shaped burrow in sand and carries out feeding movements every 6 to 7 minute. This rhythmic feeding behaviour has no apparent external stimulus nor internal physiological stimulus. It appears that the feeding pattern rhythm is regulated by a biological 'clock' mechanism dependent, in this case, on a 'pace maker' originating in the pharynx and transmitted through the worm by the ventral nerve cord. The biorhythm in women that help bring life to earth are complex and time bound. The menstrual cycle is a monthly sequence of changes that prepares the female body for conception and pregnancy. This cycle repeats itself about every 28 days until either conception occurs or the child bearing years end the menopause at about the age of fifty. This rhythm is also regulated by a biological clock.

267

Rhythms involving a biological clock or pace maker are known as endogenous rhythm, as opposed to exogenous rhythm which are controlled by external factors. Apart from examples such as the feeding behaviour of *Arenicola* and menstrual cycle of women, most biological rhythms are a blend of endogenous and exogenous rhythms.

In many cases the major external factor regulating the rhythmic activity is photoperiod, the relative lengths of day and night. This is the only factor which can provide a reliable indicator of time of year and is used to 'set the clock'. The exact nature of the clock is unknown but the clock work mechanism is decidedly physiological and involve two different but related systems of co-ordination : the nervous system and the endocrine system. The effect of photoperiod has been studied extensively in relation to behaviour in insects, birds and mammals and, whilst it is evidently important in activities such as diapause in insects, migration in birds and preparation for hibernation in mammals, it is not the only external factor regulating biological rhythms.

The behaviour of many completely terrestrial insects appears to be controlled by endogenous rhythms related to periods of light and dark. For example, *Drosophila* emerge from pupae at dawn. Cockroaches are most active at the onset of darkness and just before dawn. These regularly occurring biological rhythms, exhibiting a periodicity of about 24 hour, are known as *circadian* rhythm or *diurnal* rhythm.

Circadian rhythms have many species specific adaptive significances and one of these involves orientation. Animals such as fish, turtles, birds and some insects which migrate over long distances use the sun and stars as a compass. Honeybees, ants and sandhoppers use the sun as a compass in locating food and their homes. Compass orientation by sun or moon is only accurate if organisms using it possess some means of registering time so that allowances can be made for the daily movement of the sun and moon. The concept of 'jetlag' is an example of a situation where the human internal physiological circadian rhythm is out of gear with the day-and-night rhythms of the destination.

Lunar rhythms, too, can influence activity in certain species, such as the palolo worm of Samoa. The polychaete worm swarms and mates throughout the whole South Pacific on one day of the year, the first day of the last lunar quarter of the year, on average 2nd November. The influence of lunar rhythms on tidal variations is well known, and there are two exogenous factors which have been shown to impose a rhythmic behaviour pattern on the midge *Clunio maritimus*. The larvae of *clunio* feed on red algae growing at the extreme lower tidal limit, a point only uncovered by the tide twice each lunar month. Under natural conditions these larvae hatch, the adults mate and lay eggs in their two-hour-long life during which they are uncovered by the tide. In laboratory conditions of a constant 12 h light–12 h dark photoperiod the larvae continued to hatch at about 15-day intervals, demonstrating the existence of an endogenous clock programmed to an approximately semi-lunar rhythm coinciding with the 14.8 day tidal cycle.

Rhythmic events are so prominently expressed in the behaviour of an animal that Biological rhythms or biorhythms make an integral part of ethology.

HISTORICAL PERSPECTIVE

Rhythmicity or periodicity of various kind in the living world have remained a matter of keen interest for humans. In the year 1729, scientists observed that the extreme downward position of leaves of plants were frequently a few hours after midnight. On the basis of this observation they came to the conclusion that the time of day was the major factor affecting the movements of leaves and thus started the work on the effect of time on behaviour of organisms. It was also found by De Mairan, an astronomer that these movements continue even in the absence of any external cues of any sort and it proved the endogenous nature of these rhythms. There is so much synchronisation of the phenological behaviour of the plant species and the different factors of the environment that plants are spoken as biological clock or ecological clocks. Fig. 9.1 explains the different stages of the ecological life cycle of a plant species. Biological clocks couple environmental (external timing hypothesis) and physiological rhythms and enable the organisms to anticipate daily, seasonal and other rhythmicities in light, temperature, tides etc.

After a gap of about hundred years i.e., in the last decade of nineteenth century Kaisel did some work on animals and found daily fluctuation in pigment patterns in arthropods. Quinke was the first to measure the rhythmic pattern in the urinary excretion, pulse frequencies, temperature in human beings. The major break through in the study of human circadian rhythm came with the work of Kleitman (1939) who reported a definite pattern of sleep and wakefulness at a certain time of day.

Different plant species differ in respect of their response to interacting climatic factors at different stages of their life

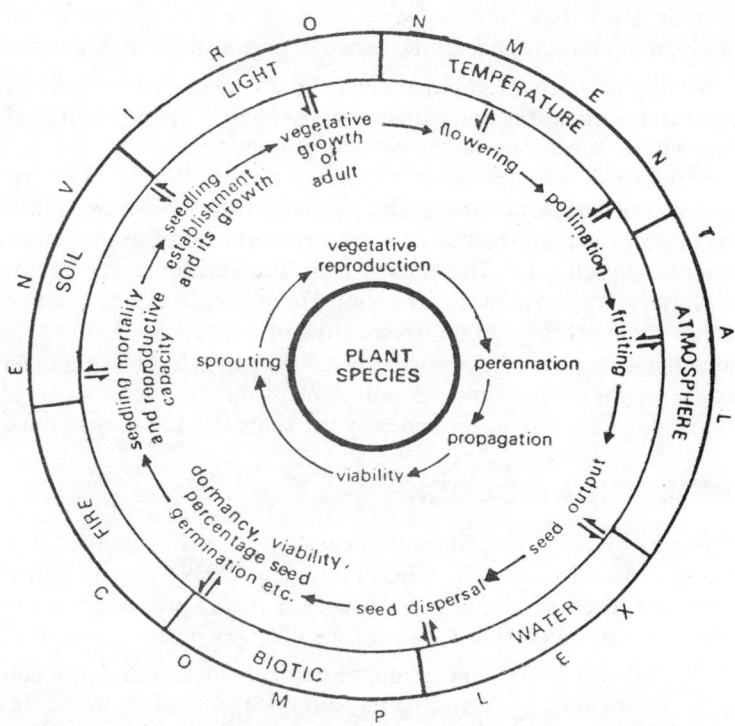

Fig. 9.1. Ecological life cycle of a Plant or biological clock. Each stage in the life cycle is influenced by many factors opening in conjunctions as an environmental complex and not, as shown in the diagram, that only one particular factor influences particular stage (s) of the life cycle of a plant.

cycles. Each species has a definite period (month, season) in the year during which its seeds will germinate, its seedlings will grow, it will show vegetative growth, and will flower and fruit. Study of all these periodic behaviour of a specie is called its *Phenology*. Since each species has a definite period for a particular stage of its life cycle, presence of the species in that particular stage will indicate the time (month, season) of the year. Each species in other words is able to tell a particular time of year hence plant species are said to be *biological clocks*.

Exogenous rhythm and Endogenous rhythm

Up to beginning of twentieth century scientists could not recognise the importance of behaviours occurring periodically (without regard to changes of environmental factors) a kind of innate rhythm of behaviour. A German botanist Erwin Bunning (1936), on the basis of his own investigations and those of others, was able to state that organisms have an in built and automatic rhythms which are independent of environmental rhythms.

The study of periodicity in behaviour opens an interesting field of biology known as *chronobiology*. The term "chronobiology" was coined by F. Hallberg in the beginning of the 20th century. It is made up of two words '*chrono*' means *related to time* and '*biology*' means *science of life*. Thus chronobiology may be defined as "*study of science of life related to time*". The science of life related to time means study of "in built time keeping sense of organisms" i.e. biological clock of organisms.

An Indian scientist Sirohi and two American scientists Hammer and Hoshizaki went to Antarctica and carried few plants (Fungi, hamster and been plants) and animals (Fruit flies) to study rhythmicity in their behaviour. These organisms were kept on a turning table. The table rotated in such a fashion that it nullified the rotation of earth which is minimum at poles. The organisms were kept in constant darkness and at constant temperature. The plants and animals showed their usual rhythmic behaviour at the pole and there was no influence of earth's rotation either. Both plants and animals maintained their 12 hour sleep/wake schedule. The eggs of fruit flies hatched every 24 hours and fungi in petridish showed light dark rings of growth every 24 hours. These simple experiments on poles indicated that once the biological clock is set they go on irrespective of exogenous rhythms. Experiments have showed that animals and plants maintain their biorhythms even when the relevant external stimuli were either removed artificially or when organisms were displaced from their habitat and placed in conditions of constant light or dark, they continue to show nearly the same rhythm they maintained in their natural habitat.

BIOLOGICAL CLOCK

Different behavioural, physiological and physical rhythms of an organism remain linked together to form a clock like system called biological clock. The biological clock of an organism does not only expresses the periodicity in behaviour, but also programmes the entire drama of a particular phenomenon. It also predicts the onset of the changes in environment.

Prasad S. tried to make a mini biological clock taking into consideration some of the parameters of a fish *Macrognathus,* exhibiting physiological annual rhythms. He observed that studied parameters were repeated in successive year in control cases (Fig. 9.2).

A human being's clock becomes evident after we fly to another continent through changing time zones. "*Jet lag*" are fatigue, lack of concentration and motivation, disorientation and fuzziness. 'Jet lag' happens when we cross quickly from one time zone into another sitting in a boeing. Yet "Jet lag" remains one of the most persistent curses of modern jet travel where long-haul flights across varying time zones disturbs the body clock enough for it to need several days to readjust. One needs one day for every time zone crossed, to regain normal rhythm and energy levels. So a five-hour time difference means one requires five days to get back to normal. Crossing time zones can cause one to wake during the night and then want to fall asleep during the day. Menstrual cycles of air hostesses get affected because their hormonal rhythm is thrown out of gear constantly.

There are medicines to combat "Jet lag". Currently the pills used most frequently remain the allopathic *maltonin* or "*no jet lag*", consisting of a cerebral hormone, or the homeopathic "no jet lag", consisting of ingredients like Arnica, Ipecac, Lycopodium, Chamomilla and Bellis perenis.

The above discussion explains that organisms possess internal clock that controls the rhythm in behaviour, and keep it along with the help of internal physiology while external stimuli serve only to set and reset this clock periodically. J. Aschoff (1960) coined a term *Zeitgebers* (a German term meaning time giver) for the environmental agent that entrains the behaviour of organisms to the external environment. Another German Scientist Von Buttel Reeper proposed a new tern *Zeitgedachtnis* (time sense) to express for animals having internal biological clock.

Origin and evolution of Biological clock

Rhythmic events occur every where in the environment. The *sun rises and sets* forming *days and nights* (circadian cycle). The *moon moves* through its phases forming lunar cycle. The *tides get high and low* regularly constituting *tidal rhythms*. The orbit around the *sun rotation of earth* creates *seasons*. It has been a subject of keen interest whether periodicity in an organism is determined by external environmental stimuli (exogenous) or controlled through physiological factors within the animal itself (endogenous).

Initially to set the clock and run it, external daily or annual or seasonal or lunar phase or tidal cycle played main role, but after very long period, the biological clock of the individuals is maintained and run by internal body physiology. In other words we can say that during the process of organic evolution, organisms have acquired a variety of endogenous rhythms, their periods are matched with rhythmic events occurring in the environment. Some rhythms are matched to about 24 hour cycle of light and dark (circadian), and 29 day (circalunar), and yearly seasons (circannual).

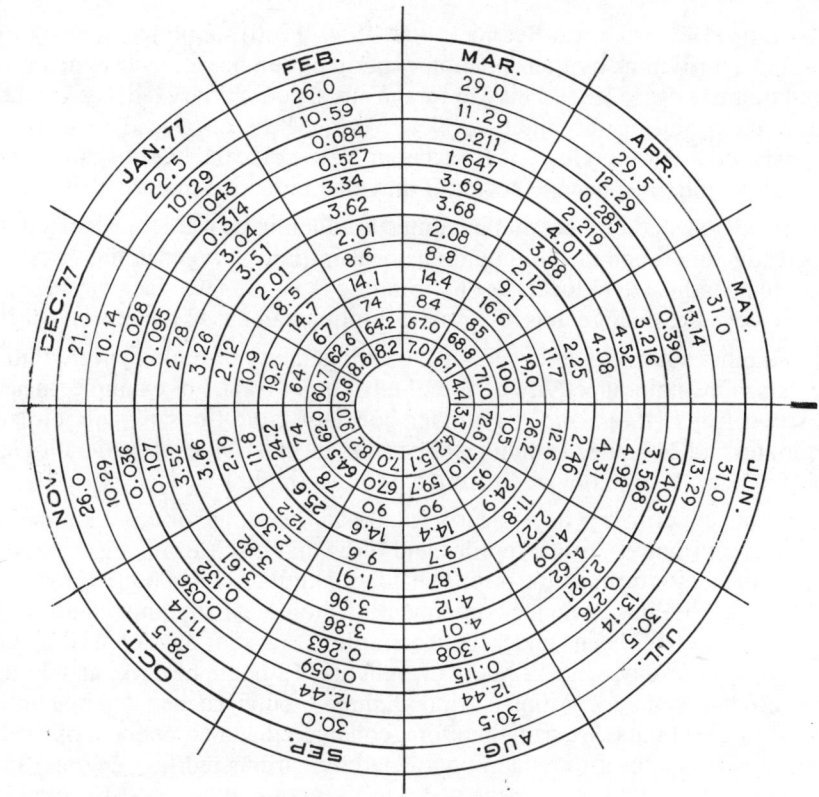

Fig. 9.2. Annual rhythm of some of the parameters of a fish. M. aculeatus constituting a kind of mini-biological clock. 1. Months : Jan. '77 to Dec. 77; 2. Water tempe-rature; 3. Day length; 4. GSI: Male; 5. GSI: Female; 6. Cell height of thyroid follicle; 7. Mean nuclear diameter of interrenal cell of adrenal; 8. R.B.C. (millions); 9. H.b.%; 10. P.C.V.%; 11. Oxygen consumption; 12. Water % body; 13. Lipid % body. (Sequence of the No. follows from periphery to the centre).

The physiological rhythms of an individual become linked together to make a time sense endogenous clock. The endogenous rhythms remain well adapted with that of the exogenous cycle (such as day-night, annual or seasonal changes) and ultimately become innate and independent. In general, it is apparent that many species of animals, ranging from the single-celled to the complex multicellular animals, have evolved a time sense endogenous clock.

Following examples show how endogenous rhythms (Biological clock) work independently after deviating from the influence of exogenous cycles. Honeybee native to Brazil use the sun as a compass in foraging. They were trained to search food in a particular compass direction and when they were moved from one locality to another, they continued to forage in the same compass direction, irrespective of the local time of the day. Thus, bees native to Brazil are capable of compensating for the anti clockwise motion of the sun. However, northern hemisphere bees transported to Brazil are initially unable to make the appropriate compensation. In the northern hemisphere the sun appears to move in a clockwise direction and the bees have to learn to adjust to the changed conditions in Brazil (Lindauer, 1960 ; Saunders, 1976). Hasler and Sehwassmann (1960) observed similar abilities in fishes and Schmidt-

Koening (1979) in birds. Renner (1957, 1959, 1960) supported the hypothesis of endogenous control of biological rhythms by translocation experiment on bees. He designed a room with constant conditions and trained bees to leave a hive to forage at a specific time each day. He trained the bees in Paris and then flew them, during the night, to New York, where he placed them in a similar enclosed room with constant conditions. On their first day in New York, the bees began to forage at a time identical to that which would have been expected if they had remained in Paris that is 24 hours after their foraging.

In related studies, bees that inhabited outdoor hives were translocated from Long Island to California. Investigators found that, although the bees initially foraged at the same time as at the original site, they gradually adjusted to local time by foraging later and later each day. This experiment suggest that while the clocks are endogenous, external condition can cause the biological rhythms to be reset.

Another source of evidence for the endogenicity of biological rhythm comes from the variation that exists in the natural activity period of most organisms. For example, measurement of the activity period of two frogs (*Rana pipiens*) under constant conditions reveals circadian rhythm of 23 hours, 10 minutes and 24 hours, 33 minutes. The animals must have internal biological clock that, due to individual differences, lead to deviation from a 24 hour rhythm.

Some experiments have clearly ruled out "learning" or other similar influences as a mechanism for biological rhythms. Some reptiles and birds that hatch from eggs can be kept under constant condition in an incubator from a time prior to hatching until after hatching. If the newly hatched organisms exhibit circadian rhythms, a major component of biological rhythms would appear to be inherited. Hoffman (1959) kept lizard eggs under three conditions, 18 hour days consisting of 9 hour of light and 9 hours of dark; 24 hour day, with 12 hours of light and 12 hours of dark; and 36 hour day with 18 hours of light and 18 hours of dark. Animals from all three groups hatched and maintained running activity periods of 23.4 to 23.9 hours. We can, therefore, conclude that a component of the biological clock mechanism in these lizards appear to remain unaffected by various rearing regimes, and is thus endogenous.

Rhythm gene

Biological clock is specified by genes or not is a debatable question. Some studies support the view that organisms bear rhythm gene that help to maintain periodicity in activities of animals. *Drosophila* is excellent for studies of circadian rhythms — the *eclosion rhythm* (concerning the time of day when they will complete metamorphosis and emerge from the pupal cases), and the *locomotor activity rhythm* (concerning the time of the day they will be active and the time they will rest). *Drosophila* ecloses very early in the morning, at about 4 a.m. They thus have sufficient time to stretch and harden their cuticles and begin to fly about before their predators become active. They too have a circadian clock that permits them to eclose.

Ronald Konopka and Benzer generated mutant *Drosophila* bearing a gene *per*. These flies had abnormal circadian rhythms. The various forms or alleles of the *per* locus make the flies different having clocks that have cycles of about 16 hours, about 19 hours or about 28 hours instead of the usual "about" 24 hours and one form even makes the fruit flies arhythmic. Incidentally the defect is seen not only in the eclosion rhythm but also in the locomotor activity rhythm.

The *per* gene protein is made in brain cells but its exact job is not known. But it is known that the levels of per messenger RNA as well as per protein oscillate in the brain cells with a periodicity that mirrors other rhythmic functions. Thus the per messenger RNA and protein oscillate with a periodicity of 24 hours in normal and mutant flies entrained to the normal circadian cycles. The molecules oscillations have a periodicity of about 24 hours in normal flies deprived of environmental cues, and a periodicity of the appropriate 16, 19, or 28 hours in mutants deprived of environmental cues. The messenger RNA and protein do not oscillate in the arhythmic mutant when it is deprived of environmental cues.

We are not definite whether *per* is the clock itself or whether *per* is only the part of the clock, and some other master control gene has yet to be discovered. But it is definite that *per* takes part for such complex behaviours as the timing of eclosion and the locomotor activity cycles of *Drosophila*.

Hajima Tei at Human Genome Centre in the University Tokyo has identified human and mouse gene that produce peptides similar to the product of *Drosophila's per gene*. Their finding might lead to the identification of molecules that constitute the biological clock. This would help in better understanding of how the clock works in mammals, including humans. Recent studies have shown that two genes are responsible for circadian rhythms in humans. The first gene acts as an independent timer, like a clock spring, while the other gene is gear log which keeps the clock running.

ENDOGENOUS RHYTHMECIES

Most of the organisms show periodicity in behaviour through various endogenous rhythms. Various types of endogenous rhythms are as follows :

I. CIRCADIAN RHYTHM

Among all rhythms, circadian rhythms have been widely studied. The term circadian is originated from the Latin word, *circa* = about, *dian* = a day. It has been defined as an approximately 24 hours physiological pattern that exhibits daily changes in activities. In other words ability to time and repeat functions falling short of a 24 hour interval even in the absence of the conspicuous diurnal clues such as light, is known as circadian rhythm. It is easy to study circadian rhythms as they recur within 24 hours in the activity of an individual.

Patra (1994) studied circadian rhythm in Vo$_2$ consumption in three air breathing fishes (Anabas, Channa and Clarias), and observed a rhythm in their metabolism. These fishes were most active during the morning, when they moved actively in search of food and from afternoon onwards they became inactive. This rhythmicity is closely interrelated with the diurnal fluctuation of dissolved oxygen.

A few birds and smaller mammals, inspite of being homeothermal, show diurnal variations in their body temperature and this is correlated with their changed metabolic activity during day and night.

Different organisms of a community exhibit different time in circadian rhythm. Some are active during night (mosquitoes, cockroaches, owl etc.) other during the day (man and most mammals, houseflies, etc.), and still others only during twilight period (Sandfly).

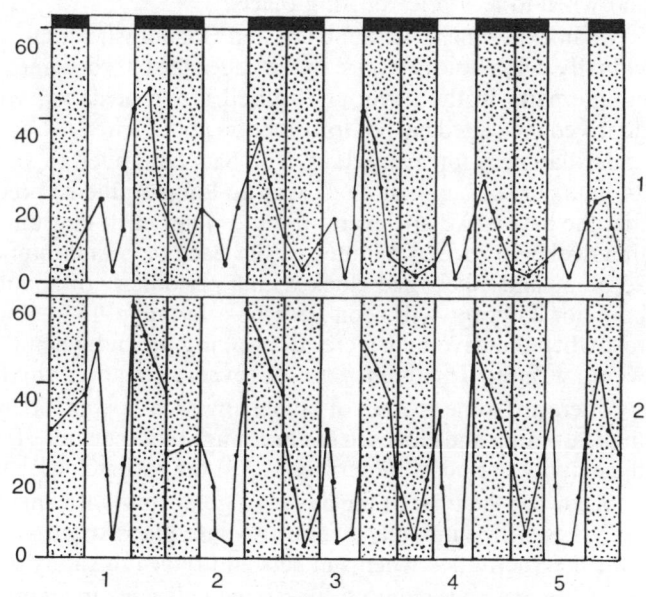

Fig. 9.3. Periodic activity of two mice (Mus *muscularis*) on a 24 hour light/dark schedule (Circadian rhythm) in the laboratory.

To study the circadian rhythm of mouse, a cage outfitted with a device that recorded all movements of the mouse, was used. When the records are summarized in the form of a graph with appropriate units for the time axis, the graphs reveals a cycle of activity which often reaches a major peak just after sunset and a minor peak around sunrise. There is little activity in the middle of the day (Fig. 9.3). Studies on rats have shown that rat hypophysis shows a circadian periodicity in TSH ovulation. Hormone is secreted by the hypophysis according to diurnal rhythm.

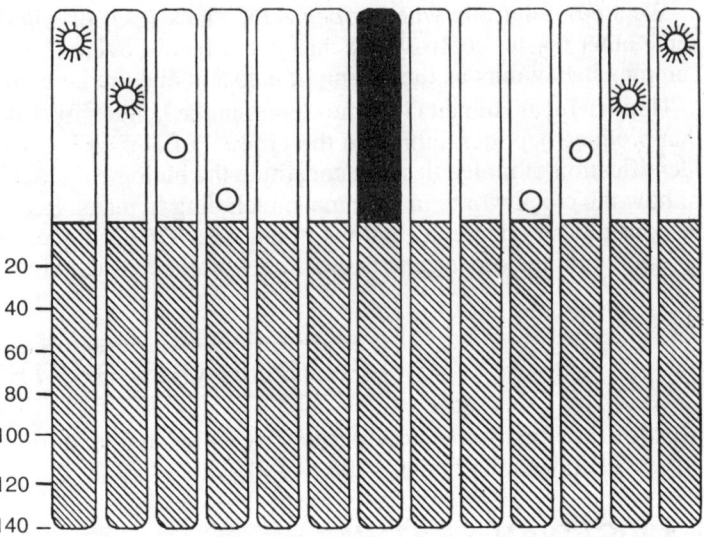

Fig. 9.4. Vertical day-night migration of three species of zooplankton in a pond.

Circadian periodicity in aquatic habitats is found in the vertical migration of zooplantons which regularly occurs in both lakes and oceans. Copepods, Cladocerans, larval forms of crustacea etc., which make up the vast floating life in the open waters, generally move upwards the surface at night and downward during the daylight.

M.K. Chandrashekharan and his students at Madurai Kamraj University (Tamilnadu, India) have established an array of research activities in an attempt to understand how the bats know when to leave and when to return to roosting place.

In an experiment, R. Subbaraj and Chandrashekaran captured some of the bats and kept them individually in laboratory cages. In the cages the bats became restless and tried to fly about at dusk, like their counterparts in the cave, and quited down at dawn, when the free bats returns to the cave. They deprived the caged bats of information about when it was dusk and when it was dawn, by keeping them under darkness for many days. The bats continued to show the same periodic bursts of activity every 24 hours or so, but their clock was no longer quite so precise. Sometimes their clock was a bit slow, so that the bats woke up several minutes later each day, and sometimes their clock was a bit fast, so that they woke up several minutes earlier each day. Thus some bats had a clock with a periodicity of about 23 hours and others had clock with a periodicity of about 25 hours. Obviously bats with a clock of 23 hours or 25 hours will soon become arhythmic. In about 12 days the experimental bats were ready to rest when the cave bats were just waking up and when the cave bats were going for rest the cage bats were awaking. This is the case of reverse circadian rhythm.

There are some species of plants of which flowers open in the morning and close at night; some open in the evening and closes in the morning. Most species of moths fly during night and rest in daytime. But the activity period of butterflies is just the reverse, it fly in day time and rest at night.

Knowing the time of the day is of great survival value to animals. Diurnal animals need to start their activities with sunrise and return to safe place when sun sets. Conversely, nocturnal animals need to start their activities when sun sets and return to safety with sun rise.

Migratory birds show striking punctuality in circannual rhythm for emigration and immigration. The arrival time (month and even day) of certain birds (Cranes) from Baikal Lake of Siberia to Keoladeo National Park (Rajasthan, India), can be predicted with 100% accuracy. The purple martins return to their homeland on the same day and same locality.

Honeybees have great power to know the time. Some flowers blossom once in a day (once in 24 hours) in a specific time. Honeybees reach to these flowers at the same time with the help of alarm of its own biological clock. Light compass response (Menotaxes, *Meno* = I remain) shown by ants while returning to nest is the interesting example of time keeping sense (Fig. 2.4c).

The microfilarae of African eye worm (*Loa-Loa*) appear in the peripheral circulation of the host (men) in day time only, going deeper during night. *Wuchereria bancrofti* (causing filaria to man) show nocturnal periodicity. The microfilarae of Wuchereria live by day time chiefly in large deep seated blood vessels. But at night they come to small superficial vessels in the skin. Pinworm (*Enterobius vermicularis*) live in the colon of small intestine of *Homo sapiens* in day time. The gravid females of this worm migrate to perianal region at late night to deposit eggs in the skin folds about the anus. These all are examples of Circadian periodicity in some behaviour of free living and parasitic animals.

Human circadian rhythm

Numerous physiological activities such as hormone levels, blood pressure, EEG, ECG, activity—rest cycle, body temperature etc. in humans show a periodicity of 24 hours. The secretion of various hormones from different endocrine glands show rhythmic pattern. Pineal gland is the most important gland for this rhythmic pattern. The secretion of *serotonin* hormone from this gland is highest in the noon and lowest in the mid night, whereas the secretion of *melatonin* hormone, is highest in the night and it stops in the early hours of morning. Brik and Boyt in their book, "stay young with the melatonin way" have suggested that the increased secretion of melatonin hormone makes a person lazy. Hastings found this hormone is responsible for "Monday Morning Blues" because on Saturday and Sunday mornings we get up late in the morning and it works as jet lag. "Because nothing has reset our clock, it will be running and make us run at first one, then two hours slow". He also suggested that for those working in shifts, it is best to move from the morning to afternoon to the night shift than the other way. If a dose of melatonin is given early in the Monday morning it would put the clock back.

Pituitary gland is an important gland controlling the circadian organization of body. Increase in pituitary hormone during the day time increases the body temperature, pulse rate, blood pressure and oxygen consumption. The pituitary ACTH rhythm is strongly influenced by hypothalamus, which functions as a light absorbing function. There is also a 24 hours rhythm in the excretion of 17-Ketosteroids as a function controlled by these rhythms.

Different mental activities are differently affected by the time of day they are performed. In several studies it was found that performance on a calculation task, vigilance task, sensory and motor performance, threshold, correct signal detection etc. was high in the afternoon and early evening, and low in the night and early morning, but performance on digit span was best in the morning. On the basis of his study Calguhoun (1971) suggested that "tasks with a large memory load component may perhaps be expected to show an inverse relation to temperature while those demanding a more immediate processing or information will follow the more typical direct relationship."

Higher mental process, like thinking, also have rhythmic pattern. It was found that thinking skills slow down at night and increase in the morning.

Human circadian rhythms are not merely physiological in nature. A number of other factors, such as compulsory or elective activity, financial or prestigious incentives, social condition and personality also influence these thythms.

Two types of persons have been identified on the basis of these rhythms, morning types and evening types. Morning types are at their best in the morning and evening types in the evening. If they try to change their life style, they found it quite difficult to change. It has a practical implication in industries.

To morning types should be given morning shifts and evening types evening shift, it is likely to increase their performance.

This "morningness" and "eveningness" was found related to personality type. Introverts are found to be morning types and extroverts evening types. They have different body temperature pattern throughout the day. Introverts have higher temperature in the morning than extroverts, while extroverts have higher temperature in the evening than introverts. It is because the introverts are more aroused in the morning and extroverts in the evening.

Bernard Gittelson, on the basis of some practical work, claimed that a doctor by knowing his patient's biorhythm, would be better able to administer safe and effective health care. Likewise, by knowing the biorhythm of workers in an industry, the rate of accidents can be decreased. He distinguished three types of biorhythms. *Physical rhythms*, which make individual feel very active or very sluggish. *Emotional rhythms*, which control the emotional cycle of an individual and *Intelectual rhythms* which is responsible for intellectual alertness and dullness. Gittelson asserted that on the basis of the date of birth of an individual three different charts of these three rhythms can be plotted and if the individual worked according to this chart, he would be benefited to a greater extent. When all these cycles are at their high then the maximum performance would be expected. In this way, we can conclude that circadian rhythms affect our day to day performance and by knowing his pattern of circadian rhythm, the individual can achieve his best.

MECHANISM OF CIRCADIAN RHYTHM

Three components are supposed to operate circadian rhythm. These are :

1. An Oscillator

Since circadian rhythm is observed among acellular organism too, it is supposed that the oscillator of biological clock resides in the cell. There are three theories that are put forth for precise identification of the clock :

(i) **The plasma membrane** : Giese (1989) is of the opinion that since permeability of membrane changes at different times in 24 hours periodically hence physiology is changed in circadian way.

(ii) **The nucleus** : Rhythm is absent in prokaryotes and hence it is supposed that the clock resides in the nucleus and acts by changing levels of macromolecular synthesis.

(iii) **Geophysical variables** : It is believed that some geophysical variables change function of a cell membrane or nucleus or both.

2. A Receptor

The input to the oscillator is made by certain receptor. Most probably the photo-receptors present either in the eyes or pineal gland or in the brain itself.

3. A Coupling Device

The device that couples the receptor to the oscillator is supposed to be chemical. Truman and Riddiford's (1990) experiment with two species of silkworm showed that the eclosion (emergence) of moths is controlled by a chemical (hormone) in the brain which can be used in inducing eclosion in another species of silkworms. The coupling device does not seem to be species specific.

II. CIRCANNUAL OR CIRCASYNODIC RHYTHM

The term circannual is originated from the latin word *circa* = about, annual = year. This has been defined as an approximately 365 days physiological pattern that regulates annual changes in activities. Circannual rhythm may also be represented in terms of seasonal rhythms (spring, summer, autumn, and winter). In India Spring lies between March-May, Summer between June-September, Autumn between September-November and Winter between November-February. Circannual rhythms are widespread amongst animals and plants. Different physiological annual rhythms of animals may be studied as follows :

BREEDING CYCLE

Onset of the breeding cycle in many birds and mammals are examples of cicannual rhythm. In spring, a male *Chaffinch*, alone in an aviary, will begin to sing, and will continue singing for some minutes at a regular rate some three songs per minute. This song rhythm of chaffinch is independent of any external environmental factor. Nice, in her study of the American song sparrow observed that the tendency for males to sing gradually increased during early spring. Innate urge to sing increases through January and February and decreases in extreme cold. Birds at middle and high latitudes have a seasonal reproductive pattern in which the eggs are usually laid during the spring, a pattern that enables the young to mature sufficiently to withstand the winter conditions or to endure a migratory flight. Sandpipers breed in Arctic regions and they nest and incubate in spring when the snow is still on the ground. The eggs usually hatch when the snow melts and there is an abundance of insect life to provide food for the young (West and Norton, 1975). Several sea birds, including the brown booby (*Sula leucoaster*), the sooty tern (*Sterna fuscata*), and the lesser noddy tern (*Anaus tenuirostris*) breed at intervals of 8-10 months.

HIBERNATION

In parts of the world where climate is seasonal, animals may have to adjust to prolonged periods of unfavourable weather. Some animals are able to survive unfavourable periods by entering a prolonged phase of dormancy, called *hibernation* at low temperature and *aestivation* at high temperature. Phenomena of hibernation in winter and aestivation in summer are found in Indian frogs (*Rana tigerina*) periodically. Some desert rodents, such as ground squirrels (*Citellus*) become inactive during the summer and enter aestivation state in which the body temperature falls and a general reduction in physiological activity occurs. Many species of *European earthworms* become dormant during the summer. Some mammals including the *golden-mantled ground squirrel* (*Citellus laterailis*) and the *woodchuck* (*Marmata monax*), have a marked circannual rhythm underlying their seasonal hibernation. Many species of Humming birds sink into a torpor of laziness during which their body temperature falls to that of the environment. Torpor usually lasts only a few hours in birds, and seasonal dormancy is known only in a single family of birds, the *goatsuckers* (*Caprimul gider*).

DIAPAUSE

A period of dormancy in response to unfavourable climate occurs among insects known as diapause. Some insects can avoid freezing by supercooling and can survive very cold condition in diapause, in which the body fluids freeze at temperature well below 0°C. *Baracon cephi*, a Canadian wasp, may lower its body fluid below freezing point to –46°C by increasing the concentration of glycerol in the blood. Larva of *pink cotton ballworm* of South America undergoes diapause during September and October. They remain in this condition for the whole winter season. On the arrival of spring season (when day length increases) they get rid of diapause and metamorphose into adult.

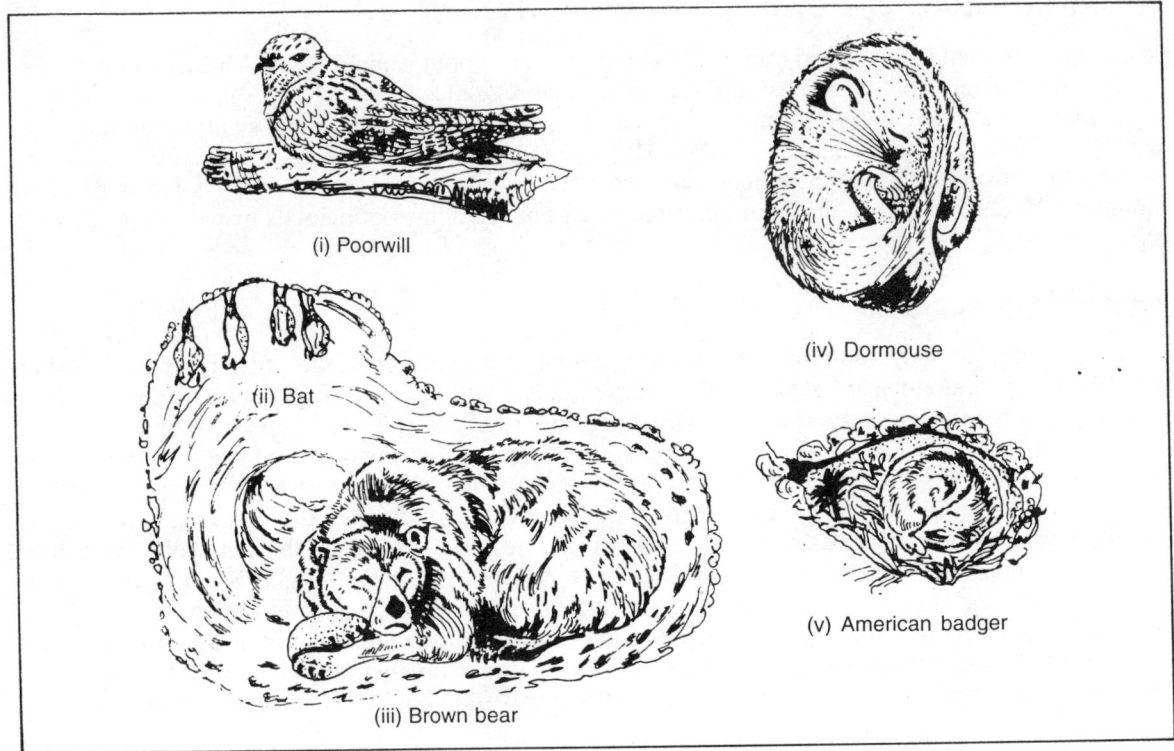

(i) Poorwill

(iv) Dormouse

(ii) Bat

(v) American badger

(iii) Brown bear

Fig. 9.5. Some hibernating animals.

MIGRATION

Migration between two different habitats, once in a year, takes place by many species of animals including Butterflies, Locusts, Petromyzon, Eels, Indian shad (*Hilsa*), Salmon, birds and mammals (lemming, bats and antelopes). Migration is initiated by endogenous biological clock of the individual.

Some seasonal migrants initiate their migration mainly on the basis of circannual rhythm rather than in response to changes in environmental conditions. In the typical long-distance migrants such as *garden Warbler* (S. borin), the *Subalpine Warbler* (*S. cantillans*), and *Willow Warbler* (*P. trochilus*) there are marked changes in body weight, moult, testis size, nocturnal restlessness, food preferences etc., once in a season. The European populations of these species winter in Africa and migrate across the Sahara Desert annually. When they are maintained under constant laboratory conditions in Europe, having been hand raised from a few days after hatching, the events that are known to be seasonal in free living birds appear as seasonal events in caged members of the same species.

To reach the destination, a migratory bird must travel not only in the right direction and distance but also in a definite time. Eberhand Gwinner (1972) calculated the distances travelled on the first migration by juvenile warblers unaccompanied by adults. The evidence suggests that the birds have an endogenous clock that induces as many hours of flight as necessary. There is good correlation between the number of hours of migratory restlessness of caged birds and the distance normally travelled during migration (Berthold, 1973). The distance travelled by the birds that is equivalent to an hour of restlessness can be estimated by comparing the behaviour of caged and migrating birds from the same population. From knowledge of the speed of flight of migrating birds Gwinner calculated the distance of his caged birds would have covered had they been going in the right direction. His calculations gave results close to those obtained by observations of freely migrating birds from the same population.

It is interesting to know that biological clock, control not only the onset of migratory activity but also its pattern. Many species have specific migratory routes characteristic of particular breeding populations. For example, *white storks* (*Ciconia ciconia*) that breed in western Europe fly to their wintering ground in Africa by a westerly route over Spain and Gibraltar, whereas those that breed in eastern Europe take a south easterly route. Young storks of eastern Europe kept in captivity, and released in western Europe, flew in the easterly direction characteristic of storks of eastern Europe (Shiiz, 1963). Similar experiments with other species indicate that the direction of migration is controlled by biological clock.

SEMILUNAR OR CIRCASYZYGICK RHYTHM

Lunar rhythm is a cyclic rhythm of about 15 days. It coincides with the rotation of the moon around the earth. This cycle is of 29 days having two phases. Full moon phase and a new moon phase. Each phase is of about 14.5 days. On full moon and new moon days the sun, the moon and the earth are in a single line. Many animals exhibit lunar rhythm in their behaviour. Most striking lunar rhythm is shown by the palolo worm, grunion fish and marine alga.

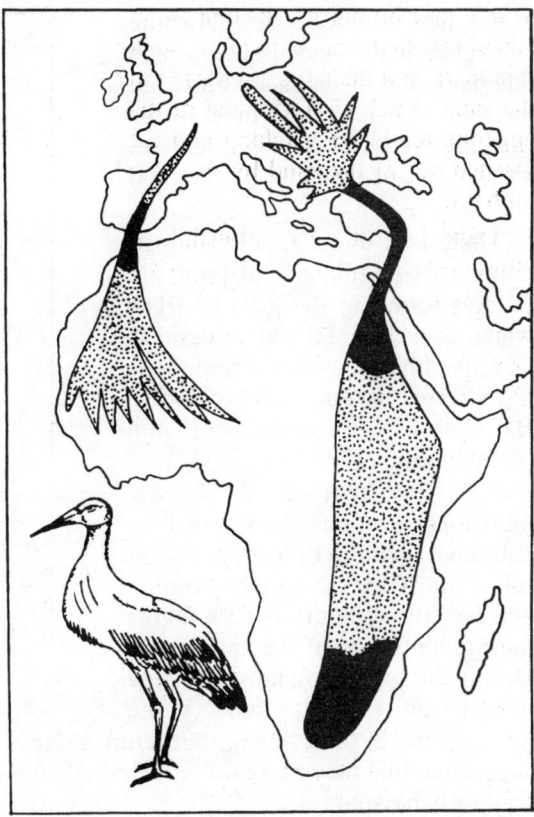

Fig. 9.6. Biological clock controlling migratory activity and migratory patterns. Migratory routes of the eastern and western European populations of the white stork (Ciconia ciconia).

SWARMING OF PALOLO WORM

The palolo worm (*Eunice*) of the Pacific ocean (southern hemisphere) rises to the surface to spawn in great numbers when the moon is full during October/November but the Atlantic palolo worm in the northern hemisphere spawns at the surface about the last quarter of the moon in July. As illustrated in Fig. 9.7 the posterior part of the worm, containing the genital organs, becomes detached from the anterior part and swims to the surface of the water, where the eggs and sperms are shed (Korringa, 1947). Worm isolated in the laboratory produce their gametes at the correct time, showing that this activity is controlled by biological clock of the palolo worm.

GRUNION FISH

The Grunion fish exhibits lunar rhythm. It breeds on full moon days. It is the only fish which breeds on land. The species *Leuresthes temuis* assemble near the bank of southern California coast to spawn from March to July each year on full or dark moon. The fish rides the high waves upto the beach where day to day tide do not reach. Spawning takes place in the sand just below high tide mark and the eggs are buried in the sand. After 15 days most of the eggs are ready for hatching and are washed out of the sand by the next high tide.

There is a direct relationship of number of conjugants of parasitic ciliates found in the gills of fresh water mussels and the lunar periodicity, maximum number is found one day after regular appearance of moon. Barmuda Cire worm swarm in full moon night.

Some terrestrial animals also exhibit lunar rhythms. Jamaican fruit bats have a pattern of feeding during full moon. They roost in the evening and feed throughout the dark nights during the period of the new moon. During the full moon, however, they depart from their day roost at the

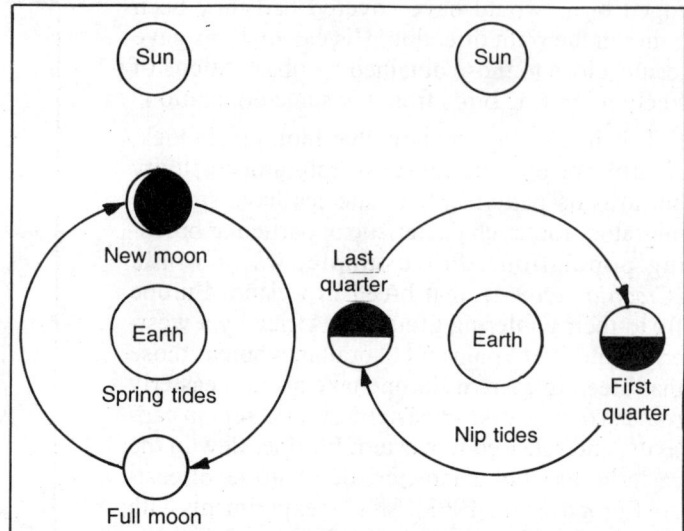

Fig. 9.7. Theoretical relationship of Earth, Moon and Sun in producing aquatic tides. At neap tide the attraction of the sun does not actually produce a sun tide. It merely reduces the moon tide.

normal time in the evening, but return there when the moon is high, even when obscured by clouds, suggesting that they make use of a biological clock (endogenous lunar clock) to time their foraging and feeding behaviour.

DICTYOTA

A marine alga *Dictyota* produces gametes only on full moon days.

DISEASES

Children are more susceptible to diseases like cold, cough, etc. on full moon and new moon days.

TIDAL RHYTHM

Many marine animals show rhythms of behaviour that coincide with the tidal cycle and have been shown to be operated by endogenous clock. For example, the Shore crab (*Carcinus maenas*) and Fiddler crabs (*Uca*) have a daily rhythm of activity that is superimposed upon a tidal rhythm. The crabs emerge from their burrows at low tide and actively forage, court, etc. As the tide floods, they retreat back into their burrows, rhythm of shore crab and Fiddler crabs persist under constant laboratory conditions for a week and upto 5 weeks respectively. This rhythm fades away after a week in case of shore crabs and after 5 weeks in case of Fiddler crabs, but this Faded tidal rhythm can be restored by putting them into almost freezing point for about six hours. The cold shock appears to restart the tidal clock (Palmer, 1973)

Superposition of circadian and tidal rhythms can enable an animal to adapt to the irregular changes of high and low tides that occur in some parts of the world. On the coast of California, for example, a period of 13.80 hours between high tide is followed by one of 10.43 hours. The intertidal crustacean *Synchelidium* has a pattern of swimming activity that closely follows this tidal pattern. This swimming pattern continues for several days even under constant laboratory conditions.

Relationship of exogenous cycles and endogenous rhythms (biological clock) of organisms

Ethologists, geneticists, physiologists, neurologists etc. have worked together and have come to the conclusion that both exogenous and endogenous rhythms are interrelated. Their intimate relationship was brought to notice as early as 1960 by Lorenz. Endogenous rhythm is not quite independent in controlling behaviour through biological clock. It is the intricate interaction between the two together to set the clock and run it. External environmental factors : day length, lunar phases, tides, cloudy weather etc., play the most important role but after lapse of required time the clock is maintained and run by internal stimuli controlled by body physiology. New born baby sleep and awake according to his own clock and irrespective to day/night cycle. Gradually and gradually he/she becomes diurnal.

Since endogenous rhythms tend to gradually coincide with that of the exogenous cycle, an organism must have a means synchronising its endogenous rhythms with the cycles of external events.

Study of exogenous rhythms and biological clocks suggests us to consider two important aspects :

1. Functional mechanisms of exogenous rhythms on biological clocks, and
2. Regulatory aspects of exogenous rhythms on biological clock.

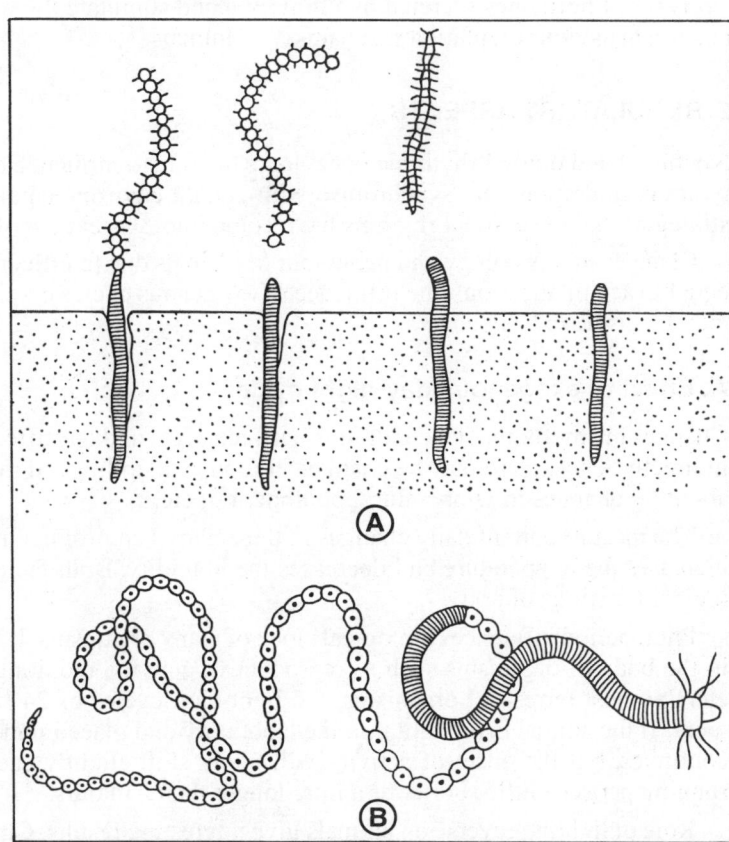

Fig. 9.8. (A) The mating routine of the palolo worm. (B) Palolo worms breed in large numbers on the full moon day.

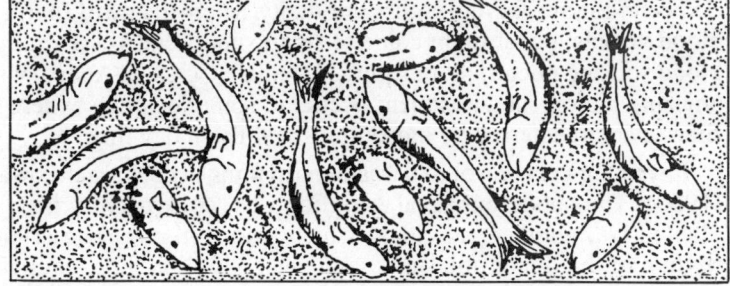

Fig. 9.9. Grunion, a California fish, breeds on the sandy shore on full moon days.

1. FUNCTIONAL MECHANISMS

Exogenous cycles influence and regulate biological clock of organisms through nervous system in higher animals. They receive information of environmental changes through sense organs. Changes received by sense organs are converted into electro-chemical massages by neuro-secretory cells which act upon hypothalamus. Hypothalamus secrete neuro-hormones which influence pituitary gland. Different types of hormones secreted by pituitary gland stimulate the whole endocrine system of body which act as a behaviour regulation mechanism in animals.

2. REGULATORY ASPECTS

Nocturnal and diurnal rhythmic behaviours are due to influence of day-night rhythm. Hibernation, aestivation, migration, etc. synchronise with annual environmental cycle. Diverse ways of reproductive strategies due to seasonal rhythms have come into existence in different groups of animals.

Changes in physiology and behaviour of animals due to influence of exogenous cycles are somewhat equal to acclimatization. The influence of exogenous cycles on physiology and behaviour of organisms may be discussed as below :

A. Effect of exogenous day-night cycle

Changes in environmental conditions between night and day affect animals and plants both directly and indirectly. Thus, there may be changes in food availability and in numbers of predators, which brought about by changes in temperature, photoperiod, etc.

The most important daily changes in the external environment is the photoperiod. Long photoperiod increases the temperature and decreases the humidity. Both factors have definite influence on physiological functions of body.

Photoperiod influences biological clock of many organisms. It determines the physiological sequence in the body of organisms such as reproductive activity, moulting, fat deposition, migration, breeding, etc. For most terrestrial organisms, the light-dark cycles of 24 hours are the critical cues for entrainment. If the animal is brought into the laboratory and placed under constant darkness, the daily rhythm continues, but the onset of activity will likely shift slightly each day, indicating a persistent or free running period a little shorter or a little longer than 24 hours.

Role of lighting reverse on animals give interesting results. Chipmunk (*Tamias striatus*) brought into the laboratory with artificial lighting reverse the light and dark positions of the chipmunk's natural cycle. The animals shift their activity phase to the light portion of the cycle within a few days. An interesting case of lighting reverse is found in parasitic worms. In the blood of infected man, the microfilarae of *Wuchereia* show day and night periodicity. Microfilarae of filaria live by day chiefly in large deep-seated blood vessels, but at night come to small superficial vessel in the skin, to be sucked by certain kind of blood sucking nocturnal mosquitoes (female Culex or Aedes) which serve as the intermediate host. An amazing biological adjustment occurs in some localities where the opposite occurs so that the microfilariae are transferred by mosquitoes that fly in day time.

Physiological control of Circadian rhythms in cockroaches was studied by Harker (1956) and Robert (1960). The suboesophageal ganglion of a cockroach, with a certain circadian rhythms was transplanted into another individual which was arythmic. The arythmic cockroach took up the circadian rhythm of the donor, the suboesophageal ganglion thus maintains a circadian rhythm of activity. The groups of neurosecretory cells in the ganglion responsible for the activity cycles have been located. These cells receive material from nerosecretory bodies the *Corpora Cardiaca*, by way of a small nerve. If this nerve is cut the circadian rhythm fails, even in a normal light-dark cycle. It is possible that the substance responsible for rhythmicity may be proteinaceous neurohormone released through axons (Arechiga, 1987).

B. Effect of seasonal cycle

The tilt of earth's axis along with its annual revolution around the sun produces different seasons. Seasonal periodicities are nearly universal in communities and often result in an almost complete change in the community structure during the annual cycle. The role of temperature, photoperiod, humidity and seasons regulate community structure and function.

One of the important aspects of seasonal cycles is the reproductive behaviour of different species. Generally the breeding period of a population is restricted to a species specific season of a year, when the ambient environmental conditions are favourable to the growing young one. Population of the same species inhabiting climatologically different terrains have shown differences in the reproductive cycles. Contrary to this, different species which coexist in the same environment reacted differently in having breeding periods during different seasons of a year. Consequently, many aspects of structural and functional organization of systems concerned directly or indirectly with reproductive cycles in a species manifest regular systematic changes.

H.B. Devraj Sarkar (1989) studied reproductive rhythms in Lizards. He observed cyclical changes in some biochemical parameters like lipids (cholesterol) proteins, phosphorus etc. Study of lipid accumulation and utilization provides valuable information on the role of lipids in Lizard's life histories. Cholesterol is a precursor of steroid hormones. Protein and phosphorus are involved in sythesis of yolk. These data were extrapolated to seasonal meterological data. His findings indicate that no single system or factor seem to be involved in the regulation of Lizard's reproductive cycles. Reproductive activity and reproductive cyclicity appear to be a result of consummate and concerted effort of interaction between the endogenous rhythm and the exogenous environmental factors. A balance between these two seems to be necessary to complete the reproductive cycles.

N.C. Dutta (2001) Observed the circannual rhythms of bath in birds (*Lonchura*). The month of July shows the peak of bath time in twelve months. High relative humidity, clouds, rain and intermittent light and darkness during light phase of 24 hours are entrainer in this month. Intervention of D in L phase during July (Sunny days) has got a capacity to change the bath time. This may be treated as a very strong synchroniser.

The reproductive physiology of seasonal breeding is geared to the annual cycle of environmental changes so as to anticipate either peak abundance of food of adverse climatic conditions. There are two main ways in which this is done. First, changes in surrounding temperature, day length, or other environmental clues induce physiological change at a particular time of year. Second, the physiological changes are programmed on a seasonal basis by means of an endogenous circannual clock.

The most important seasonal change in the environment is the fluctuation of day length. The *photic* stimuli are converted to chemical massages by neurosecretory cells. In some mammals the pineal body, on the dorsal surface of the brain, may act as a light transducer (Wurtman et al., 1968). The influence of light on mammalian reproduction appears to be primarily via the retina to the hypothalamus. The control of reproductive physiology involves the complex interaction of a number of hormones. In addition to seasonal cycles of sexual activity, many mammals have a much shorter estrous cycle, or "heat". Red foxes (*Vulpes vulpes*), have only one period of heat annually. Domestic dogs have two; others have more. Reproductive pattern of many species is influenced both by photo-periodic factors and by the endogenous circannual clock. Two mechanisms may interact with each other. Animals occupying dry desert environment may depend upon the beginning of rainfall to trigger the process of reproduction (Marshall, 1970). Reproductive activities (territorial defence, courtship, mating and parental care) put extra physiological burdens on the animal. Therefore, the reproduction is abandoned for the next year.

Photoperiodism in certain insects provides a sort of birth control. Long day length of late spring and early summer stimulates the brain to produce a neurohormone that brings on the production of a diapause on resting eggs that will not hatch until next spring, no matter how favourable food, temperature and other conditions are. Thus, population growth is halted before rather than after the food supply becomes critical.

Factors influencing hibernation behaviour: Penegelly and Asmundson (1947) injected, blood serum of a hibernating *ground squirrel* into a non-hibernating squirrel and found that hibernation was induced. The experiment suggests that the basic physiological mechanism responsible for controlling hibernation is driven by an endogenous factor. This has also been demonstrated in the Woodchucks, which show a circannual rhythm of hibernation. Woodchucks were transported from USA to Australia and were exposed to the prevailing light and temperature conditions. The woodchucks reversed their normal rhythm within two years, bringing it into line with local conditions, even though the animals were provided freely with food and water and had no need to hibernate.

C. Effect of lunar cycle

The moon moves along a path similar to that of the sun and rises 50 minutes later each day. The lunar cycle of 29.5 days is known to influence a variety of aspects of animal behaviour studied above.

D. Effect of tidal rhythm

The tides result from changes in the combined gravitational pull of the sun and the moon. The tide raising force of the sun is only about 5/11th of that of the moon because the distance of the sun is much greater from the earth. The moon is much closer to earth than the sun. It exerts a force twice during the lunar cycle. The gravitational pull of the sun and the moon each cause two bulges in the water of the oceans. Such bulges of water are called tides which usually consist of a regular rhythmic rise and fall of water twice a day over a range of several meters.

Tides occur on opposite sides of the earth at the same time. Intervals between successive rises of the tide are about 12 hours 251/2 minutes. This is the same interval as the average daily passage of the moon across the meridian. So it is almost certain that the moon is the principal regulator of tides.

Since a moon day is longer than a sun day, there is constant change in the relationship of moon and sun tides. Fig. 9.7 indicates that in new and full moon, the attraction of sun and moon on tides reinforce each other, and causes the tide to rise higher at high water and fall lower at low water. These are called spring tides. At first and last quarters of moon, the forces oppose each other and the daily fluctuations are much smaller due to the neutralizing effect of the force. These are called neap tides.

WHAT IS THE ENDOGENOUS SOURCE OF BIOLOGICAL CLOCK

The most vital question about biological clock is that "is there any definite point or location in the body of animals which controls biological clock." There is no definite proof of endogenous source of biological clock in all organisms but some experiments performed on cockroaches, crickets and crustaceans are mentionable. Cockroaches and crickets lose their daily rhythmicity if the connection between Lobi option (part of the brain) and rest of the brain are either cut or chemically blocked. In crustaceans the circadian rhythms could be altered by removing the eye stalks. This suggests that innate circadian rhythm is controlled by optic lobes of brain. In higher vertebrates the melatonin is produced by pineal gland. Lerner et al. showed that synthesis of melatonin is performed in presence of HIOMT (hydroxyndolo-methyl transferase) enzyme. HIOMT enzyme becomes active only during night i.e. dark. As a result of which melatonin is synthesized only in night i.e. circadian rhythmicity is implied in its synthesis. Thus pineal clock can be considered as the endogenous source of circadian and other rhythms of time giver invertebrates.

EXERCISE

1. Write concise account on biological clock.
2. What do you mean by seasonal rhythms? Write the role of seasonal rhythms on biological clock of migratory birds.
3. Write an essay on concept of biological rhythm.
4. What is biological clock? Explain its various types giving examples.
5. What do you mean by Chronobiology? Describe origin and evolution of biological clock.
6. What is rhythm gene? Describe various types of endogenous rhythms.
7. Write a short note on influence of exogenous cycles on endogenous rhythms.
8. Write a short note on bathing behaviour of Lonchura bird studied by N.C. Datta.
9. What do you mean by zeitgeber? Who coined this term? Explain it with earlier discoveries.
10. What do you mean by endogenous rhythm? Mention different kinds of rhythms shown by animals. Mention some experiments showing influence of exogenous rhythms on endogenous rhythms in crabs and cockroaches.
11. Write short note on endogenous source of biological clock.

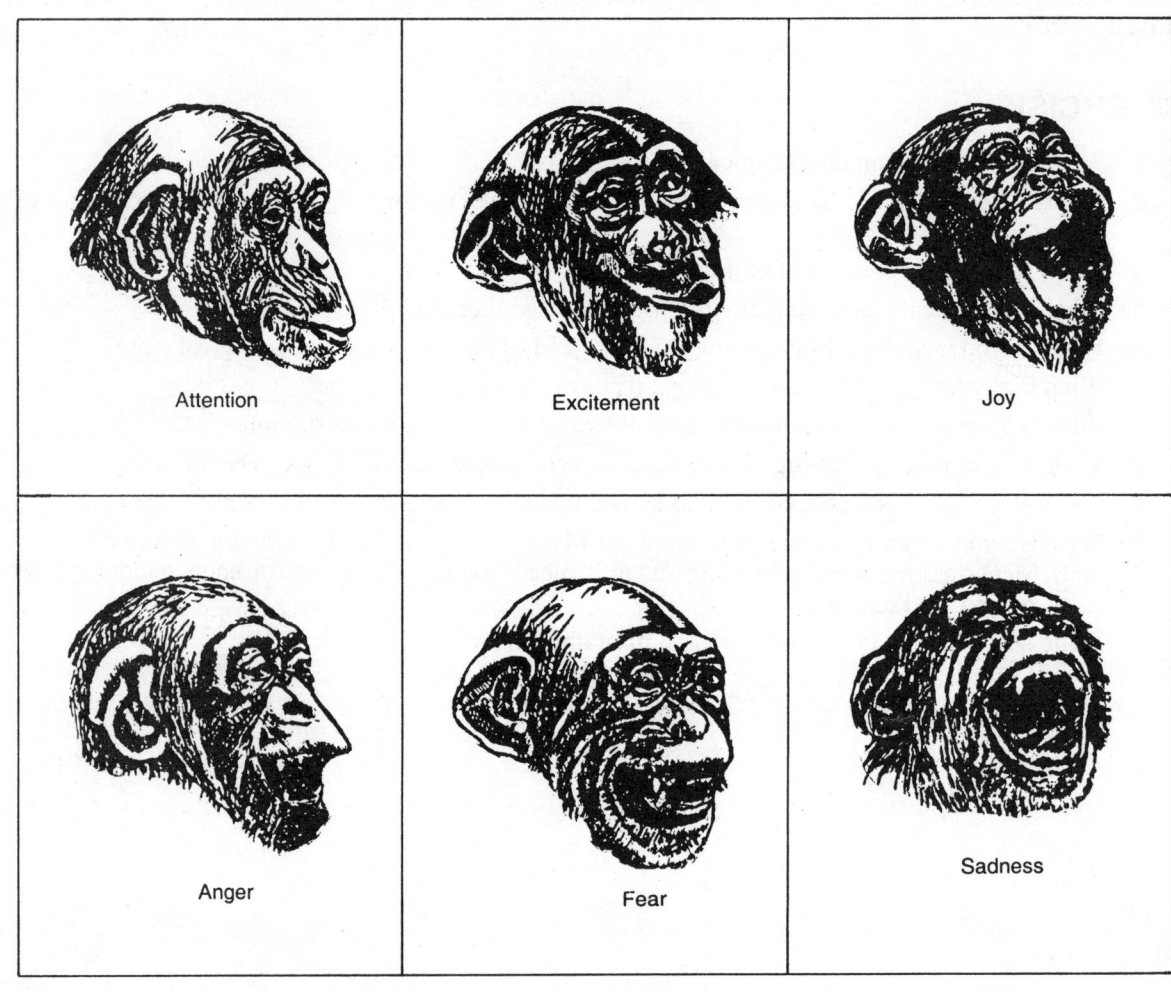

Attention

Excitement

Joy

Anger

Fear

Sadness

Transfer of information through signals between two animals is called animal communication. Communication occurs in a wide range of animals. Bees give directions about flower bed to their inmates by dance. Fish communicate through light signals. Birds communicate through songs. Mammals convey and obtain messages by smell and different rich variety of "language". Oral communication is not unique to humans; frogs croack, snakes hiss, birds chirp, lions roar. But probably humans alone have developed spoken and written language. This chapter gives an idea that how animals communicate to each other.

ANIMAL COMMUNICATION $\boxed{10}$

INTRODUCTION

Animal communication is the passage of information between two animals. The animal which sends signal is called *signaller* and the animal that receives signal is called *receiver*. Animal communication is also known as Biological communication.

Wilson (1975) defined Biological communication as "*an action on the part of an animal that alters the probable pattern of behaviour in another animal in a fashion adaptive either to one or both of the participants.*" This definition is not universally applicable because the mouse that rustles in the grass, making sound enables the owl to catch it. Here mouse is not communicating to its predator the owl. Keeping this in mind Slater (1983) very cautiously defines communication as *the transmission of a signal from one animal to another such that the sender benefits, on average, from the response of the recipient.*

Lorenz (1903-1989) laid the foundation stone of the classical ethological view of communication. He used the term *releaser* or *sign stimuli* or *signal* "for those characters exhibited by an individual of a given animals species which activate existing releasing mechanism in conspecifics and elicit certain chains of instinctive behaviour patterns". Lorenz's ethological view of communication was further developed by Niko Tinbergen.

BASIC QUESTIONS ABOUT COMMUNICATION

In context of communication five basic questions arise :
1. Whether any transfer of information can be considered to be communication?
2. Should we restrict the definition of communication to transfer of information within a species or between two or more species.

3. What is communicated?
4. How do we know when communication occur?
5. Is communication always honest?

WHETHER ANY TRANSFER OF INFORMATION CAN BE CONSIDERED TO BE COMMUNICATION?

Strictly speaking any transfer of information cannot be considered as communication. In a communication system both *signaller* and *receiver* should be benefited.

Foraging ants produce certain scent as signal for communication purpose which help other members of the colony to find the source of the food. But this signalling system in ants is also disadvantageous to them because a small predatory snake (*Leptotyphlos*) also detects the scent trails and follows them back to the ants' nest where it eat up the brood. In above example we consider the scent as a signal, evolved by the ants for communication with each other, but we cannot consider that the ants communicate with the snake.

SHOULD WE RESTRICT THE DEFINITION OF COMMUNICATION TO TRANSFER OF INFORMATION WITHIN A SPECIES OR BETWEEN TWO OR MORE SPECIES

We cannot restrict definition of communication within a species. Animals communicate both of their own and different species. A sphinix moth that suddenly displays the vivid eye-spots on its hind wings in response to a light touch is actually signalling to a potential predator. Here moth and predator are two different species and moth is communicating the predator that frightens the predator and signaller is escaped. Honeybees are attracted towards nectar of flowers and in turn flowers are benefited by being pollinated, so both signaller (flower emitting scent) and receiver (honeybees) – both belonging to two different groups – are benefited.

WHAT IS COMMUNICATED?

Vervet monkeys communicate not just the presence of danger to other members of their troop but also what sort of predator is threatening them. One alarm call consists of a series of relatively long tonal units and is given in response to mammalian predators, particularly *leopards*. Other monkeys hearing this 'leopard' alarm call will run up into a tree. A second alarm call, the '*eagle*' consists of short tonal units. In response to this alarm call all monkeys group together. Seyfarth et al. (1980) observed that if this call is given the response of other vervet monkeys is to look up into the sky and hide in bushes. A third alarm call, the '*snake alarm*' consists of a series of short, widely spaced sounds and on hearing it monkeys look down on to the ground. Other animals, including ground squirrels (Leger and Owings, 1978) and chickens (Colias and Joos, 1953) have also been shown to convey information about the type of predator they have seen (Fig. 10.1).

Honey-bees and Chickens (Marler et al. 1986) can communicate information to the members of their colony about the quality of a food source. Cockerels have a special call that they give when they have found food, and that causes hens to come and feed. The food calls are produced at a higher rate with highly preferred food is discovered.

A very interesting category of signals arises when animals come into conflict over a food source or access to mates. Under such circumstances they may give 'threat' signals to one another, before they come to physical combat.

Male anole lizards give threat signals to competitor male by bobbing head and changing body colour while defending its territory. Rival male lizards judge strength of each other by bobbing head and decide to stay and fight or escape. During the autumn rutting season the stags challenge one another for ownership of harem. These challenges sometimes result in damaging fights, in which one or both stags are injured, but they almost always begin with a 'roaring march', in which the stags signal to each other with roars, giving gradually greater and greater numbers of roars per minute (Clutton - Brock and Albon, 1979). Roaring is an exhausting signal to give and the ability to roar at a high rate means that a stag will be stronger enough to fight long and hard. If a stag is 'out-roared' by another, he may well decide to abandon his challenge altogether (Fig. 10.2). If, on the other hand, both stags can roar at the same rate, they then proceed to the next stage of the conflict, the 'parallel walk'. In parallel walk both contestants walk up and down, eying each other and apparently trying to judge the other's strength in more detail. The result is that real fight occurs only between stags of almost equal fighting ability that each has estimated that it may be able to win.

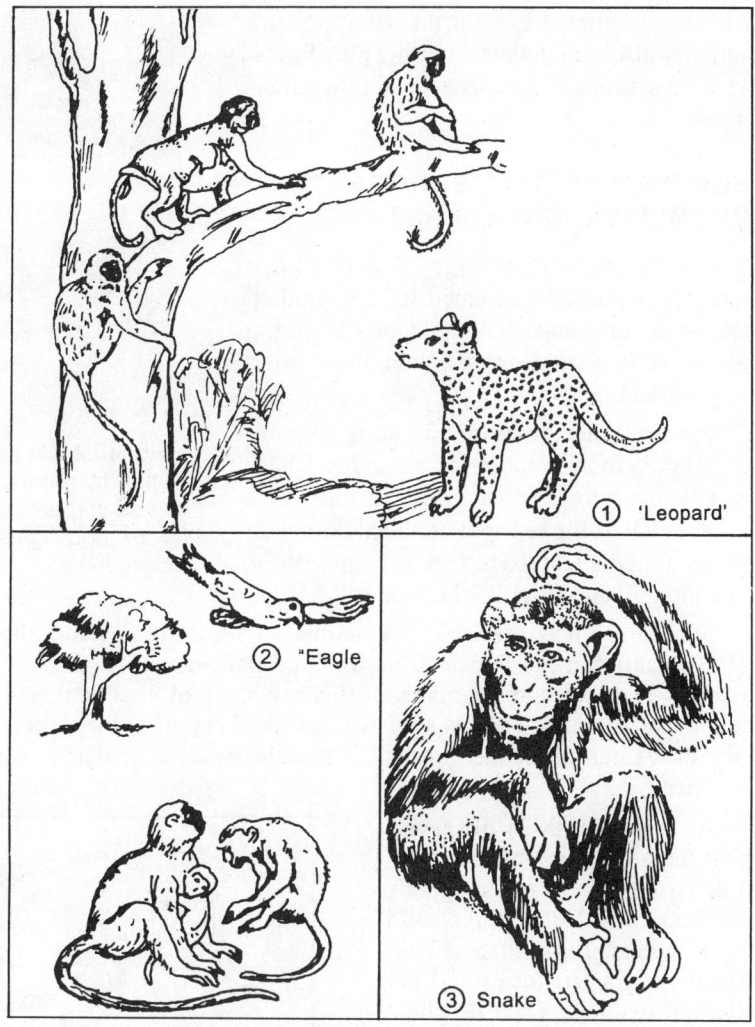

Fig. 10.1. Vervet monkey conveying the sort of predator threatening them.

One of the aspects that animals convey to each other during courtship is what species and sex they are. Different species of crickets emit different mating calls, different firefly species pulse light in different patterns in time. Fiddler crabs wave their claws in different ways that differ from species to species, and lizards have species-specific pattern of head-bobbing. Pheromones are another way some animals have of identifying the species of its own.

A kind of communication called *metacommunication* is interesting to note. The function of this signal is not only to communicate information in itself, but to qualify other signals that follow it. Metacommunication phenomenon is best known from play situations in carnivores and monkeys. Fig. 10.3 shows an adult male lion inviting a cub to play. His posture with forequarters lowered is not seen in any other context and its message is that all aggressive movements that follow are play. Dogs and wolves use almost exactly the same posture and may also wag their tails during play fights. Monkeys adopt a 'play face' in similar situations.

HOW WE INVESTIGATE WHETHER COMMUNICATION OCCURS?

We have discussed that "signal" given by one individual being "responded to" by another. But to be sure that communication is taking place, we have to use systematic observation and experiment.

Powerful method of investigating communication is to use models or dummies. These can be used to reveal the key features of a signal such as the red spot on the abdomen of three-spined stickleback fish, bill spot of the herring gull etc. (Fig. 2.7 iii, iv).

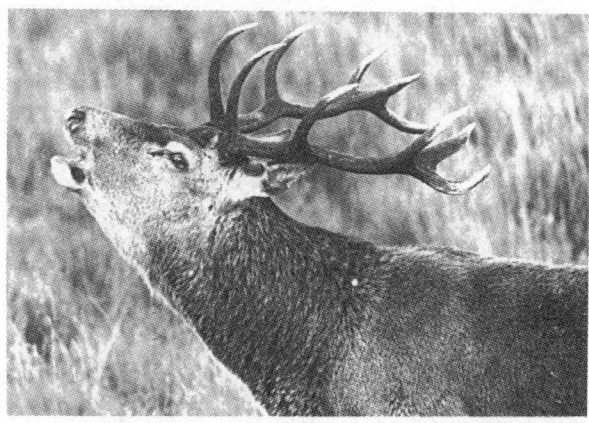

Fig. 10.2. Contests of red deer stags challenge each other by roaring. Two equally strong stags established through roaring try to show their dominance by parallel walk and fights. Each parallel line represents one encounter.

Sometimes it is easy to 'fool' animals with dummies and alternation of their morphology. Noble (1936) captured the female from a mated pair of yellow-shafted flickers, a type of American woodpecker. The males and females of this species look identical, except that the male has a black moustache. Noble stuck a moustache of black feathers on to the female and the male promptly attacked her and drove her out of the territory. When the moustache was removed she was once more accepted by her mate.

Anderson (1982) observed that female widow-birds are attracted to the long sweeping tails of the males. He captured wild male widow-birds that had already set up territories and cut the tail feathers. Then he glued tail feathers back on, making the tail longer than before, shorter than before and the same length. He found that longer tailed males attracted more females. Moller (1988) performed similar experiment with swallows and found that long tails are an important signal to the females.

Sometimes the stimuli used by animals to communicate with each other are so subtle that sophisticated instrument is needed to pick them up. Different types of mating calls given by differ-

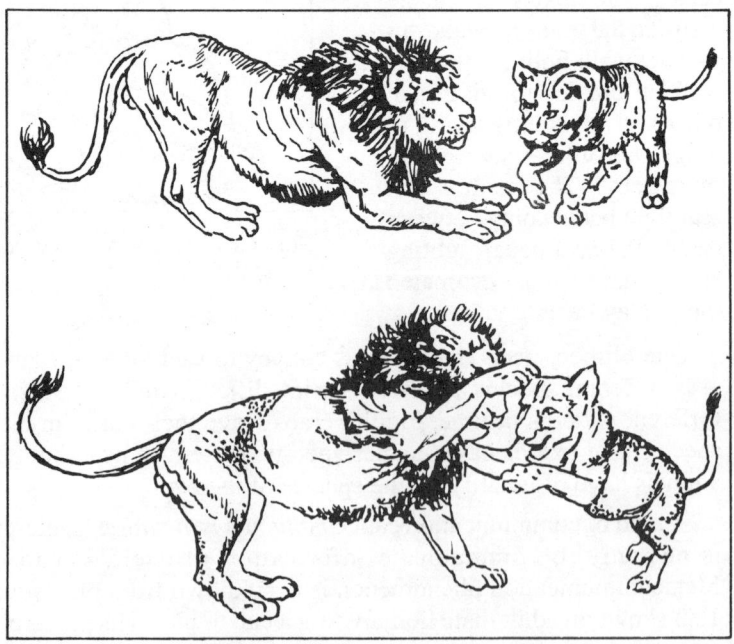

Fig. 10.3. Metacommunication in lions.

ent species of male crickets; different signal call given by vervet monkeys for different kinds of enemies; talk of elephants through infrasonic sounds etc. are beyond the human sensory organs to perceive. By recording mating calls of different species of male crickets and grunts of Verbet monkeys and playing them through a sound spectrograph we become able to detect and distinguish them (Fig. 3.3).

IS COMMUNICATION ALWAYS HONEST?

Most of the communications are clearly of benefit to both the signaller and receiver. But some of the communications seem to be manipulated; that is, the sender appears to influence the behaviour of the receiver for its own ends.

Holldobler (1971) observed an interesting case of dishonest communication by some species of beetle. These beetle live parasitically in the nests of ants (*Myrmecophiles*) and befool the ants in carrying them into the nest by mimicking the signals given by an ant larva. Females of predatory fireflies (*Photuris*) can flash in two ways. They can either flash in their own specific pattern to attract males of its own species or mimic the flash pattern of another smaller species of the genus *Photinus*. When the *Photinus* males approach in response, fireflies kill and eat them. Some ground-nesting birds, such as plovers, lure predators away from their nest by feigning a broken wing (Fig. 7.21).

Zahavi (1987) and Grafen (1990) believe that animal signals are essentially honest. But many ethologists believe that there are many examples of dishonest communication. How can ethologists reconcile the opposite views ? Are signals 'honest' or 'dishonest' ? Magnard Smith and Harper (1988) suggest that it is better to divide signals into two categories : assessment signals, which are always honest and conventional signals that sometimes allow cheating.

BASIC COMPONENTS OF COMMUNICATION

According to Ewsbury (1978), in a communicating system the following seven essential components are seen :

1. *Signaller* : An individual which emits signal.
2. *Receiver* : An individual which receives the signal.
3. *Message* : The behaviour emitted by the signaller.
4. *Channels* : A pathway through which normally a signal travels. These are vocal, auditory, olfactory, electrical, surface vibrations etc. where different sensory receptors are involved.
5. *Noise* : This is a background activity in the channel which is not related to the signal.
6. *Contacts* : The setup under which a signal is emitted and received.
7. *Code* : A possible complete set of signals and contacts.

SIGNAL

The basic general characteristic of common concept of communication includes a signal (coded information or message). The sender gives the signal and receiver receives the message. The sender and receiver must possess the appropriate structures respectively to send and receive the message.

The distance travelled by a signal and duration of existence of a signal varies considerably. Small amount of sex attractants of many insects produced by a female can be detected by a number of males several kilometers downwind. Visual displays operate over much shorter distances. Alarm signals, through chemicals produced by many invertebrates, may have a localized, short-term effect and fade out rapidly. Signals such as the male secondary sexual characteristics in polygynous species can last for long periods of time. Information about reproductive status, like the bright red vulva region of female rhesus monkeys or the antlers of male deer in oestrus, is communicated during the breeding season. In some cases the information conveyed by animals may be simple. Sometimes animals couple two or more signals for effective communication.

CHANNELS OF COMMUNICATION

Messages are communicated among animals via signals which are dependent on various sensory modalities. Animals communicate through the use of *Visual*, *Auditory*, *Tactile*, *Chemical* (odour), *Electrical*, *Surface vibration*, *Language* means etc.

VISUAL COMMUNICATION

Information transmitted by visual means is called visual communication. The visual signals may be given by various means like colour identification, posture or shape of the body, movement, light etc.

Visual signals are most often used by species that are active during the day. Most animals are sensitive to light and can therefore receive visual signals at night. Visual signals have been extensively studied in crabs, bees, reptiles, birds and mammals.

Fiddler crabs (*Uca annulipes*) found on tropical beaches, communicate with one another by means of visual signals. Each individual signals to announce its own presence and marks out its personal territory by waving its enlarged pincer like a flag. Male fiddler crab have one pincer or claw considerably larger than the other. This greatly enlarged pincer is used to signal to other males as warning and to female for invitation (Fig. 10.4).

LANGUAGE OF BEES

The dance language of honeybees was decoded by Karl von Frisch (1965). He revealed that worker bees communicate the location of nectar sources to one another by means of a complex dance language. As soon as a worker has discovered a food-source, it returns to the hive and alights on her comb to perform a ritualized dance. Each movement of this "dance language" has a very precise meaning.

If the source of nectar is less than about 100 meters away, the honeybee performs a "round dance". Other workers from the hive also move round. They also get message by rubbing their antennae against guide dancing bee. After this performance has continued for a few minutes, the dancer stops and regurgitates a small amount of the nectar collected from the source. From all of this, the other worker bees can know the exact direction and distance of their location as well as assess the quality and identify the flowers involved.

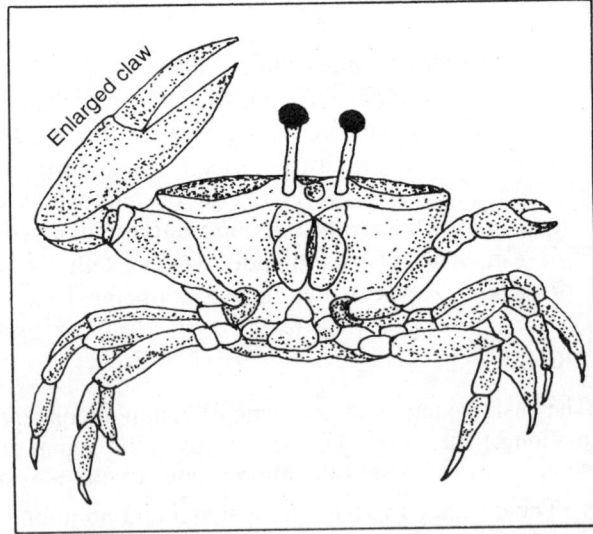

Fig. 10.4. Male fiddler crabs have one claw greatly enlarged and use it to signal to other males as warning signal and to females as invitation signal. They give signal by waving their pincers in the air after the tide has receded.

If the source of nectar is more than 100 meters away from the hive, the returning worker communicate their identity, distance and direction by performing a complex dance. In this complex dance, a figure of eight pattern is followed with the two loops separated from one another by a straight line running down the middle. As it dances, the bees waggles its abdomen in a rhythmic sequence of movements and hence called **"waggle dance"**. The rhythm and duration of the movements, together with the intensity of the humming sound produced, constitute a message which enables the other bees in the hive to fly to the food source. The identity of the flowers concerned is usually indicated by the odour of the regurgitated nectar, but it has been observed that flowers without a particular scent are indicated by pheromones secreted from glands on the posterior part of the dancing bee's abdomen.

Fig. 10.5 illustrates the language of the bees. The round dance is performed by scout bees when the food source is quite close (less than about 100 meters away) to the hive. Dance performed in a figure of eight with waggling movements of the abdomen indicates a distant food source (more than 100 meters away) from the hive. The angle against the vertical formed by the straight line in the middle of the figure of 8 corresponds to the angle formed between the position of the sun and the food source, in relation to the hive.

The rhythm of the dance corresponds to the distance between the hive and the food source. For example a food source 100 meters, 500 meters, 1500 meters away ; a bee will carry 36 to 40, 24 and 16 circuits respectively will be performed. The humming sound produced during the dance come from varying degrees of vibration flowing out from the stomach muscles, while the wings are kept in the resting position. A system of visual, auditory and olfactory stimuli help bees to communicate to one another the location of food source.

Bees are able to navigate according to the sun, using a kind of internal compass. Since they can see ultraviolet light and can also respond to polarized light, they are able to navigate even in cloudy days.

Honeybees can travel long distances in order to gather their nectar and pollen. Usually they forage within a radius of 2-10 kilometers. D. H. Janzen (1971) reported that South American bees of genera *Euplusia, Euplaema* and *Euglossa* can cover a radius of 23 kilometers. Bees of species *Euplusia surinamensis* were able to cover a radius of 20 kilometers in an hour.

Pheromones play major role in social life of honeybees. Queenbee regulate the reproductive cycle of the colony by secreting a pheromone (9- ketodecanoic acid) from her mandibular gland. Development of ovaries is inhibited in workers which absorb this substance. The same pheromone is used by the queen to attract males during her nuptial flight.

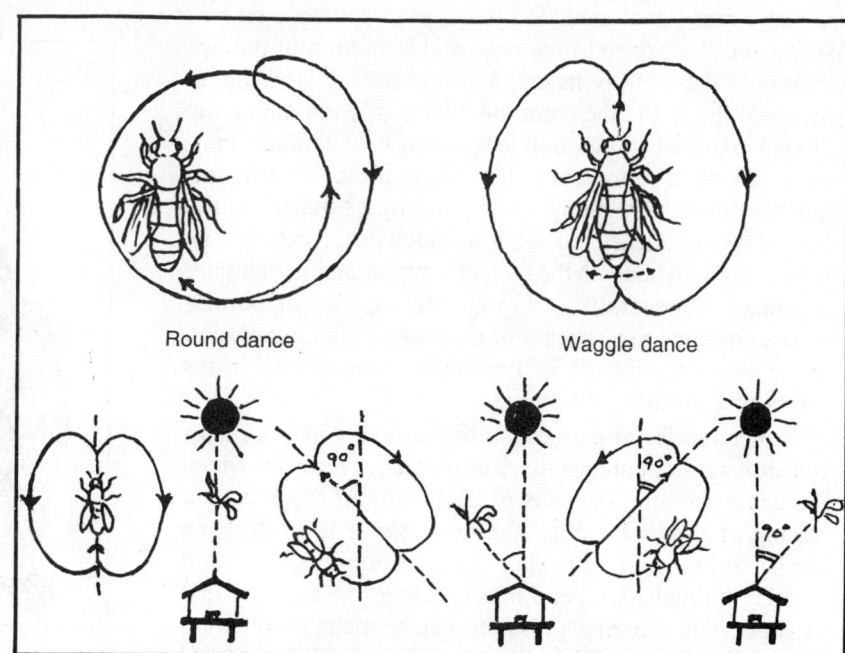

Round dance   Waggle dance

Fig. 10.5. Communication in honeybee.

It is of common observation that when bees attack a human-being, their attentions are often directed to one specific spot. Why it is so ? This can be explained by the fact that the bees deposits on the victim's skin a pheromone called *isoamyl actuate* at the moment that the sting is used. This substance, attracts other bees and directs their attacks to that particular victim on the same spot.

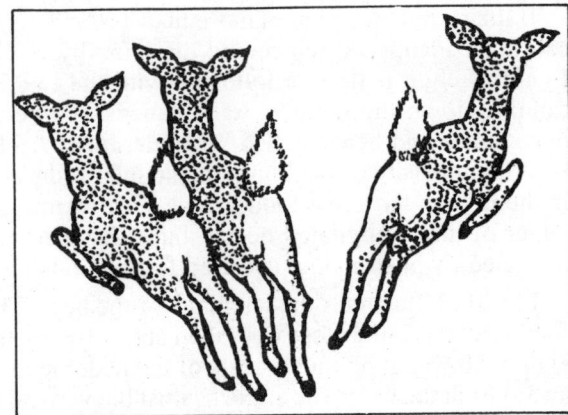

Fig. 10.6. The alarm signal of white-tailed deer. As the deer leap away, the tail is elevated, revealing its brilliant white underside and the white hair of the rump.

Many invertebrates and fishes are capable of changing colour within seconds. The most spectacular in this regard is the octopus, waves of colour advance and recede according to the animal's mood. Usually visual displays are coupled with other modes of communication. The redwing spreads its tail, lowers its wings and raises its epaulette (a decoration of the shoulder) while singing a song.

In many cases, visual signals involve special colour patches which the animal displays in a particular situation. The most striking example is provided by the white-tailed deer. They have a patch of long white erectile hairs around the anal region. The white hairs are raised, whenever danger threatens them. This alarm signal of white-tailed deer can be seen from a long distance. This alarm signal immediately provokes the entire heard to run away (Fig. 10.6).

Some mammal species, particularly the cat family (felidae) and the dog family (canidae), give specific signals by the position adopted by the head, ears and tail. Wolves keep its ear picked up and tail raised when threatened. Flattened ears symbols fear or suspicion. Wrinkling of the nose and retraction of the lips to expose the teeth represent a threat display. The movements of the tail is the common means of communication among mammals. Side-to-side wagging of tail of pets indicates complete submission. This is the posture that is frequently adopted by a dog when greeting its master. If the animal is very uneasy indeed, it will tuck its tail between its legs and hold it beneath the belly. Communication in higher mammals is generally elaborate and capable of putting across complex messages. For example, facial expression along with vocalization in primates communicate various forms of emotions and messages.

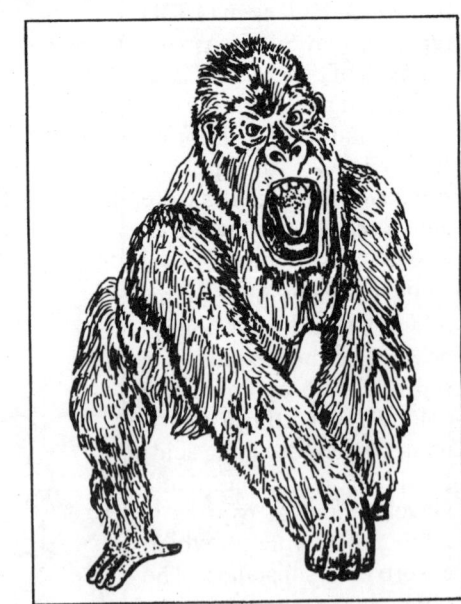

Fig. 10.7. The expression of Emotions in chimpanzee.

Protective facial expression of mammals play a major role in visual communication. The protective reflexes, which include narrowing of the eyes, flattening of the ears, and raising of the hair around the neck, serve to protect the animal at moments of danger. Such responses give signal to other animals, who can interpret them as signs of fear or anger. Thus facial expressions can be made more effective by exaggeration, by accompanying vocalization, and by distinctive markings that draw attention to the face in

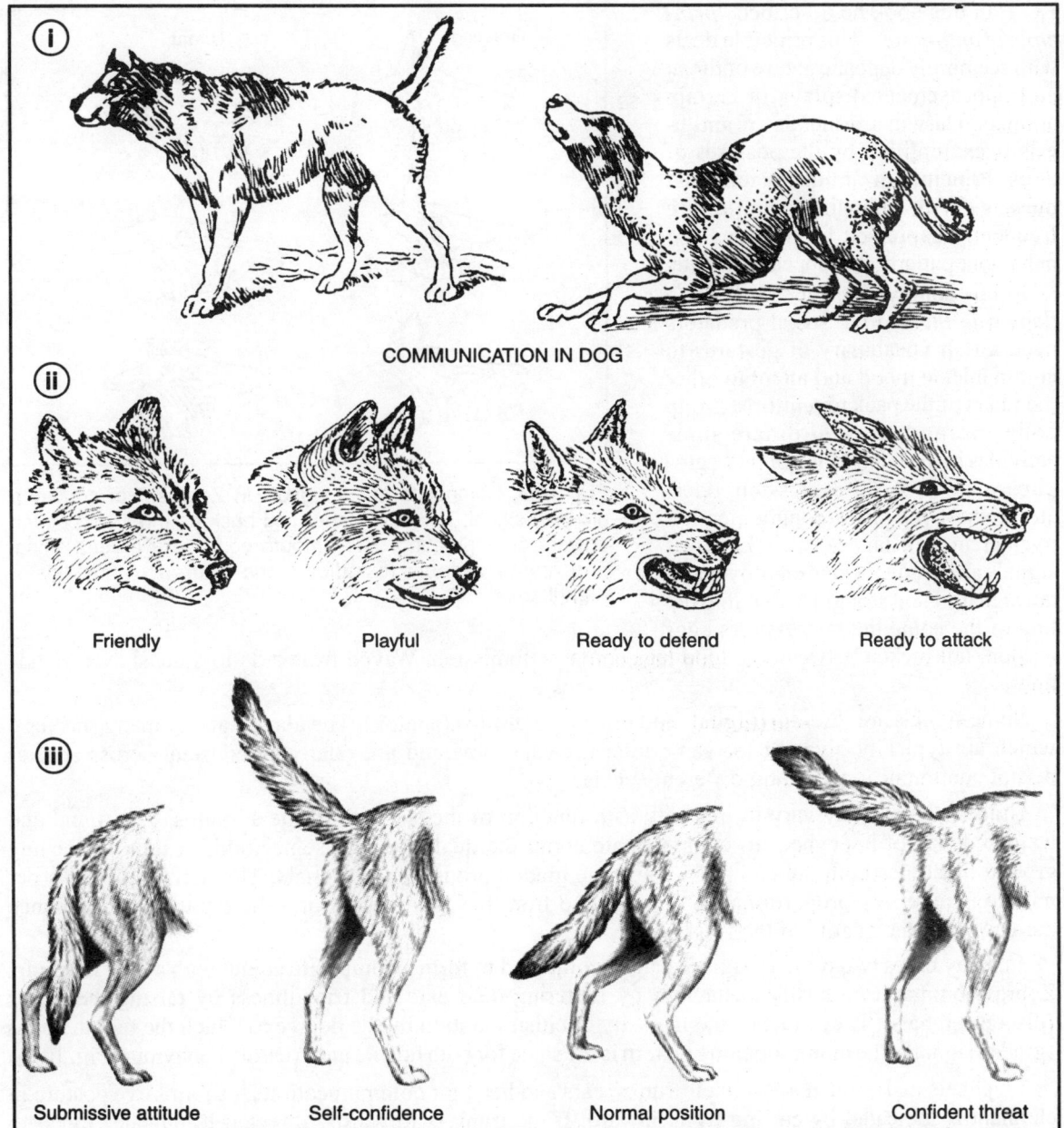

COMMUNICATION IN DOG

Friendly   Playful   Ready to defend   Ready to attack

Submissive attitude   Self-confidence   Normal position   Confident threat

Fig. 10.8. (i) Darwin's principle of antithesis illustrated by postures of a dog when friendly (left) and angry (right); (ii) Facial expressions of wolf - friendly, playful, ready to defend and ready to attack; (iii) Tail positions and different behaviours of Alsation dog.

facial expression. The absence of hair on parts of the human face draws attention to the main features used in communication.

Charles Darwin published a book *"The Expression of the Emotions in Man and Animals"* in the year

1872. In this book he described "*principle of antithesis*". This principle deals with seemingly opposite nature of threat and appeasement displays in certain animals. Darwin's principle of antithesis is examplified by the postures of dogs. Principle of antithesis tells that message with opposite meaning are frequently expressed by postures and behaviour patterns that appear opposite.

In this context one can ask *Why do dogs wag their tails*? Social predators need a rich vocabulary of gestures to communicate mood and intent to other members of the pack to reinforce group cohesion and to co-ordinate their activities in the hunt. Many of these gestures, such as facial expression, operate at short range. In communication over greater distances other kinds of signals are needed. Dogs employ many tail signals. Held straight, extending the line of the spine the tail, express aggression; tail tucked between the hind legs convey submission. Waved from side-to-side, shows friendliness.

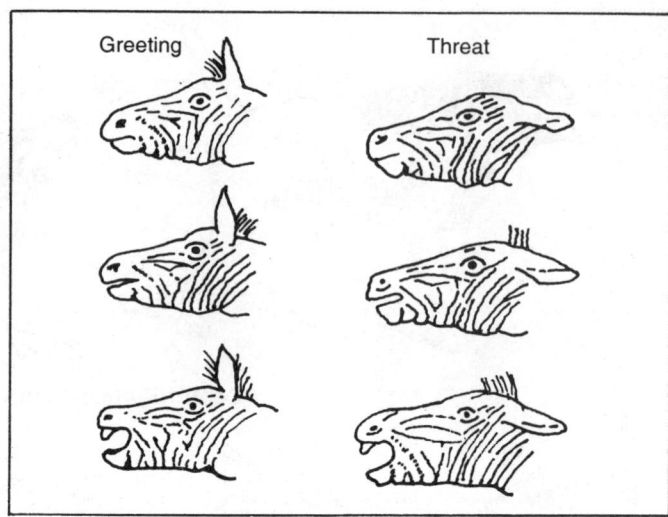

Fig. 10.9. Composite facial signals in Zebras. Ear convey a discrete signal. They are either laid back as threat or pointed upward as a greeting. Their mouth conveys a graded signal and opens variably to indicate the degree of hostility or friendliness.

Some signals are *discrete* (digital) and others are *graded* (analog). The alarm calls of many species – which are typically given at the same intensity each time and are relatively constant across species permit communication among different species.

Graded signals may vary in intensity as a function of the strength of the stimulus. The round and waggle dance of honeybees to communicate about the quality plus distance and location of feeding ground illustrates both the complexity and the graded properties of signals. The number of turns per minute is inversely proportional to the distance from the food source and the duration of the dance increase with the quality of the food.

In many cases two or more signals can be combined to form a composite signal with a new meaning. Zebras communicate hostile behaviour by flattering their ears and friendliness by raising their eyes (discrete signals). They indicate the intensity of either emotion by the degree to which the mouth opens (graded signal). The mouth-opening pattern is the same for both hostile and friendly behaviour (Fig. 10.9)..

Elephants make much use of their trunks, ears and head for communication. A submissive posture in elephant is indicated by curling trunk inward. If the trunk is forwardly directed it indicates threat to enemy. Aggressiveness is indicated by raising his ear of head. Hippopotamuses have territorial displays that include mouth opening.

Altmann (1962) and Hindi and Rowell (1962) studied social communication in rhesus monkey and attempted to describe their visual signals. Members of a rhesus monkey troop will respond to a range of diverse stimuli from the dominant male. His general body posture and manner of walking will convey information quite apart from any signal, such as threat movements, he may make. Almost every feature of his body when moving or at rest is strong contrast to that of a subordinate male.

Visual signals in mammals often involve movement of extension of body, such as ears, legs and tails. Behaviourists have now developed the process of communication with Gorilla through signs. 26 year old female Gorilla named Koko understands and responds to 500 signals and through these she expresses her feelings and experiences. She could express her choice about drink, her relationship with pet cats, with humans and also about her dreams. She blushed and covered her face with hands when she was asked if she would like to be a mother. However she did not make any response to the proposal of her marriage offered to her.

Male sticklebacks, preferentially court large females with distended abdomens, which indicates that they have a lot of eggs to invest. Rowland (1989) showed that, when presented with two dummy females, a male would first detect his courtship to the larger and fatter one.

The Peacock displays its plumage coloration by dancing during breeding season. Visual alarms are seen in birds which flock together. They flash their wings and tail feathers when there is danger.

SIGNALLING WITH LIGHTS

One of the most remarkable forms of visual communication is that involving bioluminescence (light of biological origin), where particular species generate their own light signals. Certain insects and deep-sea fish make use of this spectacular technique.

Luminous insects

Luminous insects are the glow-worms and their relatives the fireflies. Springtails (*Collembola*), flies (*Diptera*) and homopterans are light producing insects. Among beetles bioluminescence is the most widely distributed. Fly larva of the species *Arachnocampa luminosa* (found on the walls of caves in New Zealand) emit light to attract the tiny insects which they feed upon.

Communication by means of light signal is closely linked to sexual behaviour and serves almost exclusively the function of recognition and mutual attraction between individuals of opposite sexes for the purpose of mating. In certain beetle species, it is the female which emits the light signal. Any male flying around her are attracted to the spot so that mating can take place. Male firefly *(Luciola lusitanica)* performs a series of loops and somersaults in the air above the female before landing beside her. The males of two Trinidad cucuyos, *Pyrophorus pellucens* and *Pyrophorus extinctus*, manage to distinguish females of their own species by differences in the light intensity emitted and variation in the pulses of light. Though we have entered in new millennium but we still have a lot to learn about the use of light of biological origin as signals in the insect and fish world.

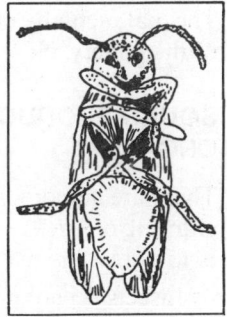

Fig. 10.10. The male glow worm, *Lampyrus noctiluca* signals his presence by alternately switching on and off his abdominal light organs.

Bioluminescent fish

Most light-producing fish live at the bottom of the sea, where there is almost complete darkness. Light producing fish bear special organ known as photophores which are arranged in series along the length of the body. Among fish of the family *Myctophidae* (lantern-fish) the photophores are aligned in rows along the flanks, whereas in bristle-mouths the photophores are arranged in rows along the belly as well as on the flanks. The micro-anatomical structure of the photophores is well-known, but no study has yet been complete in the aspect of light "languages" in the ocean fishes. Grescitell (1958) revealed that bathypelagic fish possess eyes which are sensitive to a spectrum of light ranging from red through violet to blue, which is the range covered by luminous organs. It can therefore be concluded that fish can communicate with one another by means of light signal in the extreme darkness of the abyssal depths. Light signal also play a part in sexual relationships between members of a given species, facilitating the location of suitable partners. It is not known whether such light emissions are involved in aggressive or territorial behaviour.

AUDITORY COMMUNICATION (BIO-ACOUSTIC MEANS)

Sending information from one member to another by sound production is called auditory signal or bio-acoustic signal. In a number of Invertebrate and Vertebrate species, bio-acoustic means of transmitting information is the chief means of communication. Sound is good means for communicating over long distances both in air and water. Auditory communication or acoustic signals may have a vocal origin or it may be produced by other organs.

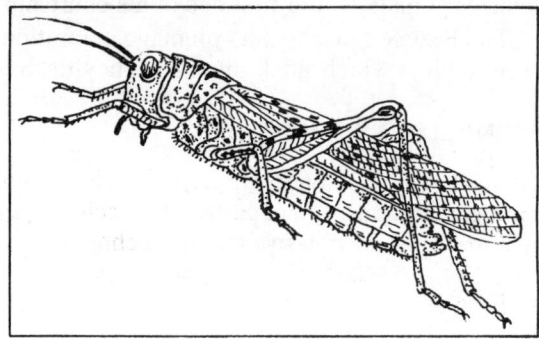

According to the species and exact nature of the sound produced, these signals can have a variety of functions. Calls of mammals and birds have a vocal origin but sound produced by **Cicadas** and **Crickets** is rhythmic oscillation of forewings. Sound is more effective signal at night and in darkness. Sound can go around obstacles that would interfere with visual signals. Sound is better than visual signal at getting the attention of a receiver. Sound may be transmitted by the air or water or via the substrate.

Fig. 10.11. Grasshoppers 'sing' by rubbing their legs against wings.

SOUND PRODUCING BARNACLE AND SHRIMP

Barnacles produce sonorous grating noises. These underwater noises can serve a variety of functions. Some shrimp species produce loud noises, by clicking their pincers.

Clicking sounds produced by the male wood boring deathwatch beetle (*Xestobium rufovillosum*) attract females during the breeding season. The male actually makes the sound by striking his head against the floor of the gallery, close to its opening (Fig. 10.12).

SOUND PRODUCING INSECTS AND SOUND RECEPTION ORGANS

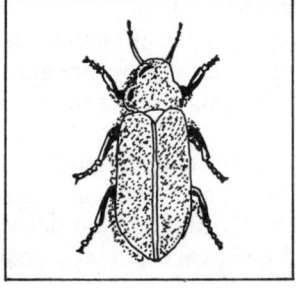

There are numerous sound producing insects. The song of *cicadas* and chirping of *crickets* is well known. Usually sound production in insects is to attract his mate.

Fig. 10.12. Death watch beetle signal to each other by tapping their heads against the wood.

Insects do not possess "ears" like us then how do they receive sounds and vibrations ? There are a number of different organs adapted for sound reception in insects. The sense organs involved range from simple sensory hairs on the cuticle to fully developed ear on leg or abdomen. Sound is received in the form of a sequence of vibrations, which are converted to nerve impulses prior to interpretation by the nervous system. The most rudimentary "ears" consist of sensory hairs, which may be located anywhere on the body. Johnson's *organ* is a step towards a more elaborate auditory organ. This sound receiving organ is located near the base of the antenna and is extremely well developed in lepidopterans (moths and butterflies), hymenopterans (ants, wasps and bees) and dipterans (flies and mosquitoes).

The antennae receive vibrations, concentrate the vibrations at their bases where they are converted to nerve impulses and transmitted to the central nervous system. Fully developed tympanic organs (like our own ear-drum) which act as true ears may be located in a variety of places. Some grasshoppers have a pair of well-developed tympanic organ located on the base of the abdomen. Grasshoppers and crickets bear tympanic organs on the tibial segments of their forelegs. Owlet moths and hawk moths bear tympanic organs located on the thorax. Geometrid moths have tympanic organs on their abdomens.

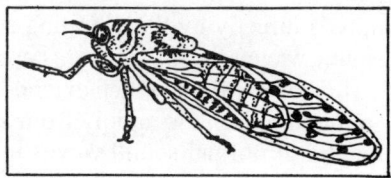

Fig. 10.13. Cicadas : There are several hundred cicada species. The drumming organ of the cicada – which gives rise to the well-known stridulations – is located close to the abdomen within a cavity which acts as a resonating chamber. The sound is further intensified by means of a large air sac, which is located in the abdomen and displaces all the other organs upwards.

Some insects produce "accidental" sounds. Everyone is familiar with the humming sound of the bee and with the irritating noise produced by the beating of wings of a mosquito searching for a human victim. These sounds play no part in communication. Some locusts, grasshoppers, moths and butterflies emit crackling sound while in flight, but these are incidental noises produced by the wings striking against one another. No communication between individuals is produced by these wing vibrations. In mosquitoes, the acoustic vibrations from the wings may help to establish contact between the sexes. Males produce a high pitched-noise with 430–470 wing beats/second. Wing vibrations in male mosquito of one genus *Forcipomaya* goes as high as 1000 per second. Female mosquitoes produce deeper sound with 260 to 340 wing-beats/second.

SOUND COMMUNICATION IN ANTS

Although ants communicate mainly by exuding chemical signals – 'smells' but they also exchange sounds that are barely audible to the human ear. They produce sound by moving head and rubbing one part of their bodies against another. This activity is called 'stridulation'. They hear each other's whispers with their antennae.

Because ants seem to be entirely unresponsive to normal noise, it has been assumed that they detect, not the sound waves in air, but the vibrations that stridulation creates and transmits through the ground.

Acoustics expert Robert Hickling of the University of Mississippi, and ant biologist Richard Brown of Mississippi State University, have studied stridulation in the black fire ant *Solenopsis richteri*, and their findings challenge conventional thinking on ant conversation.

Ants stridulate just as musicians play their washboards : by rubbing set of ridges attached to the posterior abdomen. Hickling and Brown find that the insects can thus create a range of different sounds that convey different messages such as '*attack*' or '*watch out*!" or "*I'm distressed!*" (Ant talk is invariably exclamatory).

Many insects detect sound waves in air by using hairlike sense organs called *trichoid sensilla*, rather like the sound sensors in our ear. It seems likely that ants do the same as their antennae are covered with such hairs. Moreover, it would be hard for an ant to adapt its stridulations to transmission through the wide range of materials it encounters – leaves, wood, soil, animal tissue – rather than simply using the air in every case.

But if ants do indeed send sound signals through the air, why do they apparently not hear much louder sounds? Hickling and Brown suggest that they don't sense propagating sound waves, but instead the 'near-field' sound pressure that radiates very close to a sound source. In this region the air is being moved directly by the vibrating source rather than by the pressure of the adjacent peaks of a moving sound wave.

In the near field, which extends perhaps ten centimeters or so from a stridulating ant, the speed of the sound impulse falls rapidly from a high value very close to the source to the lower value that is characteristic of normal sound waves in air. Hickling and Brown say that this sharp change in sound speed might be easier for another ant's trichoid sensilla to detect than is a normal sound wave moving at constant speed, which needs more sensitive apparatus.

They propose that an ant might in fact not be detecting the pressure of the moving air at all (as our ears do), but instead the difference in sound speed at each of its two antennae. This difference is appreciable in the near field, even for antenna tips spaced just a few millimeters apart; but it falls rapidly to zero beyond the near-field region. Sensing sound in this way would give ants excellent hearing for sound sources close to them (such as other ants), while making them deaf to more distant sounds, however loud.

The researchers point out that the imported fire ant, so called because it invaded the USA from South America, causes widespread damage to animal and plant life. They hope that, by learning how these insects communicate, it might become possible to control them by non-chemical methods.

SOUND PRODUCING FISHES

You may wonder to hear that there are a number of sound producing fish species. Many marine fish species produces sounds by rubbing together parts of their body, such as individual fin rays. Others produce dull grunting noises by vibrating their swim-bladders by muscle contraction as a resonating chamber. Still others grind their teeth together to make sounds, as does the sunfish. Numerous species produce anguished distress calls when they are wounded or threatened by some danger. The sea horse (*Hippocampus*) produces musical rattling noise when it shakes its head.

Three Mediterranean fish species are well known for their sound producing abilities : the caprus (catfish), the lyra (piper : *Trigla lyra*) and the chalcis.

Fish perceive sounds either by means of the internal ear, which receives high frequency noises, or through the "lateral line system", composed of a large number of sense organs. Fish respond to vibrations emitted through the water as a result of the variation in the pressure exerted on the fish's sides. In fact, it operates rather like radar, notifying the fish of the presence of an obstacle or of a predator. Thus, the fish is able to find its way without difficulty even when the water is cloudy or during the night. Recent researches reveals that fishes are found to communicate with one another with an unexpectedly wide range of grunting and crackling noises.

The codfish produces low-frequency noises during the spawning season, while the male toad-fish (*Opsanus*) produces whistles to attract a receptive female. The "song" of certain fish species is known to play an important role in their sexual behaviour. Tavolga (1955) studied the song of gobies and blennies. There are several fish species which exhibit "singing" in chorus, as in the case with the piper (also known as the "sea-robin"). Some marine catfish produce veritable choruses at night.

The electric fish, *Eigenmannia virescens* has an unusual short range signal : the male discharges its electric organ in a series of "chirps". Hagedorn and Heiligenberg (1985), having transposed them into sound for our ears, describe as "short and abrupt during aggressive encounters" and "with a softer and more raspy quality during courtship".

SOUND PRODUCTION IN FROGS AND TOADS

One can distinguish different frog species with the help of bio-acoustics. Bergert (1960), Blair and Duellmen (1963) discovered that it is possible to identify different tree frog species by their calls, since these calls remain absolutely constant within each species.

Frogs utter a variety of calls (the distress call, the fear call, the territorial croaking call, the rain call etc.) but the most common type is the *mating call* of the male. This call is of great biological importance, since it constitutes the mechanism by which frog species are reproductively isolated from one another. Each female only responds to the call of a male of her own species. Recording of the calls (by sound spectrogram) can be used for reliable identification of any frog species, even if its external appearance is difficult to distinguish from that of a related species.

In tree frogs and toads, the vocal sac is expanded to form a balloon beneath the throat, whereas many frog species have resonance sacs distributed elsewhere on the head. The volume and frequency of croaking calls are directly linked to ambient temperature levels as was studied by Zeifel (1959) in the yellow bellied toad, *Bombina variegata*.

Duellman and Fouquette (1968) observed the existence of regional "dialects" in a single frog species with a wide geographical distribution. Duellman (1970) demonstrated the great importance of male mating calls as a reproductive isolating mechanism species. In fact, tree frog species which breed at the same time and in the same places never hybridize with another species. This is because the females only respond to the call of males of their own species.

21st century Zoologists have realised the importance of the croaking calls for classing and keeping a sound spectrogram identification file for each species. As a result, numerous frogs which had been classified as separate species in 20th century were actually found no more than individuals or local variants of a single species. Conversely some tree frogs which had been classified as single species have distinct croaking calls and are different species.

Barhardt (1974) observed that the calls of male green tree frogs have two peaks of sound energy – a *low one* at 900 Hz and a *high one* at about 3000 Hz. The ears of the females are tuned to pick up these two frequencies in particular. Narins and Capranica (1976) showed a remarkable sex difference in the hearing of a related species of tree frog, which accounts for the fact that males and females respond to different sign stimuli in the call of the male – a double 'co-qui'. Neurophysiological recordings revealed the truth that each sex herd only the note of relevance to itself because the neurones of the inner ear were tuned differently for males and females.

SOUND PRODUCTION IN REPTILES

We know that snakes hiss but no specific communication system by sound production has been studied in reptiles. In a rattle snake, the rattle which is a modification of the skin in the tail region vibrate to produce sound. But purpose of its sound production is not known.

BIRD SONG

Bird song has been a source of pleasure for man through the ages. Now biologists have realized the full significance of vocalizations of birds, both for the study of behaviour and for the classification of bird species.

Usually male birds sings a song during breeding season. They sing when they attain a territory and in some cases they stop singing as soon as they win the heart of a mate. Basic message of song may be "*I am an unmated adult male come on my territory*". In breeding condition, the singing bird may also be saying *where he comes from, exactly who he is and about his motive*. The chirping of bird may be matter of joy or may be song of sorrow. Still we are not aware about the basic vocabulary of language of birds.

Only a limited number of bird species utter musical sounds which can justifiably be called "songs". Birds use their songs as an extremely rich and varied means of expression and communication. Bird-song can be broadly classified into 5 categories, though there are of course a whole host of intermediate forms :-

1. A simple note, or a number of isolated notes of mediocre musical quality. Example : the sparrow.

2. A simple phrase composed of one or more notes with a certain musical quality. Examples : the cuckoo; some doves; the willow-warbler.

3. A song of longer duration, containing a dozen notes or so, permitting some degree of variation from one bird to another. Examples : yellow - hammers; the chaffinch.

4. A song containing a great variety of phrases which the bird can combine in different ways without repetition. Examples : the blackbird ; the nightingale.

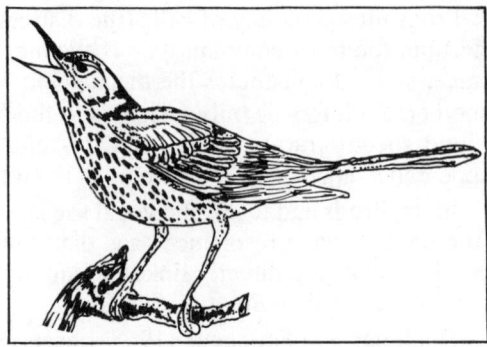

Fig. 10.14. Song birds singing to show that he has claimed a piece of land.

5. A continuous song in which virtually no repetition can be identified. This type is quite similar to the preceding one, but its rapid execution and the absence of pauses prevent identification of individual phrases. Examples : the blackcap ; the skylark.

Like musical instrument, the notes of which a bird song is composed vary in tonality, force, volume, timbre and duration. A nightingle is one of the most gifted bird singers.

Song is a signalling device related to territorial establishment and defence during the breeding season. The song typically has a sexual connotation and it is usually seasonal in character. The intensity of the song varies and reaches its peak when the pair is selecting a nest-site. There are some bird species in which the male and female sing together in duets. Duets serve to maintain a close bond between the male and the female in a pair and this form of communication is found among dense forest-living birds where the foliage does not permit clear visual contact.

Within a single species which has a wide geographical distribution, isolated populations sometimes have songs which differ from each other. The different songs within a species can be considered as dialects. In some species it has been observed that members of a single species taken from different areas are unable to understand the song of one another. For example, the alpine race of the willow tit, (*Paras montatus*) sings in a different dialects from that found tits of the same species living on the plains. The chaffinch has several local dialects. An English chaffinch cannot understand a Finnish relative and has difficulty in communicating with a central European chaffinch.

There are a number of birds which are able to imitate the songs or dialects of other species. Birds which can imitate the human voice are well-known ; parrots, mynahs, jays, ravens, magpies, blue whistling thrushes and starlings. In addition to dialects and imitation, there are often recognizable variations in the songs uttered by individuals of any bird species.

Eastern crows make mobbing calls or assembly calls to draw the different members of the group together to defend themselves. They also produce a departing call before flying off on getting the danger.

TALK OF EGGS

Readers may be surprised to know that eggs also speak. Prior to hatching, the late embryos of certain bird species communicate with one another and mother. Collias (1952) and Guyomarch (1966), and Kear (1968) studied the vocalizations of domestic chick embryos and unhatched mallard ducklings respectively. About three days before hatching, the duckling embryos become capable of producing the cheeping call and thus of communicating one another, so that they all can hatch at the same time. This phenomenon has been experimentally analyzed in ducks, quail and bobwhites.

Driver, Lind and Kirman have confirmed the existence of vocalization with late embryos of the seagull, the godwit and numerous duck species. Kear (1968) published sonogram showing that *contentment calls* are interspersed between regular clicks. Synchronization of hatching only occurs when the eggs are together in a clutch in the normal way. If the eggs are separated from one another, forty-eight hours before hatching, synchronization is no longer found and there may be gap of one or two days between the hatching times for the first and last chick. This proves that acoustic communication between the developing eggs is essential to enable them to hatch simultaneously.

SOUND PRODUCTION IN WHALES AND DOLPHINS

Whales and Dolphins possess a highly developed brain. They communicate with members of own society by means of an articulated language consisting of a large variety of sounds. They produce their sounds while under water. These mammals "speak" a language composed of whistles groans and clicks, covering a wide range of frequencies extending from low pitched sounds to ultrasonic squeaks which are inaudiable to the human ear. Such echo-locating calls constitute ultrasonic signals similar to those used by bats.

It was thought for a long time that cetaceans (Whales and Dolphins) talk by mouth like us. But in fact Whales and Dolphins speak through their 'Noses'. The sound-producing apparatus is located close to the nasal passages. The harmonious, modulated sounds of the sperm whale are indicative of a high degree of control by the brain.

M. Jacobs found that behind the nasal passage, there is a series of inflatable air sacs, the number and extent vary from species to species. The common dolphin possesses three pairs of sacs which act as reservoirs of air. These sacs are filled whenever the animal inhales and they may also receive air exhaled from the lungs when the dolphin is under water. The aperture of each sac is regulated by lips reinforced with muscles or cartilage. These sacs help in the production of sound. Jacobs inferred that the muscle fibres surrounding the air sacs are voluntarily operated by the facial nerves. In cetaceans, this nerve, which governs facial expressions in other mammals, is entirely devoted to the modulation of sounds through its control of the vocal air-sacs. In all cetaceans, facial expressions are completely lacking. The numerous little facial muscles have been transferred inside the head, to a position close to the vocal sacs. Whereas we can smile, grimace and frown, Whales and Dolphins always have the same fixed expression. We are familiar with the mocking "smile" of the dolphin, but the animal is never able to change this expression because it lacks the appropriate facial muscles.

In 1971 a group of American scientists picked up vocalizations from the blue whale off the coast of Chile, at a distance of 160 kilometers. Four of these giant whales, were communicating with one another by means of series of short, high-pitched calls with little modulation. The call of seals and other pinnipeds (Sealions and Walruses) are just as variable as those of whales and dolphins. They range from the deep, bell-like calls of the Walrus to the short, high pitched vocalizations of Weddell seals.

The language of cetaceans is difficult to decipher since the call sequence is extremely rapid. They are of very short duration, lasting only 1/1000 to 1/25000 of a second ; and their frequency can be as high as 150 kilocycles/second, whereas the human ear is unable to detect sounds higher than 20 kilocycles/second.

BAT'S LANGUAGE

Like many other mammals, bats communicate with one another by means of vocalizations and maintain contact by acoustic means.

Bats live in large aggregations. Colonies are known in which there are more than a million individuals. Bats possess an exceptional acoustic communication system, which help them to maintain close social contact. It is known that the young call to their mothers and mother recognise her own offspring among tens of thousands of other helpless mites, suspended upside-down from the ceilings of caves. Nelson observed that with Australian fruit-bats of the species *Pteropus poliocephalus* there are more than twenty different signals exchanged between the mother and her infant. It seems that a large number of calls and ultrasonic pulses involved in echolocation are also used for communication between individuals.

Use of "sonar" to locate their prey by bats cannot be considered under the heading of "communication". This is an echolocation system of the kind used by some marine mammals and certain birds, and it has no direct link with the topic of communication or language.

The echolocation system used by bats is, in fact, a natural form of sonar. While in flight, the animals emit high frequency sound pulses (higher than 20 kilocycles/second – inaudible to the adult human ear) and a part of the sound energy is reflected back by any obstacle encountered, to be received by the ear.

WOODCHUCK'S LANGUAGE

Woodchuck advertise their territories and communicate with one another by means of high-pitched squeaks and whistles. The American woodchuck *Marmota monax,* utters short whistles like those of their close relative the alpine marmot, but it can also sing. American woodchucks can emit a melodious babble rather like bird-song. The call, which is composed of soft trills, is produced when the animal is in restful state, at the entrance of its burrow, or when it is sitting on top of a mound and looking around. However, the exact purpose of the call is not known.

PRIMATES

The siamang, *Symphalangus syndactylus,* is arboreal apes. It inhabits the forests of South-east Asia and lives in small groups of about four individuals, dominated by an adult pair. Every morning, the adult male gives a "concert" in which the other members of the group all play a part. The exceptional power of the siamang's call is due to the animal's capacity to inflate its larynx, which acts as a large resonating chamber. When a siamang is singing, the throat is inflated and the vocal sac expands to become a balloon. The sound which is produced can travel from 5 to 8 kilometers through the forest. The daily concerts produced by siamang family serve two purposes :

1. Communication between them
2. Territorial advertisement and notification of group composition.

Chimpanzees, in addition to a great variety of calls – such as *hooting* related to feeding and *rhythmic howls* linked to displays of strength – have a rich repertoire of facial expressions. Their highly mobile faces permit them to express different moods. A grimace (a contortion of the face in pain or amusement) in which the teeth are exposed signifies fear, while a similar grimace without exposure of the teeth represents an invitation to play.

Gorillas communicate with one another by means of a variety of grunting calls. The males beat their chests with their cupped hands and produce loud sound when they are excited or in order to intimidate an enemy.

Orang-utans communicate with one another by means of resonant sounds, interspersed with low-pitched noises. In the evening and just before dawn (at the time of roosting), males utter low, drawn-out howls, perhaps in order to maintain cohesion among the scattered groups.

Examples of non-vocal auditory signals are also there. Certain woodpeckers produce sound by drumming tree trunks. The tail-beating performed by beavers on the water surface, and the drumming produced by rabbits with rapid stamping movements of their hindlimbs are non-vocal auditory signals.

Information can be conveyed by both low and high sound frequency. Low frequency sounds travel great distances and are used by animals with large home ranges. Howler monkeys (*Alouatta*) live in Central and South American forest. They produce low frequency sound which can be herd over a distance of 3 kilometres. Howler monkeys have a repertoire of 15 to 20 different vocalization which elicit specific behavioural responses from other members of the group : gurgling noise, loud howls, grunts, groans, and so on. Usually animals with smaller home ranges use higher frequency sounds. Squirrel monkeys (*Saimiri sciureus*) use high frequency sounds which dissipate rapidly. High frequency sounds are also used by a variety of animals. Human speeches and bird songs are most complex auditory communication.

The calls produced by many other animals are not necessarily audible to the human ear. This is particularly the case with high frequency sounds such as those emitted by dolphins and infrasonic sound produced by elephants. Female elephant call musth elephant through infrasonic sound signal during breeding season. Echo-locating bats emit bursts of ultrasonic sound pulses of short duration (5-15 milli seconds) and high frequency (20-120 khz.), which are beyond the auditory range of humans. Dogs can hear very low frequency sound which are not audible to human ears.

Crying is the most powerful way human beings, especially babies, can communicate their needs. Babies have patterns of crying : 1. Hunger cry, 2. Anger cry, 3. Pain cry, 4. Frustation cry, and 5. Habit cry.

Baby in distress cry louder, longer and more regularly than hungry babies.

TACTILE SIGNALS

Information transmitted in the form of physical contact (touch signal) is called tactile communication. Tactile communication is used by many Invertebrates (ants, termites, honeybees) and mammals. Antennae of ants, termites and honeybee, covered with receptors are the first part of the body to contact other objects and organisms. The honeybee performing round and waggle dance in a dark hive inform about the type and location of food by tactile communication as the worker bee's antennae contact the forager and pick up taste cues. Touch or Tactile communication is more developed in social interaction of termites where blind workers of termite colony totally depend on this phenomenon.

Use of tactile displays occur during copulation of many mammals. In many rodents and cat family stimulation of the back end of an oestrous female make concave arching of the back and immobility (lordosis).

ODOUR OR CHEMICAL COMMUNICATION

Odour is used as a factor for communication throughout the animal kingdom. Molecules used for chemical communication between individual animals are called pheromones. Pheromones can communicate very specific message that contain a great deal of information. Pheromones are involved in mate identification, spacing mechanisms, alarm and many other clues. Odour signals can transmit information in the dark, can travel long distance, can last for hours or number of days. (Detail "Role of pheromones in composing behaviour" Chapter 3 of this book).

We are familiar about the role of sex attractant *bombykol*, produced by the female silk moth. One molecule of *bombykol* triggers a nerve impulse in a receptor cell in an antenna of a male. About 200 receptor cells firing in one second lead to a response (Schneider, 1974). The male responds by flying upwind, equalising the pheromone concentration on both antenna, until he reaches the female. The olfactory signal in this case has become so important that other stimuli, even visual has become meaningless for male silkworm in finding female for the purpose of mating. When a female gypsy moth is ready to be inseminated, she releases a pheromone called *gyplure*. The male moths find the female by smelling gyplure. The scent tracts left behind by herbivorous mammals and a few birds can attract the attention of predators. This can be seen with hunting member of cat family (Felidae), dog family (Canidae) when it has picked up a trail. All the special odours of animals are produced by glands on the body surface which give each species its characteristic smell, as with pigs or cows. In addition, each individual within a species has its own special odour. A beaver, for example, is able to tell from deposit of faecal matter whether it has been produced by a member of the family groups or by a stranger.

CHEMICAL SIGNAL IN INSECTS

Chemical communication is the most primitive type of communication system. The communication system in insects is mostly based on chemical signal in combination with visual and auditory signals.

Pheromones are secreted by exocrine gland of insects and act to regulate the external environment by influencing other individuals. Pheromones are perceived by other members of the species and they elicit behavioural responses such as those involved in sexual reproduction. A single female moth or butterfly can produce enough pheromone to excite all males of the territory. In order to spread out her pheromones effectively, the female rapidly beats her wings after secreting the pheromone to ensure that it evaporates. The pheromone molecules are then carried and dispersed by the wind.

Males receive this chemical message with their antennae and fly upwind in search of the female. They move towards the source of odour. The scent concentration increases as the male approaches the female. Schneider experimentally proved that just 300 molecules are enough to stimulate sexual activity in a male silk-moth and to excite him to fly off in search of a female. The nervous system of moths and butterflies is so sensitive that a single molecule striking upon one of the receptors on the antennae is enough to produce a nerve impulse which is transmitted to the brain.

In fact, pheromone system alone is not only effective for successful mating, additional mechanisms are also required to ensure that females only mate with males of their own species. Now we have come to know that the female is not the only one to possess pheromones ; males, too emit chemical signals. An entomologist E. Priesner (1970) revealed that the number of different pheromones are less than the number of known species which produce them. He estimated that there are only about 2000 pheromones, whereas the total number of moth and butterfly species is more than one hundred thousand. In this situation it is clear that a combination of male and female pheromones is required for mating and continuation of race. Further, it has been observed that species which have the same scents 'transmit' at different times of the day to avoid confusion in insect world. Moreover, each moth or butterfly species show a specific annual cycle, and this provides one of the means to keep species isolated.

COMMUNICATION BY ODOUR IN ANTS

In the ant species *Solenopsis saevissima,* the pheromone stimulate workers to work. Pheromone can also be used as one of the alarm signals produced by workers in distress. Glands of Dufour, located on the hind part of the abdomen of ants secrete chemical trail. The ant alternately extends its sting to the ground and retracts it again, depositing the pheromone. The deposited chemical attracts other workers which deposit a chemical trace in their turn.

The "trail scent" pheromone is very volatile and disappears in less than two minutes. The rapid evaporation of the pheromone is obviously an asset and avoids continued use of "false trails". Each species of ant has a highly specific pheromone which does not evoke responses from ants of other species. Thus, each ant's nest possesses its own particular "language" and its own path code.

The agitated ant emits a pheromone secreted by the large mandibular gland on its jaws. Alarm pheromones are extremely volatile and dissipates within 35 seconds. But, collective secretion of pheromone in the vicinity attracts other ants in the colony to the site of the alarm. The more acute the danger, the greater the number of ants attracted to the spot. Numerous other pheromones have been identified in ants which play vital role in their social relationship. Edward Wilson (1963) observed that about a dozen different pheromones in finely - balanced combinations govern the complex society in an ant's nest. Ants produce a pheromone after death. Odour of this pheromone immediately provokes workers to remove the corpse from the nest.

OLFACTORY COMMUNICATION AMONG FISH

Some fish species possess developed sense of smell. Olfactory organ is well developed among deep-sea male anglerfish (*Ceratias, Cyclothone, Lophius* and *Oneirodes*) but absent in female fish. Some freshwater fish species possess a very sensitive olfactory organ. Hasler maintained that the eel has the same degree of olfactory sensitivity as the most sensitive dog. Fish possess a chemical alarm signal and this pheromone secreted by the skin when a fish is injured.

A kind of fish Minnows have an extraordinary sensitivity to chemicals from their own species. If a minnow is wounded and some of its blood gets into the water, other minnows show panic flight. They show far less fear when the blood of other types of fish is shed. This fear substance put into an aquarium sparks off general panic among a group of minnows.

THE CHEMICAL LANGUAGE OF MAMMALS

Scent glands remain located in a variety of places on a mammal's body. In the ungulates alone, there are glands near the eyes, in the *groin* (the part of the body where the tops of the legs meet, containing the sexual organs), at the base of the horns, at the back of the head, on the tail, on the *prepuce* (head of penis), on the hocks (the middle joint of an animal's back leg), on the soles of the feet or at the bases of the hooves. The secretions from the glands may be deposited in the course of normal bodily contact (if on the feet or on the hocks, for instance) or by a special act of rubbing against branches and other objects. In some species, such as the beaver, the scent is sprayed as it squats on a hillock of mud or sand.

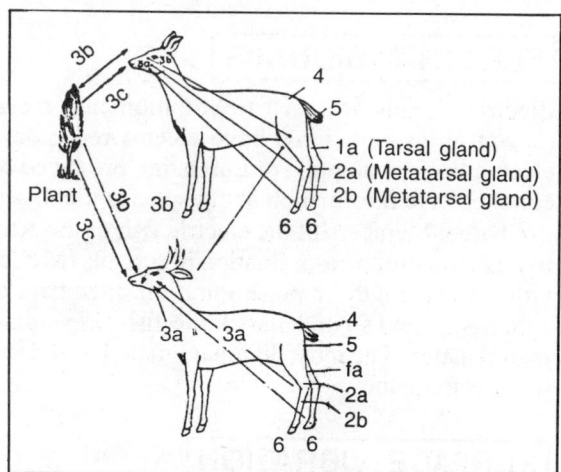

Mammals with poorly developed sense of smell are called *microsmatic* and with well-developed olfactory system are called *macrosmatic*. Human being is microsmatic whereas most mammals are macrosmatic. Macrosmatic mammals make a great deal of use of olfactory communication, employing an enormous variety of olfactory signals incorporated in urine, faeces or the secretions of a wide range of skin glands.

Various mammals produce pheromones from their anal or facial glands which are rubbed into

Fig. 10.15. Odour play an important role in communication in the world of deer. Pheromone producing glands in black-tailed deer.

trees or rocks to mark the territories of individual animals as seen in the case of a male dik-dik deer which mark its territory by depositing secretions from an eye gland on to the twigs.

Hoofed mammals (ungulates) have glands between their toes which leave a scent behind where ever they go. Voles, shrews, moles and hamsters bear glands on the flanks. The peccaries of South America and the African hyraxes have a scent-gland on their backs. Deer and a number of antelope species have an antorbital scent-gland located beneath each eye. Other species carry marking glands on their horns.

In primates, including man axillary and inguinal glands are present in the armpits and the groin. A number of mammal species bear glands beneath the tail or in the perineal region. Civet cats, Skunks, Musk deer and several other mammals are well known for their odours.

Olfactory marking of the territory is one of the most widely distributed forms of communication among mammals. Olfactory signals in mammals can be used in situations where danger threatens for individual recognition; and for attraction between the sexes. As a general rule, it is the dominant animal which marks the territory and his marking frequency will increase if he feels threatened by a rival or if he detects the presence of any intruder to his own group.

In mice, the urine of males contains a pheromone which increases the aggressiveness of other males. If several female mice are forced to live together in a relatively small cage, disruption of their reproductive cycles results, and they may even become infertile. However, the cycles return to normal once the females are isolated from one another. W.K. Whitten observed that the presence of a male in a caged group of females suppressed the "Lee-Boot effect" and that reproduction took place normally. Further, Helen Bruce discovered that the simple presence of a strange male is enough to block pregnancy in a female. Pregnancy will normally proceed if she continues to be impregnated with odour by the male with which she originally mated. It was found that the strange male's odour will suppress the secretion of the hormone prolactin in the female. Colhoun believes that pheromones play an important role in the complex mechanisms which operate to maintain relatively steady population levels in various mammal species. Six main scent substances have been identified in mammals, of which *civetone* and *muscone* have proved to be particularly important in sexual behaviour.

Lions, tigers, cats and dogs urinate to mark the edges of their territory. Species specific sex pheromones are released by many female mammals like lioness, tigress, bitch etc. when they are in heat for attracting males.

ELECTRIC SIGNALS

Electric signals are used to communicate messages in fishes. Torpedo (Electric ray), and sharks (*Scyliorhinus caniculus*) have electro receptors that they use in communication. Sharks detect the electric field by ampulla of Lorenzini, produced by prey flatfish that are buried in the sand. Electric fish communicate information about species identity and sex by modulating the shape of the electric organ discharge. Members of the electric fish of the African family mormyridae use electric organ discharges to maintain group co-ordination in schools (Moller, 1976). Bullock (1973) demonstrated that by altering either wavelength or pulse duration, members of family mormyridae communicate threat, warning, submission and so on. Glass knife fish (*Elgenmannia*) males emit electric current of lower frequencies than females. The most dominant male has the lowest frequency and the most dominant female has the highest frequency.

SURFACE VIBRATION

In some animals information may be communicated by patterns of surface vibrations. Males of *Gerris remigis* (water spider) send out ripples of a certain frequency, and receptive females respond by moving toward the source. On getting female mate the male stops sending courtship ripples (Wilcox, 1972).

Cannibalistic male spiders vibrate threads of web of his prospective partner i.e., female spider in a special fashion communicating her *"I am your lover not the prey"*.

Elephants pickup vibrations through foot stamping and low frequency rumbling generate seismic waves in the ground that can travel nearly 32 Kilometers along the surface of the earth. According to a study in the Journal of the Acoustical Society of America (JASA), elephants may be able to sense vibrations through their feet and interpret them as warning signals of a distant danger. Seismic wave could travel from their feet to the ear via bone conduction, or through somatosensory receptors in the foot similar to ones found in the trunk. Scientists think it may be a combination of both.

In the early 90's O'Connell-Rodwell began to suspect there was more to long-distance elephant communication than airbone rumblings alone. She points out that mock charges generate airbone and seismic signals with frequencies of about 20 hz. ideal for long-distance communication. "Based on our mathematical models, we estimate that seismic signals produced by elephants can travel between 16 and 32 kilometers in the ground, while acoustic signals have the potential of traveling only about 8 km through the air".

"Elephants may be able to sense the environment better than we realise," O'Connell-Rodwell contends, pointing to studies showing that elephants can detect and move toward thunder-storms from great distances.

Other creatures also produce seismic signals. Among them the golden mole, the elephant seal (no relation to terrestrial elephants) and a variety of insects, amphibians, reptiles and fish communicate by this process.

Fin whales produce calls that carry hundreds of kilometres underwater at a frequency of 20 hertz – a range so low that it is barely audible to the human ear. In the late 1980's researchers discovered that elephants also produce strong, low-frequency 20 herz rumbles that can travel up to nine km through the air under ideal weather conditions. Studies indicated that elephants use these low-frequency vocalizations to co-ordinate movements with other far-off herds.

HUMAN LANGUAGE

Oral communication is not unique to humans. Frogs croak, snakes hiss, birds chirp, lions roar but humans alone have developed spoken and written languages which are used to facilitate intraspecific communication and formulate abstract concepts of art, science, philosophy and religion. We assume that development of language in humans was associated with co-operative hunting. Whatever may be the origins, the basic anatomical structures associated with speech had to be present in our ancestors. These include the lips, tongue and larynx and three areas of brain, the speech motor cortical area (controlling the delivery of speech) and two further areas also in the left side of the cerebrum. One of these areas stores auditory, visual and verbal information and, the other is concerned in formulating statements and response, that is putting words together.

There are approximately two thousand human languages and dialects spoken in the world, but the most strangest and unusual of all is silbo. Silbo is used by Shepherds of Gomera in the canary Islands archipelago is a form of communication entirely based on whistles. The island is extremely hilly and the inhabitants have learned to communicate with one another between mountain crests. By means of modulated series of whistles, shepherds of Gomera island exchange information over distances of 3 to 10 kilometers. The modulation of the whistles is achieved by special movements made with the fingers on the tongue; the lips are not involved, in the language of silbadores. The sounds involved range across three octaves and they are of great tonal purity. Every individual has his own "vocal" style, so one silbadore can recognise another member of his island.

Some non-verbal forms of communication is also recognised, and they are equally important in human social life. In non-verbal forms of communication, man shares a number of similarities with Savanna - living chimpanzees in Africa (George Schaller, 1963 and Jane van Lewick-Goodall, 1967). These non-verbal social signals are very similar to those of higher primates. Some description of human non-verbal communication system is described in 11th chapter viz. human behaviour of this book.

RITUALS OF RECONCILIATION AND SOLACE

Ethologists discussed in *"Biology of benevolence congress"* the rituals of reconciliation and solace that chimpanzees and other non-human primates engage in after a nasty fight that threatens social ties ; gestures like holding out hand to shake and make up or hugging and grooming or mouth-to-mouth kissing. They explored instances of humans who are unable to love or connect with others. The sorrowful outcome of neuropsychiatric disorders like *autism* (a serious mental condition that develops during childhood in which one becomes unable to communicate or form relationship with others), and schizophrenia. Afflictive behaviour requires a hormonal and neural substrate, an activation of circuit by every bit as intricate as the mechanisms controlling the body's ability to fight an opponent or flee from danger. Ethologists considered the neural and hormonal differences between the rodent species that form inseparable pairs and those that prefer to go it alone.

Dr. Kerstin displayed on graph, one of the fierce, snarling battle-ready man, fists cocked, and the other of a nursing virgin Mary, she of the exposed breast and benign mien. The warrior's so called stress circuitry is indicated and labelled. The levels of fight hormones like cortisol and epinephrine are surging, his heart rate has accelerated, his blood pressure and blood sugar are soaring and any gastro-intestinal activity that could divert energy from his muscles has ceased. All in all, he is in a state of physiological catabolism, a mobilisation and breaking down of the body's energy stores for the business of attacking an enemy.

From a sociability point of view the flight-to-flight response has been shown as a strengthening of the distinction between self and the others–a tightening of the body's response mechanism like springs compressed into a box–the nurturing circuitry suggests an opening up, and expansion of self towards others, and trading of anxiety for at least, a momentary state of quiet joy.

COMMUNICATION BETWEEN HUMANS AND OTHER SPECIES

Animals living in close association with humans often behave as if humans were members of their own species. Owner of a pet tortoise realized that the animal was making repeated attempts to court his shoe. In zoos the male kangaroos may behave as if the upright posture of the keeper were a challenge to fight. If the keeper adopts the bowed posture characteristic of peaceful kangaroos, then the confrontation can be avoided (Hediger, 1964). People talk to their pets in human language and they obey their master. Circus masters order wild animals (Lion, Leopard, Tiger, Elephant, Sea-lion etc.) to do tedious actions in human language and body posture and they follow him like obedient servant.

EXERCISE

1. Give a brief introduction of biological communication.
2. What do you mean by Signals ? Describe about protective facial expression of mammals in communication. Mention Darwin's principle of antithesis.
3. Describe composite signals given by Zebras.

4. Describe in brief different channels of communication in animal's world.

5. Write short notes on rituals of reconciliation in Chimpanzees and primates.

6. Write short notes on : Signal, Signaller, Receiver/Message and Complex signal.

7. Write short notes on communication between humans and other species.

8. Write short notes on "simple signals" and "composite signals".

9. Write short notes on communication system in ants.

10. Write short notes on echolocating system of bat.

11. Any transfer of information through signal can be considered as signal or not ? Justify your statement.

12. Should we restrict the definition of communication to transfer of information within a species or between two species ?

13. Describe the Verbet monkey's communication when they spot three kinds of enemies – leopard, eagle and snake – respectively.

14. Is communication always honest ? Give few examples of dishonest signals in biological communication system. How one can rationalize between honest and dishonest communication.

15. What are basic components of communication. Explain each component in two or three lines.

16. Describe Visual communication in Fiddler crabs and Bees.

17. Describe communication through Bioluminescence in animal world.

18. Describe visual communication among birds and mammals.

19. Describe auditory communication in insects, barnacle shrimps and wood boring deathwatch beetle.

20. Describe sound communication in insects.

21. What do you understand by bio-acoustic ? Describe communication system in fish, frog and bird.

22. Describe auditory communication among whales and dolphins.

23. Is there any role of odour in animal world or not? If yes describe chemical signal in insects specially ants.

24. Describe olfactory communication among deep sea fishes.

25. Describe the chemical language of mammals.

26. Describe electric vibration signal used by Torpedo and Sharks.

27. Describe surface vibration used as signal for communication among some spiders. How this system helps male spiders to survive.

28. Language ? Describe strangest languages of *Homo sapiens*.

29. Write short notes on Rituals and reconciliation and solace.

30. Describe communication between humans and other species.

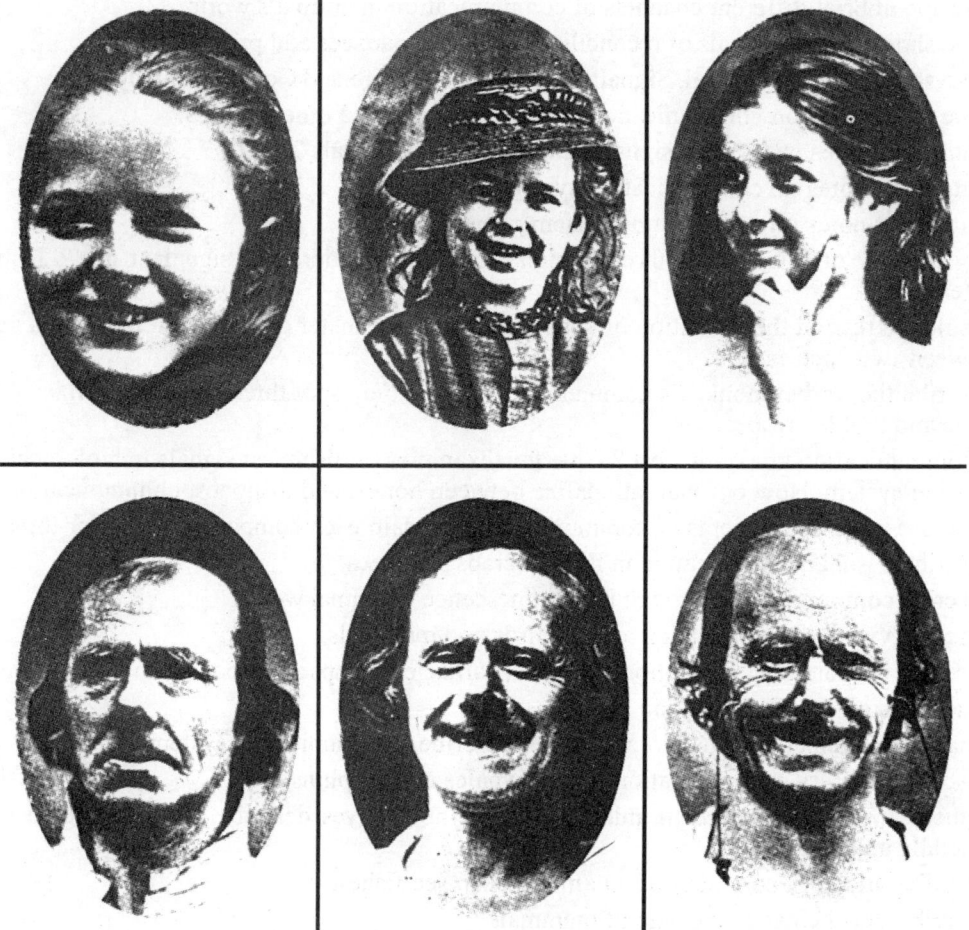

*H*uman beings exhibit almost all basic behaviours like many other animals but human behaviour is varied, complex and a little different from any other animal species. There are two aspects of human behaviour. The brighter aspect is that humans have great power of reasoning, insight and ability of cognition. The darker aspect is that superstition, blind faith, abhorrence, greed, nepotism, lust of power and wealth etc. are perhaps found only in human beings. Most notable point is that animals are not tagged with religion but we have shed much blood in the name of religion since last ten thousand years. Due to different ways of life and different complex behaviours present in human beings ethologists feel difficulty in framing general laws governing all human behaviours. However, different aspects of human behaviour has been studied extensively by psychologists, anthropologists, sociologists and ethologists. This chapter describes important human behaviours.

HUMAN BEHAVIOUR

INTRODUCTION

Ethologists feel difficulty in framing general laws governing all human behaviours because human behaviour is modified very quickly by experience and other factors. Even if we are able to have a framework for animal behaviour, it is doubtful whether one can be able to place all behaviours of humans within that framework. The reason is that man is the only species which has developed taboos, mania, phobias, complexes, tremendous power of speech, reasoning, greed of power and wealth, feeling of hatred or abhorrence, jealousy, ability of telling a lie etc. Man adopts unsuitable ways of achieving comparable goals as he has highly developed brain and great power for reasoning. To achieve genuine or ingenuine goals, he can adopt unreasonable and unsuitable ways, which may be detrimental to mankind.

Different aspects of human behaviour has been studied extensively by psychologists, anthropologists and ethologists. Anthropologists such as Lee (1979), carry out systematic studies of primitive man in their natural environment, and psychologists such as Passingham, (1982) study behavioural differences among primates, including humans, in relation to differences in brain structure and function. Evolutionary biologists explored those aspects of human behaviour that are thought to have a genetic and evolutionary basis. Different disciplines complement each other in giving different dimensions of human behaviour.

Mother baby relationship has been studied in last few decades of 20th century. Brown et al. (1975) studied mother baby relationship during breast feeding (i) infant activity and (ii) maternal care giving. The frequencies of these two behaviour patterns are positively correlated, which could mean that infant activity elicits care giving and vice versa. The conditional probability of both acts increases, following performance of the other, indicating that these have mutual stimulatory effects. However, the probability

313

levels are highest for infant activity following a bout of care giving, indicating that the effect of maternal behaviour on the child is the stronger influence.

IMPRINTING

Imprinting is the result of a predisposition towards learning [Second Chapter of this book]. It is the readiness of an organism's nervous system to acquire certain informations during a brief critical period in early life elicited by particular stimuli.

Like other creatures imprinting also happens in human new borns. The infant recognises mother primarily by smell. The British psychologist John Bowlby (1951) pointed out the importance of the mother-baby bond. The infant and parent are biologically predisposed to becoming attached to each other. Such attachment is essential for proper growth of the baby. According to Ainsworth (1979) attachment is "an essential part of the ground plan of human species for an infant to become attached to a mother".

Sensitive period of imprinting is in case of human being between birth to 5 years. Psychologists have found that if a child is not sent to social gatherings like school, playing ground (park) in childhood (2 to 6 years) they become shy and unsocial. Imprinting plays profound role in cultural inheritance. We follow rituals and exhibit behaviour based on fear and superstition due to imprinted ideals learnt in 'sensitive period' of childhood. Idea of God, Ghost, Sin etc. are result of imprinted learning.

In sexual behaviour, role of imprinting was studied and by various experiments the existence of imprinting was revealed. In humans, satisfactory marriages are not formed between couples who spend their early childhood together. Studies of Taiwanese arranged marriages and Israeli Kibbutzim indicate a lack of sexual attraction between people who spend their childhood together. The reason of failure of these marriages is imprinted memories as a non-sexual partner. Human relationships are intricate due to social convention and taboo. The evidence for some biologically based negative imprinting need extensive research. In humans some of the common examples of imprinting are language learning, sanitary habits etc.

Grandfather or grandmother tell about the happenings of their childhood to their grandchildren not due to memory only, but due to imprinted ideas commonly called nostalgia. People develop strong friendship in early stage of life only due to imprinting. Childhood association of things or people or happenings get imprinted and remain in memory life long.

INSTINCT

Instinct is an innate behaviour mechanism expressed in ordered movement sequences. A fixed action patterns (FAP) is a type of instinct also found in all members of *Homo sapiens* (stereotype). A FAP is a specific and stereotyped sequence of activities that is triggered by a specific stimulus called a sign stimulus or releaser. Releasers open a instinctive behaviour in humans in the same way as in other animals.

RELEASERS FOR INSTINCTIVE BEHAVIOUR

VISUAL RELEASERS

First thing, which is done socially as a human being is smile. The first time the baby smiles, mother, father, grandmother, grandfather, sisters, brothers, the whole family as a whole smiles back at the baby. For the rest of the life the baby will smile more frequently to a smiling face than to any other facial expressions.

Numerous facial expressions studied by Charles Darwin are a few example of visual releasers and FAP. The smile is a universal gesture among humans, signaling appeasement and friendliness. The grimace (a sign of threat or anger) is exhibited by all races of human beings. Children born blind have the same set of facial expressions as sighted children, although they have never seen a face.

AUDITORY RELEASERS

Sound is very important in human life. Evolution of language is quite recent and well organised language is found only in human beings. Language is important for human communication and tone of voice communicates emotion. Music and musical rhythms are interesting sources of human sound production. Hindi songs in India is just as soothing to a Russian or German.

ODOUR RELEASERS

Humans produce pheromones which affect our behaviours like other animals. Axillary hair (hair in the armpits), pubic hair (hair on the part of the body near the sexual organs) and hair on our scalps have a specialized kind of sweat glands. The secretions of these glands have more proteins and oil than that of other sweat glands. They release more oil in males than in females. The secretions cling to hair, creating scent traps. It is significant that sites of these hair patches are located where scents can best be perceived during mating by apes. Dr. George Dodd identified human pheromone in male sweat. It is identified as X-androsknol. A perfume called Androm costs $1000 for an ounce. Frequent bathing with soap or shampoo removes body odour which reduces the sex attractant chemicals in humans.

Women are sensitive to the smell of musk. Sexually mature women at the time of ovulation are highly sensitive to the smell of musk. This suggests that in past our ancestors produced a sex pheromone that stimulated receptive females. Young, prepuberscent girls are not sensitive to musk but like sweet, fruity smells. The body odour of humans is commonly referred to as B.O. Every individual has a definite kind of body odour. By the 6th week baby recognises its own mother not by sight but by mother's body odour.

The prepuce of the male penis and the female vulva bear preputial glands which secrete a semisolid curd like substance called *smegma*. This substance produces a smell which may be associated with sexual attraction. Vaginal secretions from human females have been a potential source of pheromones attracting males for mating. Human vaginal smears contain a mixture of six acids. This mixture of acids has been identified as copulins in female rhesus monkeys. Mc. Clintock suggested the existence of copulins in human female vaginal secretions which stimulates males for mounting and mating.

Interesting cases of pheromones influencing menstrual cycle have been studied. Data obtained showed that menstrual cycles changed from an average of 8 days apart to only 5 days among young women living in dormitories and sororities. 'Acsynchrony pheromone' is thought to be secreted with underarm perspiration.

SLEEP

Sleep can be considered as extreme state of inactivity. Prolonged wakefulness causes fatigue, and urge to sleep. Though actual cause of origin of sleep is not clear but Allison and Van Twyver (1970) proposed that sleep behaviour must have evolved independently among birds and mammals. *Paradoxical sleep* in mammals developed after slow wave sleep, a proposed divergence of eutherians from non-eutherians.

Sleep has been studied most extensively in mammals, particularly in humans. Several lines of evidence suggest the existence of sleep inducing chemical in the brain. Normal sleep consists of two components : non-rapid eye movement (NREM) sleep and rapid eye movement (REM) sleep. NREM sleep comprises four sequential stages, each characterized by different kinds of EEG (electroencephalograph) activities.

Stage 1 is a transition stage between wakefulness and sleep that normally lasts 1–7 minutes. The person is relaxed with eyes closed and has quick thoughts.

Stage 2 or light sleep is the first stage of true sleep. In this stage, a person is a little more difficult to awaken. Fragments of dreams may be experienced and eyes may slowly roll from side to side.

Stage 3 is a period of moderately deep sleep. Blood pressure and body temperature falls. It is difficult to awaken the person. This stage occurs about 20 minutes after falling asleep.

Stage 4 is the slow wave sleep or deepest level of sleep. The person responds slowly if awakened. The EEG is dominated by slow, large amplitude delta waves. Brain metabolism decreases significantly during slow wave sleep.

REM is also known as active sleep, rhombencephalic sleep, paradoxical sleep, fast or dreaming sleep. This sleep is the time of dreaming. Usually total amount of dreaming each night is about 1½ to 2 hours. Dreams vary among individuals and between the sexes and apparently depend on much on what goes on in an individual's life.

REM and NREM sleep goes on alternately throughout the night. As a person ages, the average total time spent in sleeping decreases; moreover the percentage of REM sleep declines. As much as 50% of an infant's sleep is REM, as opposed to 35% for 2 years old children and 20% for adults. Complete understanding of the function of REM sleep is not known, but the high percentage of REM sleep in infant's and children is thought to be important for the proper maturation of the brain.

LEARNING AND MEMORY

Learning is an adaptive change in individual behaviour as a result of previous experience. Memory is the ability to store and recall the effects of experience and without it learning is not possible. For an experience to become part of memory, it must produce persistent use of the brain. This capability for change associated with learning is termed plasticity.

In humans memory may be short lived or long lived. Short term memory is the temporary ability to recall a few pieces of information. Memory of exercise during examination is short lived. The ability to carry out coordinated motor activities such as swimming, riding a bicycle, toilet training etc. lasts throughout the life.

Long term memory has three main components : *Episodic memory, Semantic memory* and *Procedural memory* :-

(i) *Episodic memory* : It is linked to specific events. We retrieve an item from our "mental diary" by reconstructing the original experience in our mind.

(ii) *Semantic memory* : It is like a "mental encyclopedia". It holds knowledge of geographical locations, social customs, historical facts, meaning of words and the like. This memory does not depend on remembering when and where something was learned; it shows little decline with age.

(iii) *Procedural memory or Implicit memory* : It includes motor skills, habits and ways of doing things that can often be recalled without conscious effort. Remembering how to ride a vehicle is an example of procedural memory.

TERRITORIALITY

History of man tells that much blood has been shed mainly for three reasons– women, land and religion. Early humans moved about in small groups and frequently set up temporary camps or territories. These areas became their home range. Like any other animal species home range is also defended by human tribes. This brought competition for the sanctity of their home range.

Are we territorial in a modern society? Certainly, as we protect our homes, food stores, family members, and personal belongings. Is our defensive behaviour learned from our culture, or is it a biological characteristic of being human? Comparison of modern and primitive cultures indicate that all humans regardless of culture, display the same territorial behaviour. So it must be partly biological and partly cultural.

Tribal Territory

Countrymen of an organization, or a race constitutes tribal territoriality. The territorial boundaries of all countries are defined but sometimes disputes arise between two countries over piece of land in the border area.

Family Territory

Our home range is family territory for which we remain most defensive. Our home territories are also breeding territories, because breeding and other sexual activities are performed in a home territory. The centre of the home territory is the bedroom—often of the second floor. One feels most secured in his bed room. Feeding, grooming, and parental activities occur in other parts of the family territory.

Personal Territory

Every human have individual space like any other species. This territory moves with the person everywhere. There are different levels of individual space.

(a) *Intimate space* : Space reserved near our bodies for intimate relations which involve physical contact. Intimate space is reserved for mate, siblings and parents. Others who attempt to intrude this space are discouraged and physically expelled.

(b) *Casual space* : Space extending around us about one arm length. This distance is maintained with family members.

(c) *Social space* : A large space around us for interacting with colleagues, friends and known persons. This distance is usually 2 metres or more from our bodies.

AGGRESSION

Like other higher animals humans also have displays of threat. The most obvious facial expression of anger is the grimace. This includes partial exposure of the teeth, often more pronounced on one side of the face than on the other. The tooth exposure is created by curling the lip upward. The muscles along with nosed contract, forming ridges and furrows. The eyebrows are brought downwards and closer together, creating a furrow that extends upwards onto the forehead. The sides of the forehead become wrinkled. The eyes stare straight ahead or at the person who is responsible for the anger.

CHIN DISPLAY

Man stick its chins when he threatens someone. This behaviour is called chin display. The chin display shown as intention to bite. Modern humans do not bite but they have the chin display. Young children bite but restrain this behaviour by training.

THREAT DISPLAY

During threat, man holds its body more erect and åttempt to increase height. He stretches his leg and muscles pulling knees into a locked position. Deep inhalation of air cause the chest to increase in dimension. Inhalation also causes the shoulders to elevate upward. The total effect is to look larger. Simultaneously man use arm gestures to communicate his mood. It is common during threat to place the hands on the hips. When provoked further, and a confrontation is anticipated, then hands become clinched into fists, and people hold their arms outward, above and in front of the face. This posture warns "I am ready to fight".

CONFRONTATION

Human confrontation prior to the manufacture of weapons was probably just that a grappling or wrestling match. Natural and ritualistic form of human confrontation is to strike the opponent with the open palm, like a slap. To show the strength, the person attempt to hold the hands of the person who did the striking. This kind of manoeuvre may lead to neck and body grappling, also the tests of strength. It is only by training that a man can "punch out" another man with his fists.

Sports is a form of ritualized aggression. Rules of sports prevent serious injury to the participants. One can observe ritualized nature of the aggression in any sports. In matter of aggression mankind is different from all other species. First, we have group aggression. Group of humans as teams, tribes or battalions attack another group of humans, a behaviour not known for other animals. Second, human confrontation often ends in the death of the either of the opponent.

APPEASEMENT

A strong appeasement gesture is the smile. Greeting some one combine the smile with the eyebrow flash. Many other appeasement gestures are reverse of threat gestures. Throughout the world, the open palm is a signal of appeasement, although its use may vary from culture to culture. People wave their palm vigorously or flash it quickly when they say "hi". We use our palm as a signal of "good-bye", and appeasing mood. All religions demand appeasement postures to the god or goddess being worshipped.

Signalling appeasement by standing with shoulders thrown forward, arms and hands hanging beside the sides of body, knees flexed etc. are also common in humans.

SEXUAL BEHAVIOUR

Sexual behaviour of humans can be divided into four units :

1. MALE SELECTION OR PAIRING

Humans are sexually dimorphic. Male and female differ in body weight, hair colour, skeletal characteristics, and secondary sexual characteristics. Some of the differences between the sexes are due to different roles of males and females. The differences between the skeletons of male and female humans are primarily due to the greater muscularity of the man and to the fact that the female pelvis is designed to enable her to give birth to an infant with a large head.

Both men and women select mating partners, that are suitable to enhance their reproductive success and race continuation. Sexual releasers help them to select suitable partners.

(a) Male sexual releasers

Strong body and high status male are sexual releasers for women. They choose strong and high status male who can provide material resources that help her to raise her offspring. The secondary sexual characters also act as sexual releasers. The secondary sexual characteristics of humans include the different body hairs of the man, the change in the male voice that occurs at puberty. Puberty refers to the changes that take place in boys and girls to bring about sexual maturity. In modern society new kind of dress and fashion also act as sexual releaser.

(b) Female sexual releasers

Receptive, fecund and characteristics that suggest she will be a successful mother are female sexual releasers. A man chooses woman having these characteristics.

The hips of young sexually receptive female becomes wider and fleshy, making them more prominent. The pelvis widens and rotates backward, causing a more pronounced protrusion of the buttocks. This posture makes a woman walk differently from a man. The rear view of a walking women is a sexual releaser that attracts the man for mating.

Singh (1993) presents evidence indicating that body fat distribution, as measured by the waist-to-hip ratio, is correlated with good health and high fecundity. Her studies exhibit that men prefer female figures with a low waist-to-hip ratio, and judge them to be more attractive and have higher reproductive potential that those with a higher ratio

The secondary sexual characteristics of women include the protruding and rounded breasts. Crook (1972) believes that attractiveness of female breasts may be a cultural phenomenon, since it is apparently not a feature of sexual behaviour in all human societies.

Although it may be true that strong or high status, men may be sexually attractive to women and that female body shape, especially wider and fleshy hips, is attractive to men, this does not necessarily mean that sexual selection is responsible for these features only. Even in the total absence of sexual selection, it may be that these male and female features have no relevance to reproductive activity.

It is the custom in all human societies that people marry. In humans three patterns of association are prevalent. The first is a partnership between a man and a woman which lasts for their lifetime. Such strict monogamy, is probably not very common in many societies. The second is serial monogamy in which one person is married to several partners in succession. This may happen due to separation, divorce or the death of the partner. The third is polygamy – one man having many wives.

EXPERIENCE

Girls develop faster and become sexually mature earlier than boys. First menstruation occurs on the average during the twelfth year. Pair bonds occurred between males and females of different ages, the males being two or three years older. The difference in age and experience suggests that women evolved as the subordinate sex, men as the dominant sex.

VOICE

The tone of our voice is an vocal signal and inform about mood than what was spoken. During pair bonding, the soft, whispering sound of the voice as it speaks of love and loving is most likely an sexual releaser.

SEXUALLY SENSITIVE PARTS OF BODY

Though the entire body is involved in mating but some parts of body are sexually sensitive zones called erogenous zones. These are lips, nipples, breasts, buttocks, genitals, genital areas etc. But these parts are not sexual releasers in the usual sense. Their premature exposure or in different psychological state may 'turn off' the drive of sexual act. Exposure of genitals out of context is rude and threatening or embarrassing. Genital displays and genital manipulation plays major role in sexual behaviour but not during pairing.

2. COURTSHIP

Courtship displays of humans are slightly different from other animals. In Hindi movies, hero plays all sorts of courtship behaviour in melodrama form. Men display dominance during courtship, women display more appeasements and diversionary behaviour. It is pertinent for a woman to be attracted by some combination of male sexual releaser but are frightened enough not to approach and make her intentions known.

Courting humans can be recognized easily. They are those pair walking around holding hands/clinching bodies while staring into each other's eyes. Women show many postures of appeasement; such as standing, sitting or moving in a lazy way before the man. She gazes into his eyes, smile and turn her head downward looking at the ground. She may laugh lightly in a nervous or silly way. Cover her face, or suck her fingers. In response man stand close, grasp her chin and pull her head upward so that their eyes meet.

Kissing is one of the most frequent behavioural exchanges between courting humans. Kissing does not only have to be lip-to-lip. In fact, lip contact with nearly any part of the body commonly observed during human courtship. It is a very short step from kissing to nibbling with the teeth which is also commonly preferred between courting individuals. Courting pair feed each other. Prior to feeding, pair show begging by lip, making fold of lips, or intentional biting using the teeth.

Male sexual strategy in humans involves rivalry in acquiring women and a certain amount of aggressiveness in protecting them from other men. This may account in part for the man's greater size and strength.

3. PRECOPULATORY BEHAVIOUR

Precopulatory behaviour in humans involves close physical contact and mutual sexual stimulation. Courtship stimulates erogenous parts that elicit sexual arousal, when stimulated. The precopulatory behaviour of humans called foreplay includes, manual stimulation of various parts of the body, along with the shoulders, breasts, abdomen, thighs and genital regions. Kissing, molesting and sucking the breasts is a must precopulatory behaviour. Genital displays and genital manipulation are common. The display of the erect penis is not threatening at this stage. The penis and vulva are displayed and positioned for coitus.

4. COPULATORY BEHAVIOUR

Men and woman become physically and emotionally intimate to each other during copulation. The bond between human partners becomes more enduring during coitus. Copulation is performed in a prone· posture in partially or complete naked condition.

GENITAL DISPLAYS

Wolfgang Wickler (1966) studied the significance of penis display in some primate species and compares it with penis rituals and artifact in humans.

In papua, men of certain tribes enhance the penis with a sheath that is kept in an erect position by means of a string. By analogy with other primates, this may appear to be sign of male dominance and, therefore an important indicator of sexual selection. However, some anthropologists (Heider, 1967) are of the view that the penis sheath is not associated with social position or with erotic practices, a certain amount of doubt is there. After all, so many parts of the body are decorated by people living in different parts of the world. That it is not surprising to find some places where the penis is currently in fashion.

Wearing of cloth makes phallic displays almost impossible. Our cultural learning taught us that phallic displays is rude and even obscene. Still phallic gestures are made throughout the modern world because sexual behaviour is instinctive behaviour and instinct always dominates over learning. "Giving the finger" is no more than a phallic threat. Romans considered the middle finger their obscene finger. Arabs hold the open palm downwards with the middle finger extended and the whole hand raised and lowered quickly, they mimic the act of copulation. People of Mediterranean countries bend the arm at the elbow, clinching the fist and then jerking the arm as obscene gesture of threat. The fist mimics the penis, and the arm mimics the shaft. A person can make phallic displays by sticking out tongues even if his hands were tied.

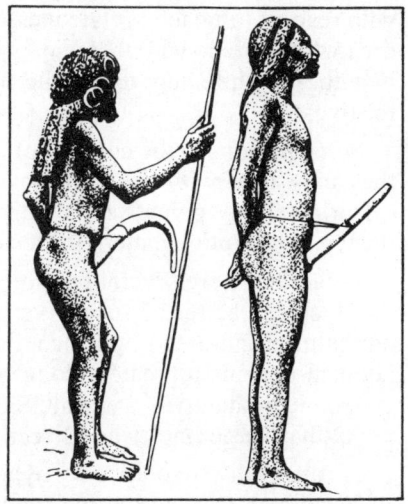

Fig. 11.1. Some tribals displaying their genitals.

PARENTAL CARE

Parental care is of highest level in humans. Not only parents but entire family and society takes care of new born baby. Birth is celebrated in almost all sects of human. Every person of the family participates in a tickling game or playing with human infant. Aunt behaviour is highly developed. Parents take care of their children for whole life. Human beings even take care of their great grandchildren. Entire family rather society becomes anxious if a child fells ill.

ADOPTION OF CHILD IN HUMANS

Why humans sometimes adopt children? In 1976, the cultural anthropologist Marshall Sahlins gave an analysis of adoption of child in Oceania, the islands of the central Pacific Ocean. In Oceania practice of adoption is to such an extent that about 30 percent of the children are adopted. Sahlins is of the opinion that the adoption practices of these cultures had no relation what so ever to kinship, demonstrating the arbitrary nature of cultural tradition and the irreverence of evolutionary theory to an understanding of human behaviour.

Sahlin was under the impression that there was only one possible sociobiological hypothesis for adoption, one based on indirect selection. He argued that this hypothesis required that adoption be a form of altruism rigidly determined by kinship relations between people. Because some persons in Oceania adopted children that were not their kin, he concluded that evolutionary theory could be discarded in context of adoption by humans.

Anthropologist has noted, the indirect selection hypothesis that adoption provides a means for individuals to raise their inclusive fitness by helping non descendents kin does not demand that every case of adoption involve closely related individuals. The indirect selection hypothesis does require that people should tend to direct their adoptive assistance to genetic relations more often than would be expected by chance alone.

John Silk analysed data on the relationship between moderately large samples of adopters and adoptees in 11 different cultures in Oceania. These data reveal that adoption was very much a nonrandom process with respect to genetic relatedness in these cultures. A substantial majority of adopters cared for children who were cousin equivalents or closer. These findings cast serious doubt on the arbitrary culture hypothesis while supporting the hypothesis that adopters tend to direct their altruism toward close relatives.

Some persons in the cultures of Oceania do adopt the children of complete strangers, youngsters that they may treat with the same love and affection that parents typically supply to their own genetic offspring. These parents apparently subsidize the genes of genetic competitors. Are these exceptions to the typical adoption pattern in Oceania impossible to explain from the sociobiological perspective?

In fact there are several possible sociobiological hypotheses for adoption among non relatives, each of which can be tested for a given case. Joan Silk observed that the parents of small families in some agricultural cultures might benefit from gaining adoptees, even if they were non relatives, if these adopted persons ultimately contributed to the family work force, enabling the family to achieve full economic productivity as a unit. Silk's prediction that small families in Oceania would be more likely to adopt than large ones was correct.

An alternative evolutionary hypothesis for adoption among non relatives recognize that some aspects of behaviour may be the maladaptive by-product of underlying proximate mechanisms that usually generate adaptive reactions. For example, adopting a non relative may be one consequence of the motivational system that causes adult human to want to have children and raise a family. According to this hypothesis although adults who adopt infant strangers may sometimes reduce their fitness, the urge to have a family and the love of children usually have fitness-raising consequences. Because these psychological mechanisms tend to elevate fitness, they are maintained in human populations even though they sometimes include people to behave maladaptively.

The maladaptive side effect hypothesis for adoption generates some testable predictions, one of which is that husband and wives who have lost an only child or who fail to produce children themselves should be especially prone to adopt strangers. Their instinct of parental care act as a proximate basis for adopting a substitute for genetic offspring.

Adoption of non-relatives sometimes also occur in non human animals when adults have lost their offspring and are presented fortuitously with a substitute. Adoption in animal world also exists as an exception. Cardinals have been known to feed gold fish. Cows have been known to feed goat or sheep.

SOCIAL BEHAVIOUR

Like many other animal species humans also live in a society. But it is true that it is an unusual species because (i) these can apply abstract intelligence to different situations (ii) these include art, religion and free- will. No other group of animal kingdom has these capability. Our brain's decision- making mechanisms were shaped by natural selection to enhance fitness, not to provide us with the capacity to monitor the fitness consequences of each and every action. Proximate mechanisms predispose and motivate individual to do things that lead to direct and indirect fitness gain. On the proximate levels humans enjoy sweet foods, fall in love, derive satisfaction from charitable actions, desire approval from others, and learn a language. Unfortunately Darwin's theory of evolution has been misunderstood and misused by some persons to defend the principle that the rich are evolutionary superior being. In terms of natural selection only that species or society is superior which has high rate of reproduction, great ability of adaptation with society and environment. In fact insect society is most superior and will dominate mammals and will rule the earth in near future.

Social behaviour in humans developed beyond pair formation and family life to the establishment of communities at the level of bands, tribes, chiefdom and states. Co-operation among humans has been òne of the important keys to its evolutionary success. Co-operation spirit caused us to share with others – but most often our 'fair share' was earned in competition. The combination of some human characteristics–territoriality, co-operation and healthy competition has led to an efficient system that reduces fighting, social chaos and unpredictable behaviour. Co-operation was necessary when our ancestors first became hunter. Skilful hunting required each member of a hunting band to have specialised job. The co-operative spirit led quickly to co-operation in matters other than hunting. Humans co-operated in maintaining ideals, taboos and group identity.

Our earlier ancestors moved about in small troops. In course of evolution troops became tribes & tribes formed super tribes. We no longer had to search for necessary resources, because our intelligence and co-operation gave us the knack to tackle nearly any environmental obstacle. One form of environmental control was agriculture. Gradually our social life travelled from agriculture to industry.

The course of the evolution of human social behaviour was intimately linked with the development of multi factors and can be summarized step-wise : Establishment of the family → Prolonged childhood association with the family and society → Development of the concepts of a home base and food sharing → Competition for food replaced by co-operation in food gathering enterprises → Increased use of speech for communication → Division of labour by age and sex, with older males hunting in bands to increase efficiency of hunting; women stay together to nurse and educate children and give protection from danger → Establishment of a broader social structure where the dominance hierarchy was replaced by kinship and prohibition of incest → Extension of geographical range by tolerance of less optimal environment → Use of simple tools and eventually manufacture of complex tools → Use of fire in cooking food and defence against animals and enemies → Development of folk wisdom, art, religion, philosophy, science and technology.

Thus need of food, sex and safety were fulfilled more efficiently by group activities based on the rapid development of culture. Indeed it can be said that current human evolution is based more on cultural development than on other factors.

Social life for human being is essential because developing children not getting opportunity to interact with family members and society may grow up into disturbed, scared, and sometimes criminals. Adults who isolate themselves from the world, are likelier to die at comparatively young age than those who cultivate companionship.

MODERN HUMAN SOCIETY

In modern human society success is measured in terms of both the individuals as well as the community. But success of other society (society of insect, monkey, baboon etc.) is measured only in terms of society and not the individual like human society. The modern city social life is almost artificial and does not represent the true human society. In true society every individual contribute maximum and take things in return only for livelihood. In our modern society every individual is trying to extract all benefits from society for itself. In apartments of big cities people do not know even their next door neighbours.

POLYVAGAL THEORY OF EMOTION AND EVOLUTION OF SOCIAL BEHAVIOUR

There are numerous theories about evolution of human social behaviour. But one theory of the evolution of social behaviour is that the nervous system evolved in mammals beyond the dorsal vagal complex below to the "*smart*" vagus, which linked emotion to the vocal and facial expressions at the heart of complex social behaviour in humans.

COMMUNICATION IN HUMANS

LANGUAGE

Humans alone have developed spoken and written language which are used to facilitate interspecific communication and formulate abstract concepts of art, science, philosophy and religion. Human brains contain a language centre. In most people, the structure, a slender inch-long piece of tissue called then *Planum temporal* (language centre), is larger in the left side of the brain than the right. This area is involved in the processing and comprehension of speech sounds and sign language. Besides language centre, the basic anatomical structures associated with speech must be present in our body. We listen to ourselves and we can tell most of the time, when we have made a mistake, and we correct it.

HUMAN NON-VERBAL COMMUNICATION

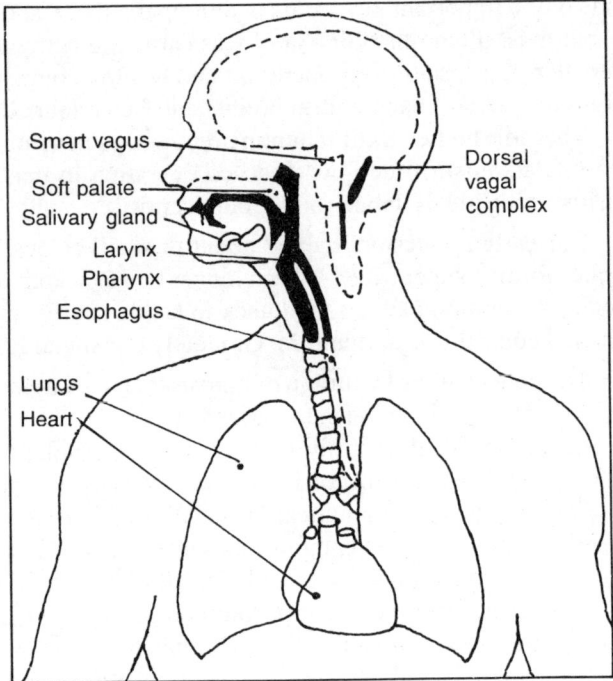

Fig. 11.2. Polyvagal theory of emotion and evolution of social behaviour in humans.

Eibl-Eibesfeldt (1970) looked at the development of reflexes in human infants, and the behaviour of children born blind and deaf-blind, and made good use of the comparative approach in his studies of human non-verbal communication. Today, scientists believe that the non-verbal aspect of communication in humans invites direct comparison with the displays of animals. But we should not forget that some aspects of human non-verbal communication are related directly to language. An obvious example is the sign language used by deaf people. However, most of the simple gestures, like the thump-up sign, are probably also derived directly from language.

One problem in studying human communication is that it may vary according to the cultural context. For example, a number of ways of signalling agreement and denial involve head movements such as nodding and partial rotation (shaking) from culture to culture. In Greece and Hyderabad state of India, 'no' is expressed by a strong backward jerk of the head. People of rest part of the globe express 'yes' by nodding their head. Some human facial expressions are universal and appear to have the same meaning in many cultures. In general, the eyebrow flash is used as a friendly form of greeting or approval, but it may be omitted by people who are reserved or suspicious (Eible-Eibesfeldt, 1970). Some basic expressions such as smiling, laughing and crying are universal. They also occur in people born deaf and blind (Eible-Eibesfeldt, 1970) and are prominent in young children (Blurton-Jones, 1972).

Analysis of human facial expressions reveals a number of basic situations that give rise to fairly stereotyped responses (von Hooff, 1972, 1976). These include alertness, surprise, fear, disgust, sadness, joy etc. *Alertness* is expressed in the relatively fixed gaze and certain tension of the facial muscles. *Surprise* is characterized by mouth. Fear is characterized by wide-open eyes and withdrawn lips. *Disgust* involves wrinkling of the nose and raising the upper lip, screwing up the eyes and turning away the face. In humans the disgust expression is ritualized, but in other primates it is merely a collection of protective responses that has no specific role in communication. *Sadness* is accompanied by arched eyebrows, retracted corners of the mouth turned downwards, and outward curling of the lips. Tears may be shed in intense cases. *Anger* takes a variety of forms, usually involving withdrawn lips and bared teeth, staring eyes and bringing eyebrows together. *Joy* is expressed by smiling and laughter, which are associated with humour. This behaviour is considered to by uniquely human. Some monkeys and apes have a relaxed open-mouth display that is associated with playfulness. It is superficially similar to human laughter. In both humans and Chimpanzees, the laughing type display is elicited by an element of surprise in the situation. In human babies and chimpanzees, this is of a purely physical nature, while in human adults it may be physical or purely intellectual.

Many other types of non-verbal communication can be classified in various ways. In addition to affect gestures, other classes of non-verbal communication can be distinguished. These include *adaptors* which serve both a communication and a non-communication function. Examples are grooming movements and intention movements. Emblems are non-verbal acts that have a verbal counterpart. They include the sign languages used by deaf people, obscene gestures and various signalling movements used at a distance like, beckoning. *Illustrators* are movements that are used to illustrate points that are also being made verbally. Gestures of emphasis, pointing etc. are included in illustrators. *Regulators* are gestures that are used to control the flow of conversation between two people. Examples are head nodding, eye-contact movements and various shifts of body posture.

The above discussion suggest that human non-verbal communication can be kept under two basic categories : firstly, communication that is ancillary to the use of language or that is part of language and secondly, communication that is independent of language and that is similar to the mode of communication employed by the majority of animals.

EMOTION

Man is highly emotional. The facial expressions of humans, and of other mammals, are usually regarded as expressions of emotions. The emotions such as anger, aggression, fear, love, hate or abhorrence, and jealousy are part of human behaviour. Human beings are supposed to have the basic emotions : pleasant or unpleasant subjective feelings such as sadness, joy and fear which motivate behaviour. People differ in their expression of a particular emotion. The emotional behaviour forms a basic elements of personality.

A baby's cry may express anger, fear, loneliness or discomfort. One can study the infant's emotions from their facial expressions as showing joy, sadness, fear and interest and to a lesser degree anger, surprise and disgust.

ART AND RELIGION

Whilst we share many aspects of behaviour with other animals there are some which are unique to the species and these include *art*, *religion* and *free-will*.

Most of the best-known *cave paintings*, such as those at Lascaux in France, are no older than 20,000 years. In some cases the art forms depicted animals and sex and these were often associated with death and birth respectively. They had no religious significance.

Religion is believed to have developed at about the same time as cave painting as evidenced by the form of burials found in various parts of the world. Religion as it is perceived today is fairly recent, the earliest shrines and temples being less than 10,000 years old.

OLD AGE BEHAVIOURAL DISORDERS

Two human behavioural disorders, sometimes associated with old age, are: Dementia and Alzheimer's disease.

DEMENTIA

It is a physiologically based behavioural deterioration characterized by confusion, forgetfullness and personality changes. Demensia is a part of aging.

ALZHEIMER'S DISEASE

Alzheimer's disease is a progressive, degenerative brain disorder that gradually destroys people's intelligence, awareness and ability to control body functions (Detail Chapter -3).

NORMAL HUMAN BEHAVIOUR VERSUS ALZHEIMER'S DISEASE

Normal behaviour	Alzheimer's disease
Forgetting things temporarily	Permanently forgetting recent events, asking the same questions repeatedly
Forgetting unusual or complex words	Forgetting simple words
Unable to do challenging work	Unable to do routine tasks with many steps, such as making and serving a meal
Get lost in a strange city	Get lost in one's own places
Occasional mood changes	Rapid, dramatic mood swings and personality

BEHAVIOUR THERAPY

Behaviour therapy is a form of psychotherapy that uses principles of learning theory. It is practiced to eliminate undesirable behaviours and develop desirable ones. Behaviour therapy is effective with children and adolescents, especially with adolescent girls. Every school must have a team of psychiatrists and behaviourists to evaluate the behaviour of disciples and guide them.

EXERCISE

1. Human behaviour? Is human behaviour different from other animals?
2. Mention similarities and differences between human behaviour and basic behaviour of other animals.
3. Describe male and female releasers to initiate human instinctive behaviour.
4. Describe Territorial behaviour in humans.
5. Imprinting? Describe imprinting in context of human behaviour.
6. Territoriality? Describe territoriality in context of human behaviour.
7. Describe different units of aggression : threat, confrontation and appeasement behaviour of humans.
8. What are the units of sexual behaviour. Describe pre-courtship and courtshipin human beings.
9. Describe precopulatory behaviour and genital displays in humans.

10. Write short notes on :
    (i) Mother baby relationship
    (ii) Synchrony pheromone
    (iii) Phallic displays
    (iv) Foreplay
    (v) Parental care in humans.

11. What are erogenous zones of human body. In what circumstances exposure of these may 'turn off' the sexual drive.

12. Describe specific human behaviours which are not found in any other animal.

13. Sleep? Describe sleep behaviour in humans.

14. Describe role of spoken and written language in human communication.

15. Write a short note on Learning and Memory in humans.

16. Write 100 lines about the behavioural disorders of human beings associated with old age.

17. What do you mean by human non-verbal communication? Describe it in 100 lines.

18. Write short notes on : Alertness, Surprise, Fear, Disgust, Sadness, Anger and Joy in humans.

19. What do you mean by Adaptors, Illustrators, and Regulators in context of human behaviour.

20. Write contributions of Eibl-Eibesfeldt, Singh, Wolfgang Wickler, Heider, Marshal Sahlins, John Silk in context of human behaviour.

GLOSSARY

Animal behaviour : All those processes by which an organism senses the external world and the internal state of its body and responds to stimulations it perceives is called animal behaviour. Thus animal behaviour may be viewed as stimulus - response relationship.

Antigravity reflex : Maintenance of equilibrium by the spinal cord and medulla oblongata.

American foulbrood : The larvae of honeybees are sometimes killed by a disease called 'American foulbrood'. To maintain a hygienic environment within the hive, the worker bees normally open the comb cells that contain diseased larvae and remove them.

Anoestrus : Unreceptive female for mating.

Animal cloning : Production of an individual from non-reproductive tissue of an adult animal by non-sexual method.

Akinesia : Muscle rigidity, involuntary tremour and inability to initiate movement is called Akinesia.

Astrocytes : It is one of the important types of brain cells surrounding blood capillaries.

Alzheimer's disease : Premature aging of brain in which loss of recent memory goes first followed by stored memory.

Aggressiveness : It refers to fighting or the act of initiating an attack.

Antagonism : On the one hand a hormone initiates a behaviour while on the other hand other hormone suppresses the same behaviour. Example : Testosteron initiates courtship behaviour while progresterone suppresses courtship. This is a case of antagonism between testosteron and progesterone.

Aggression : It refers to fighting or the act of initiating an attack.

Anthropomorphism : The interpretation of the behaviour of animals, as if they think in human terms, is called anthropomorphism.

Ad libitum sampling : A simple method of studying behaviour. One selects a group of animals and lives with them for a required period and behaviour of interest is studied and noted.

Aphagia : Loss of appetite.

Altruism : Certain species (social insects, birds, mammals) spend time and energy in rearing for other members of the society. The sacrifice of these members is called altruism. Worker bees keep the body of queen warm by covering her during winter and keep cool her during summer by fanning. In this act many workers die.

Anadromous migration : Journey of fishes from sea to fresh water (river) for spawning.

Alimental migration : Migration for the search of food.

Aestivation : Cold blooded animals enter a prolonged phase of dormancy at high temperature. This summer sleep is called aestivation.

Aggregation : To assemble many individuals of the same species due to environmental factors alone is called aggregation.

Activity period : The normal time during which animal is active, i.e. not sleeping. In species which hibernate or aestivate, time between emergence from and entrance into hibernation or aestivation is called activity period.

Activity range : The area covered by an animal in the course of its day-to-day existence.

Aggressive mimicry : Mimicry used to attract or deceive a species in order to prey upon it is called aggressive mimicry.

Agonistic behaviour : Any behaviour associated with conflict or fighting between two individuals.

Allelomimetic behaviour : Any behaviour in which animals do the same thing with some degree of mutual stimulation and consequent co-ordination.

Amicable behaviour : All specific form of behaviour which involves the association together of two or more animals and which do not involve conflict.

Avoiding learning : Learning to avoid a noxious stimulus, e.g. shock, by responding appropriately to a warning signal.

Appetitive behaviour : Chain of behaviours shown in the beginning of an instinctive behaviour.

Autism : A serious mental condition that develops during childhood, in which one becomes unable to communicate or form relationship with others.

Bioacoustics : Study of production and perception of sounds and their mechanical and physiological processes. It also includes the relationships between the vocalization of the animal and its habitat. This field helped in ascertaining the ontogeny and phylogeny of animal behaviour. Different species of cricket, very similar in their morphology, are identified by bioacoustics.

Biological rhythm : Study of periodicity of events of living organisms and their underlying processes is called biological rhythm. Rhythm may be of 24 hours (circadian), one year (circanual), 15 days (lunar) or of few minutes (tidal). Crabs emerge from their burrows at low tide and actively forage. As the tide floods they retreat back into their burrow.

Bee dance : Round and '8' shaped movement of foragers to communicate about feeding ground to their inmates is called bee dance.

Biotic isolation : Members of two opposite sex of different species do not mate due to different modes of feeding.

Bruce effect : If the male rat to which a female rat was mated is removed as soon as she becomes pregnant, and a strange male is introduced into her cage then the blastocysts inside her do not attach to the wall of the uterus. Her pregnancy is thus blocked and she comes back into oestrus - a phenomenon called the Bruce effect.

Brooding behaviour : Care of young by parents is called brooding behaviour.

Biological clock : Many internal physiological functions of body goes on in cyclic order. These physiological functions link together and constitutes a clock-like system called biological clock.

Behavioural toxicology : Study of poison is called toxicology. Altered behavioural pattern of an organism under the influence of some poison are studied in the behavioural toxicology.

Behaviour : Any response shown by an organism is considered as animal behaviour. Animal behaviour may be shown by organisms without nervous system, i.e. Protozoas and Poriferans, and animals having nervous system such as in coelenterates to mammals. Animal behaviour may be heritabled and learned.

Behaviourist : Who studies behaviour of organism is called behaviourist.

Cognition : Cognition is complex form of learning. The field of study of cognition deals with how one gains knowledge and how one uses that knowledge.

Conditioned reflexes : Reflex actions where the type of response is modified by past experiences. These reflexes are coordinated by the brain. Here innate and learnt behaviour patterns overlap.

Cranial reflexes or cerebral reflexes : This kind of reflex is carried out through the spinal and cranial nerves and are co-ordinated by the brain.

Compass orientation : The ability to head in a particular compass direction without reference to landmarks.

Courtship : The premating behaviour that stimulates one or both individuals and initiates the mating.

Components of behaviour : There are three main components of any behavioural act. (a) Anatomical (Movement of body parts). (b) Neurological involvement of Nervous System. (c) Phybiological (Metabolism).

Communication : Process of conveying feeling by symbol or sound is called communication. Human beings communicate through language. Honeybees communicate about feeding ground to their inmates by bee dance.

Cohesion : Social animals try to remain in close proximity to one another. This is called cohesion.

Climatic isolation : Different breeding season of different species keep them isolated.

Communal nesting : 1 to 4 pairs of birds build a communal nest in which all females lay eggs.

Co-operative nesting : Flocks of numerous pairs of birds build the nest and each pair has its own nesting chamber.

Catadormous migration : Migration of fishes from fresh water (river) to sea.

Chronobiology : Science of life related to time.

Circannual rhythm : The term circannual (*Circa* means about, *annual* means year) is used to refer to the endogenous rhythm that usually fall less than 365 days.

Classical conditioning : Learning that takes place when a conditional stimulus is paired with an unconditional stimulus. The well-known example is the work of Pavlov on dog. He introduced a ring of bell (CS) with introduction of meat (UCS) for salivation. After sometime salivation in dog started when only bell rang (CS) without introduction of meat (UCS).

Cultivator Ants : In South American rain forests some leaf cutter ants grow fungi on collected leaves. They use these cultivated fungi as food.

Closed society : A society in which new members are rarely admitted and the admitted member almost never voluntarily withdraws.

Comfort behaviour : Typifies a certain relaxation of tension, such as while the animal is cleaning itself, sun-bathing, feeding, embrace with opposite sex and so on.

Competition : The direct struggle between individuals for a limited supply of environmental necessities.

Consummatory act : An act which constituents the termination of a given instinctive behaviour pattern or sequence.

Critical period : Specific stage on ontogeny during which certain types of behaviour normally shaped and moulded for life.

Crowding : Refers to an excessive number of individuals, human or animal, with relation to available space.

Drive : A state of internal activity of an organism that is a necessary condition before a given stimulus will elicit a class of response, e.g. a certain level of hunger, thirst must be present before food or water will elicit an eating or drinking response.

Diodromous migration : Migration of fish from river to sea or from sea to river is called diodromous migration.

Diurnal periodicity : Migration of fish from river to sea or from sea to river is called diodromous migration.

Diurnal periodicity : Day and night cyclic activities of organisms in which organism become active during day is called Diurnal periodicity.

Diapause : A period of dormancy in response to unfavourable climate occurs among insects and this is known as diapause.

Division of labour : In context of behaviour, division of labour suggests the different functions performed by different castes of society. Perfect "division of labour" is found among social insects, because there exists highest grade of diversity of castes. Different castes among honeybee, wasps, ants and termites are queen, workers and males.

Ethology : Study of animal behaviour is known as ethology.

Ecoethology : The relationship between organisms and environment in context to behaviour is called ecoethology. Ecoethology tells us what is the biological significance of a behaviour.

Ethophysiology : Physiological basis of behaviour of organisms is studied in this field.

Ethogenetics : Study of genetic basis of behaviour is called ethogenetics.

Epigenesis : Development in gradual stages of differentiation. Each developmental event sets the stage for, but does not dictate the next. Brown 1975 suggested steps in epigenesis as $P_1 + G_1 + E_1 - P_2$, where P_1 = zygote, P_2 = Its phenotype at the next stage of development, G_1 = Genes that are active in guiding its growth and differentiation during the intervening interval. E_1 = Environment in which the development takes place.

Ethoendocrinology : Study of behavioural traits of animals, induced by endocrine system.

Epimelatic behaviour : Synonyms of maternal behaviour.

Emigration : Outward journey of individuals from homeland to breeding ground.

Endogenous rhythm : Periodicity in physiology behaviour exhibited by organisms.

Eliminative behaviour : Behaviour associated with the elimination of urine and faeces.

Estivation : The dormant condition of an organism during the summer.

Et-epimelitic behaviour : Defined as calling or signalling for care and is very widely found in animals which give some care to the young. This behaviour could be called infantile except that it also occurs in adult animals.

Focal animal sampling : A method of studying animal behaviour. In this method a particular individual of interest receives the highest priority for recording its behaviour.

Fighting : It is regarded as involving the physical contact of animals, one or each of them biting, pushing or kicking the other.

Geotropism : Orientation of part of plant towards or against the gravitation. Roots are positively geotropic i.e. grow downwards while shoots are negatively geotropic i.e. grow upwards.

Genetic memory : Behavioural traits of an organism are strictly according to its genotype. The continuation of information for behavioural trait by gene, generation to generation is called genetic memory. Genetic memory establishes a stereotyped set of responses in animals.

Genetic mosaics : Interaction of different mutant genes producing complex behaviour patterns is called genetic mosaics. When different species of *Drosophila* were exposed to radiation, these individuals showed some normal tissues and other mutant tissues. It has been seen in 'wing up' mutation. Flies with 'wing up' mutation keep their wings raised up but are unable to fly.

Gregarious : Association of members of a species neither helping nor depending on each other but living together are gregarious. High humidity under a log causes aggregation of woodlice. They form a dense aggregation but their aggregation is without much positive interaction.

Geographical isolation : Members of two opposite sexes of a species do not get a chance to mate for long due to geographical barriers and it is called geographical isolation.

Grooming : The act of removing foreign objects from the coat, using any convenient device, fingers (primates), tongue (cattle, cats), teeth (rodents) etc.

Heliotropism or diaphototropism : The vertical orientation of leaves of plants, at right angle to the source of light.

Human ethology : Study of human behaviour is called human ethology.

Habituation : The gradual reduction of responsiveness to a stimulus which are of no use or harm (at that moment) to the life of the animal is called habituation.

Hyperphagia : Desire of excessive feeding.

Hibernation : Cold blooded animals undergo as prolonged phase of dormancy at low temperature. This winter sleep is called hibernation.

Hierarchy : This term is applicable to any social rank order established through direct combat, threat, passive submission, or some combinations of these behaviour patterns.

Home range : That area which is traversed by the animal in its normal activities for food gathering, mating and caring for young.

Hypothalamus : Hypothalamus is very small part of brain forming lateral wall of third ventricle (cavity of diencephalon). It contains (1) Optic chiasma, (2) Mammilary body, (3) Tuberconeveum, (4) Infundibulum, (5) Pars nervosa. Hypothalamus also contains so many nuclei such as (1) Supra optic, (2) Paraventricular, (3) Dorsomedia, (4) Ventromedial, (5) Suprachromatic.

The activities are controlled by the neurosecretory centres of the hypothalamus. Secretions of the anterior pituitary as well as posterior pituitary are under the control of hypothalamus. Hypothalamus remains connected with anterior pituitary with a very elaborate motor system i.e. portal system.

The search for hypothalamic neuro-humours that regulate the pituitary gland has been sincerely made by many workers. Extracts from the nerohypophysis, medium eminence or hypophysed-portal vain have shown great influence on the working of the pituitary gland. There are hypophyseotropic materials which have been called releasing factors (RF) or releasing hormone (RH). Different hormones produced by hypothalamus are - CRF (corticotropin releasing factor). CRF was described by Saffran (1968) for the first time and was obtained from the extracts of the hypothalamic tissue. This stimulates the release of ACTH (Adrenocorticotropic hormone) from the tissue of the pituitary gland maintained in organ culture.

Extracts from the median eminence of the hypothalamus have been found to contain releasing factors or releasing hormones (RF or RH). There are nine such factors which include both the stimulating factors (stimulating hormones) and the inhibitory factors (inhibitory hormones). They are as follows:

TRF (Thyrotropin releasing hormone). SRF or GH-RF (Somatotropin releasing factor or Growth hormone releasing factor). MSH-IF (Melanocyte stimulating hormone inhibiting factor).

Bower et al. (1970) have prepared some synthetic hormones.

They are as follows : (1) CRF (Corticotropin releasing factor), (2) TRF (Thyrotropin releasing factor), (3) SRF (Somatotropin releasing factor). (4) FSH-RF (Follicle stimulating hormone releasing factor (FSH-RF). (5) LH-RF (Luteinizing hormone releasing factor). (6) PR-IF (Prolactin releasing inhibitory factor). (7) MSH-RF-IF (Melanocyte stimulating hormone releasing inhibiting factor).

Releasing factors secreted in certain parts of the hypothalamus reach the pituitary gland through hypophyseal portal system. The above mentioned stimulating factor stimulate the pituitary gland and the latter secretes the tropic hormones (Somatotropic hormone, Lactotropic hormones, Gonadotropic hormone, Thyrotropic hormone and Corticotropic hormone).

Now, tropic hormones will stimulate a peripheral target gland which will secrete its respective hormones according to need of the body. For example, production of thyroxine (a hormone of thyroid gland) can be cited. The hypothalamus secretes the thyrotropin releasing factor (TRF). This factor stimulate the adenohypophysis of the pituitary gland and the latter secrete the thyroid stimulating hormone (TSH). This tropic hormone will finally stimulate the thyroid gland to secrete thyroxine (T_4).

Homeostasis : Maintenance of Consistency of internal environment in the living organisms.

Irritability : It is a characteristic feature of all living organisms and involves their ability to respond to a stimulus. Considering irritability at organism level the characteristic responsiveness exhibited by an organism is called irritability.

Instinct : It is complex, inborn, stereotyped and species specific behaviour pattern of immediate adaptive survival value to the organism and are produced in response to sudden changes in the environment. Instinct forms a kind of species memory passed on from each generation to its offspring. Social behaviour of some insects and mammals; Migratory behaviour of some birds; Parental care in some fishes, amphibians, reptiles, birds and mammals are a few examples of instinctive behaviour.

Imprinting : The process of learning in the earliest stage of life is called imprinting. The process is confined to a definite brief period of the individual's early life. Once accomplished, the process is very stable and perhaps totally irreversible.

Insight : The sudden adaptive reorganisation of experiences or sudden production of a new adaptive response not arrived at by trial-and-error behaviour is called insight.

Innate behaviour : Inborn and unlearnt behaviours basically determined by genome of the individual is called innate behaviour. In other words inborn or hereditary behaviour of a species is called innate behaviour.

Incubation : The act or process of incubating (maintaining temperature of eggs by body) is found among birds and primitive mammals.

Immigration : Inward journey or return journey of animals from the breeding ground to homeland.

Ingestive behaviour : Behaviour concerned with the taking of solids and liquids into the digestive tract.

Investigative behaviour : Sensory inspection of the environment is called investigative behaviour.

Jacobson's organ : An olfactory canal in the nasal mucosa which ends in a blind pouch. It is highly developed in reptiles and vestigial in humans.

Junctional receptor : An acetylecholine receptor which occurs in clusters in a muscle membrane at the nerve - muscle junction.

Juvenile behaviour : The juvenile animal will often show behaviour is usually tailored to suit the young animal's need. The alarm behaviour of hearing gull chicks is quite different from that of adults. Many behaviours of human baby (juvenile behaviour) gives pleasure to adults.

Kinesthetic stimuli : Bodily internal cues which serve to inform the organism of its present state.

Kineses : Non-directional movement response of animals in which the rate of movement is related to the intensity of the stimulus and not the direction of the stimulus. It is the simplest form of spacial orientation and is shown by many invertebrates. The direction of movement of the tentacles of *Hydra* in search of food is random and slow, but if a prey is placed close to the *Hydra* the rate of movement of tentacles increases.

Kinesics : The body motion aspect of human communication is called kinesics.

Klinotaxes : Orientation of animals is achieved by alternate lateral movements of part or whole of the body. Intensities of stimulation between positions are compare and orientation is chosen accordingly.

Klinokinesis : Non-directional orientation movement of animals where the rate of change of direction increases in proportion to the increase in light intensity.

Kin selection : Hymenopterans have an idiosyncratic genetic system. Members of this order follow haplodiploidy during production of offsprings. Males are haploid and develop from unfertilized eggs parthenogenetically. Femals are diploid and develop from fertilized eggs. The relatedness between sisters of one family is more intimate because they share exactly the same set of genes from their father, which has only one set of genes to give. This is kin selection.

Learnt behaviour : Acquired or learnt behaviours are those which animals learn during their life time. Learning is an individual event and occurs in different ways in different species and in different contexts. Ability of learning has been demonstrated in all groups of animals except protozoans, cnidarians and echinoderms where neural organization is absent or poorly developed. Ability of learning in plants is totally absent.

Latent learning : Animals explore new surroundings or situations and learn something which may be useful at a later stage of life (hence latent).

Language : The system of sounds and words used by humans to express their thoughts and feelings.

Lunar rhythm : Lunar rhythm is a cyclic rhythm of about 15 days. It coincides with the rotation of moon around the earth.

Latency : The process which produces adaptive change in individual behaviour, as the result of experience. It is regarded as distinct from fatigue, sensory adaptations, maturation etc.

Leadership : It seems to be a case of facilitation, in which one animal sets the pace of group activity or initiates changes in it of various kinds. A leader is an individual which frequently remains at the head of a moving column and often seems to initiate a new activity. However, the emphasis in this situation should be on followership rather than leadership.

Menotaxes : Menotaxes involves orientation of animals at an angle to the direction of stimulation. An example is light-compass-response shown by homing ants.

Mnemotaxes : Involves orientation responses of animal depending on complex stimulus situations. Hunting digger wasp (*Philanthus triangulum*) uses a number of landmarks simultaneously while returning to its nest. Removal of any of the landmarks disturbs the path of hunting wasp in locating the nest.

Monosynaptic reflex : The sensory neurone synapses directly on to the motor neurone cell body. Only one synapse in the CNS is involved in a simplest reflex arc.

Motivation : Motivated behaviour is a drive that leads to goal directed behaviour and satiation. It may be measured by the intensity of rate of consummatory behaviour such as in eating, drinking and mating.

Maternal behaviour : Building nests, retrieving pups, nursing young ones etc. are maternal behaviours.

Monogamy : Mating system in which mating between one male and one female in one season or whole life takes place.

Memory : Ability to store and recall the effects of experiences.

Maze learning : Learning about maze (T-Maze, Y-Maze, complex mazes having many blind paths).

Migration : Periodic travelling (long or short journeys) of a population from feeding place to breeding place is known as migration.

Mimicry : For animals world mimicry means assumption of colour, form or behaviour patterns by one species of another species for camouflage and protection.

Mobbing : A behaviour showing habit of harassing of others, e.g. crows.

Nasties : Non-directional movement of part of a plant in response to an external stimulus is called nasties. The direction of movement is determined by the structure of the responding organ. Movement is the result of growth or a turgor change and small movements are typically amplified by the particular positioning of the responding cells. A sleep movement of certain flowers and leaves is called nictinasty. Open and close response of flowers due to light intensity is called photonasty.

Neuroethology : Study of behaviour of organisms related with nervous system is called neuroethology.

Navigation : Spacial orientation of animals in water or through the air is called navigation.

Neurones : It is one of the main types of brain cells that carry messages.

Nesting : Making nests by birds for laying eggs and incubating them is called nesting behaviour.

Nest parasitism : Some birds lay their eggs in the nest of other birds, e.g., koel lay their eggs in the nest of crow for incubation.

Nidicolous : Birds which hatch helpless, featherless underdeveloped young ones which stay in nest for sometime after hatching, e.g., pigeon, sparrow etc.

Nidifugous : Those birds which hatch well developed young ones. They leave the nest immediately, e.g., chicken and duck.

Nocturnal periodicity : Periodicity of day and night in which organism become active during night.

Ontogeny of behaviour : Study of development of behaviours in an individual is called ontogeny of behaviour.

Operant conditioning (instrumental learning) : Learning that takes place when a conditioned stimulus given by any instrument is paired with an unconditioned stimulus. Opening of box with the help of a lever by a cat when offered a fish in a box is one of the examples of operant conditioning or trial-and-error learning.

Orthokinesis : Non-directional orientation movement of animals where speed of tuning of organism from side to side is related to the intensity of stimulation.

Oligodendrocytes : It is one of the main types of brain cells making myelin, an insulating membrane that surrounds the neurones.

Oxytocin : A hormone secreted by neurohypophysis. It stimulates contraction of the uterine muscles and milk secretion.

Organising thoughts : A pattern of thinking that repeats very often and is raised to the status of a concept.

Oceanodromous migration : Long to and fro journey in sea undertaken by marine fishes is called Oceanodromous migration.

Ornithology : The biological study of birds is called Ornithology.

Psychogenic stimuli : Stimuli causing psychological drive.

Phototropism : Orientation of plants towards or against light. Shoots are positively phototropic i.e., grow upwards and roots are negatively phototropic i.e., grow downwards.

Phylogeny of behaviour : Changes of behaviour in terms of evolution is called phylogeny of behaviour.

Polysynaptic spinal reflex : This has at least two synapses situated within the CNS as a result of the inclusion of a third type of neurone in the arc : an internuncial (intermediate or relay) neurone. The synapses are found between the sensory neurone and internuncial neurone and between the internuncial neurone and the motor neurone.

Polysynaptic spinal brain reflexes : The sensory neurone synapses in the spinal cord with a second sensory neurone which passes to the brain. The latter sensory neurones are part of the ascending nerve fibre tract and have their origin in the pre-internuncial neurone synapse. The brain identifies this sensory information and stores if for further use.

Phasic reflex : It is short lived but rapid adjustment of body. Flexion response, blinking eye due to sudden strong light, withdrawal of hand due to needle pinch etc. are examples of phasic reflexes.

PKU (Phenylketonuria) : Mental retardation controlled by a single gene where patients release an odour in the urine due to presence of excess phenyl pyruvic acid.

Pilotage : Steering a course using familiar landmarks.

Parkinson's disease : Parkinson's disease is a disease of neurones. It is also called paralysis agitants. It occurs due to destruction of substantia nigra leading to less amount of dopamine secretions.

Proseptivity : Initiation of female in establishing and maintaining the sexual interaction.

Patterns of behaviour : There may be several behavioural patterns in a unit of behaviour. Courtship is one unit of behaviour which has several patterns such as dancing, singing, offering food to opposite sex, showing woven nest, showing hip and bulged vagina or colouration etc.

Perception : What we see or hear or smell or taste or feel is often determined by what we expect to see or hear or smell or taste or feel is called perception.

Periodicity : Repetition of an act such as feeding, drinking, mating etc. in a definite time frame is called periodicity.

Polygamy : A single male mating with more than one female.

Polyandry : One female bonded with several males for mating purpose.

Persuasion : Following opposite sex for mating is called persuasion.

Promendra a deus : In scorpions courtship takes the form of a dance called "Promenda a deus."

Pairing : Living of opposite sex of a species together for whole life or a seasib is called pairing.

Precocial : Young birds hatching out of egg are able to move and feed independently.

Altricial : Young birds hatched out of eggs are not capable of leading an independent life. They require greater parental care for food and shelter.

Potamodromous migration : Long journey of fishes in big river.

Pheromones : Chemical subsistences emitted by many animal species to convey information. These are secreted from exocrine glands as liquids, transmitted as liquids or gases, and smelled or tasted by other individuals of the same species. Pheromones may release immediate behavioural response or it may alter physiology of the receiving organisms, usually through the endocrine system. In many species one sex, often the female, produces a pheromone attracting the opposite sex from some distance away.

Predation : The derivation by an organism of elements essential for its existence from organism of other species which are destroyed in the process.

Psychobiology : Interactions between psychological and biological behaviour.

Queen substance : A chemical secreted by the queen bee called queen substance is very important chemical which keeps other females of its own species sterile.

Reflexes : The simplest form of irritability associated with the nervous system is reflex action. This is a rapid, automatic, stereotyped response to a stimulus. Because it is not under the conscious control of the brain, it is described as an involuntary action. Flexion due to needle pitch, narrowing of the pupil of the eye due to sudden strong light, watering of the mouth at the sight or smell of a favourite food, coughing, sneezing, yawning etc. are common examples of simple reflex.

Reasoning : Mental process of drawing inferences from two or more than two statements or happenings.

Round dance : Worker bees (foragers) convey information about the feeding place to their inmates by a circular dance when the feeding place is less than 100 metres from the hive.

Reflex arc : The neurones forming a pathway taken by the nerve impulses in reflex action make a reflex arc.

Righting reflex : It adjust first the position of hand to the earths surface, then the position of the trunk and finally position the limbs to keep the body in right position.

Receptivity : The pastural response of female in achievement of ejaculation by the male is called receptivity.

Roosting : Birds rest at night after a day of moving about and feeding. For this, they come together on trees in the evening. This is called roosting. Diurnal birds roost at night, while the nocturnal birds such as owls roost during the day. Some birds such as koels roost singly whereas bulbuls roost in small groups. Mynas roost in very large groups. Community roosting of Indian mynas, crows and parakeets can be seen very frequently on some trees. Roosting provides three main advantages to birds : (1) Receive warmth from one another. (2) Communal roosting serves as centres of information regarding good source of food that have been located by other birds. (3) If any one sees a predator, it warns others of the possible danger.

Releaser : Any specific feature or complex of features in a situation eliciting an instinctive activity or mood.

Ritualization : Many ethologists showed that display could often have been evolved from non-communicative behaviour. Moreover, the ancestral pattern often persisted, either in the same species along with the display derivative, or in another species in a similar behavioural context. This evolution of displays from non display behaviour is called ritualization or emancipation.

Spinal reflex : It occurs through spinal nerves and is controlled by the spinal cord. Flexion due to needle pinch, blinking of eye due to fall of a sand particle are common examples of spinal reflexes.

Simian cloning : Production of two monkeys from same cell by dividing the cell in the year 1997 by Dr. Don Wolf is called simian cloning.

Stimulus filtering : Animal responding only to important events and ignoring unimportant one is called stimulus filtering.

Sign stimuli : Certain specific stimuli eliciting specific behaviour is called sign stimuli.

Spatial or spacial orientation : Orientation of an individual with relation to the immediate surrounding of the area.

Sexual behaviours : Behaviour related with reproduction. In higher animals, sexual behaviour is exhibited between two opposite sexes. Components of sexual behaviour are territorial, aggression, courtship, mating etc.

Sex attractants : Pheromones bringing together members of same species at a place for mating are known as sex attractants. A pheromone called Bombykol secreted by female silk worm moth attracts male moth for mating.

Scan sampling : A method of studying animal behaviour. In this method several individuals are observed one after other in quick succession in predetermined time interval.

Skill learning : If a particular stimulus is presented and the response is rewarded then the further responses to the same stimulus will be quick and refined.

Signals : Communication through symbols is called signal. Protective facial expression of mammals play a role to in communication.

Swarming : Leaving the nest by many members to avoid over population is called swarming.

Species isolation : One sex of a species can not mate with another sex of opposite species. It is called species isolation.

Spacial isolation : Isolation between opposite sex of same members due to long distance is called spacial or spatial isolation.

Synchronization : Two opposite sex coming together and becoming physiologically ready to copulate with each other is called synchronization.

Social nesting : Members of single species or different species living in a common nest is called social nesting.

Social parasites : Certain ants lay their eggs in the nests of other ants. Workers of those nests rear the young of intruder.

Satiation : Satiation is a drive reduction. It is characterized by a reduction in activity and in willingness to work for a goal.

Sensory adaptation : Increasing or decreasing sensitivity during the course of stimulation. Example - light and dark adaptation.

Social behaviour : It refers to the reciprocal interactions of two or more animals and the resulting modification of an individuals action system.

Spatial behaviour : Reaction to an individual with relation to the immediate surrounding and including the animate and inanimate objects within that area.

Thigmotropism or haptotropism : Orientation of plants towards or against the solid surface or touch. Insectivorous plants exhibit haptoropism. Tendrils are positively haptotropic, e.g. leaves of pea plant. Central tentacles of sundew (an insectivorous plant) exhibit positive haptotropism.

Tropism : Movement of part of a plant in response to, and directed by, an external stimulus. The movement is almost always a growth movement. Tropic responses are described as positive or negative depending on whether growth is towards or away from the stimulus.

Taxes : Orientation of the whole organism in response to an external directional stimulus. Taxis movement may be towards or away from the stimulus, and are classified according to the nature of the stimulus. If stimulus is light it is called phototaxis.

Trial-and-error learning : Animals learn things in day to day life by trial-and-error method. An organism tries each alternative to achieve goal through repeated successes and failures.

Telotaxes : Directional orientation movement of animals that does not depend upon simultaneous comparison of the stimulation from two receptors (mostly the eye). It can be celled as a goal directed orientation. When there are two sources of stimulation the animal moves towards one and never in a median direction showing that the influence of one of the stimuli is inhibited.

Tropotaxes : A complete case of taxis in which orienting locomotory movement of whole body is influenced by both external stimulation and internal state of organ of animal. Such behaviour is shown by animals with paired receptors to achieve a balance in reception of the stimulus.

Tonic reflex : It is slow but long lasting adjustment that maintains equilibrium, posture muscular tone etc.

Territorial behaviour : An area selected and protected by an individual for home, courtship, mating, brooding etc. The area is protected by many defensive mechanisms and the behaviour in this context is called territorial behaviour.

Latent learning : Learning without any immediate patent reward. Thorpe (1910) for the first time recognised this type of learning through mazes.

Trophollaxis : Exchange of food between organisms, not only of the same species but also between different species, especially among social insects.

Territory : An area selected and protected by an individual for home, courtship, mating, brooding etc. is called territory.

Tidal rhythm : Rhythms of behaviours that coincides with the tidal cycle.

Threat : A posture, movement or display that signals the intention of engaging in an aggressive physical interaction.

Trophallaxis : Exchange of food between organisms, not only of the same species but between different species, especially among social insects.

Unconditioned reflex : Inborn reflexes are unconditioned reflex. Withdrawal of hand by pricking a hole in finger by a pin winking of eye in sudden strong light etc. are unconditioned reflexes.

Unit behaviour : One activity like orientation, feeding, aggression, courtship, mating, nesting, brooding etc. are units of behaviour.

Utility function : Animals behave in a way that maximizes benefit (minimizes cost). The components of cost include factors associated with the behaviour occurring at a particular time and risks associated with the animals internal state. The incubating gulls incurs physiological cost in keeping the egg warm, and it incur costs as a result of increasing hunger while on the nest.

Visceral reflex : The autonomic nervous system controlling activities of the internal environment that are normally involuntary, such as heart beat, peristalsis, sweating etc.

Viviparity : Internal incubation of eggs and giving birth to young ones is called viviparity. Few species of fishes, amphibians and eutherians are viviparous.

Wading bird : Any of the long-legged, long-necked birds composing the order ciconiiformes, including storks, herons, egrets, and ibises.

Waggle dance : Worker honeybees (foragers) convey information about the feeding site to their inmates by a dance, making a figure of '8' when the flower bed is beyond 100 meters from the hive.

Walking bird : Any bird of the order columbiformes, including the pigeons, doves, and sand grouse.

Warning display : Displays by which animals attempt to scatter off their enemies.

Whooping crane (*Grus americana*) : A member of North American migratory species of wading birds. The entire species forms a single population.

Xanthism : A colour variation in which an animal's normal colouring is largely replaced by yellow pigment. Also known as canthochroism.

X chromosome : The sex chromosome occurring in double dose in the homogametic sex and in single dose in the heterogametic sex.

X organ : A cluster of neurosecretory cells of the medulla terminals, a portion of the brain lying in the stalk of in stakked-eyed crustaceans.

Xylocopidae : A family of hairy tropical bees in the super family Apoidea.

Xenopus laevis : African clawed toad (*Xenopus laevis*). The male develops special nuptial pads on his forelimbs during the breeding season.

Yak (*Poephagus grunniens*) **:** A heavily built, long-haired mammal of the order Artiodactyla, with a shoulder hump; related to the bison, and resembles it in having 14 pairs of ribs.

Y chromosome : The sex chromosome found only in the heterogametic sex.

Young-Helmholtz theory : A theory regarding colour vision receptors that respond to short, medium, and long waves respectively. Primary colours are those that stimulate most successfully the three types of receptors. Also known as Helmholtz theory.

Yerkish : A chimpanzee was taught to read by David Premack (1976, 1978) using plastic shapes for letters. Another method was employed by Duane Rumbargh (1977), who used an artificial grammar. Called it Yerkish Glaserfeld, 1977.

Zeitgeber : It is a German term meaning "time-giver". This term was coined by J. Aschoff (1960) for the environmental agents that entraints the organism's behaviour to the external environment.

Zoology : The Science that deals with knowledge of animal life.

Zygote : 1. An organism produced by the union of two gametes. 2. The fertilized ovum before cleavage.

Zoraptera : An order of insects, related to termites, which live in decaying wood, sheltered from light; most individuals are wingless, pale in colour and blind.

Zoosemioties : The study of systems of animal communications.

Zoomorphism : The animal sometimes considers a man as one of its kind, and consequently treats him as a member of the same species. The man enters into the social organisation of the corresponding animal group.

BIBLIOGRAPHY

Alcock John : Animal Behaviour. Sinauer Associates, Inc. Publishers Sunderland, Massachusetts.

Arora, M.P. (1985) : Animal Behaviour. Himalaya Publishing House, Mumbai.

Aubrey Manning (1989) : An Introduction of Animal Behaviour. Edward Arnold (Publishers) Ltd.

Armstrong, E.A. (1947) : Courtship and Display Amongst Birds. Lindsay Drummond, London.

Austin, C.R. and Short, R.V. (1972) : Hormones in Reproduction. Cambridge University Press, London.

Austin, C.R. and Short, R.V. (1972) : Reproduction in Mammals. Cambridge University Press, London.

Baker, R.R. (1981) : Animal Migration, Cambridge University Press, Cambridge.

Bateson, P.P.G. (1971) : Importing Ontogeny of Vertebrate Behaviour. Academic Press, New York and London.

Berthold, P. (1974) : Circannual Clocks, Academic Press, New York.

Bolles, R.C. (1969) : Theory of Motivation. Harper and Row, New York.

Brown, F.A.J. (1962) : Biological Clock. George G. Harpa and Company, New York.

Brown, J.L. (1975) : The Evolution of Behaviour. W.W. Norton, New York.

Bunning, E. (1967) : The Physiological Clock. Springer-Verlag, New York.

Butler, C.G. (1974) : The Word of the Honey-bee, Collins, London.

Carr, A. (1962) : Guide Posts of Animal Navigation. George G. Harpa & Company, New York.

Church, R.M. (1978) : The Internal Clock in Cognitive Process in Animal Behaviour, Hillsale, New Yorsey.

C.A. Gupta (1989) : Animal Behaviour. Uresia Publishing House, New Delhi.

Dilger, W.C. (1962) : The Behaviour of Lovebirds, Scientific American.

Dethier, V.G. and Stellar, E. (1970) : Animal Behaviour, 3rd edition, Prentice Hall, Englwood Cliffs, New Jersey.

Ewert, J.P. (1980) : Neuroethology, Spiner - Verlag, Heldeberg.

Fraenkel, G.S. and Gunn, D.L. (1964) : The Orientation of Animals. Claredon Press, Oxford (Dovers Books, New York).

Federica Colombo (1979) : Animal Society. Burke Books, London.

Frisch, K. Von (1967) : The dance language and orientation of bees. Belknap Press of Harvard University Press, Cambridge, Massachusetts.

Felix, J. (1973) : Cage and Aviary Birds. Hamlyn, London.

Guindevia, H.S. and Singh, H.G. (1996) : Textbook of Animal Behaviour. S. Chand & Co. Ltd., Delhi.

Hinde, R.A. (1970) : Animal Behaviour. 2nd ed., McGraw Hill, New York and London.

Iersel, J.J.A. Van (1953) : An Analysis of the Parental Behaviour of the Male three-spined stickleback. Behaviour, Suppl.

I. Akimushkin. Ethology what animal do and why. Moscow.

J.L. Cloudsley-Thompson, Animal Behaviour. Oliver & Boyd, London.

John Farndon : Collins Children's Encyclopedia : Harper Collins Publishers Ltd., London.

Kingfisher first encyclopedia of Animals, Kingfisher Books Grisewood & Dempsey Ltd. Great Titchfield speet London.

Lorenz, K. (1958) : The Evolution of Behaviour, Scientific, American.

Macmillan Encyclopedia of Science, Macmillan Reference USA, Yew York.

McFarland, D. (1999) : Animal Behaviour. Pitman Publishing Ltd., London.

Max Nicholson (1972) : Looking into Organism. John Murray (Publishers), London.

Mathur, Reena (1994) : Animal Behaviour. Rastogi and Company, Meerut.

Paul Schauenberg : Animal Communication. Burke Books, London.

Pavlov, I.P. (1941) : Lectures on Conditioned Reflexes. Internation Publishers, New York.

Payne, T.L. (1974) : Pheromone Perception. In Pheromones, ed. M.C. Birch, North Holland, Amsterdam.

Ranga (1994) : Animal Behaviour. Agro Botanical Publishers (India).

Singh Harjinder (1995) : A Text Book of Animal Behaviour. Anmol Publications, Delhi.

Thorpe, W.H. Learning and Instincts in Animals, Methuen, London.

Verma and Sharma (1988) : Ecology and Animal Behaviour. Jai Prakash Nath and Company, Meerut City, U.P.

Wilson, E.O. (1965) : Chemical Communication in the Social Insects Science, New York.

Wooton, R.J. (1976) : The Biology of Sticklebacks. Academic Press, London.

Wood Fenden, G.E. (1973) : Nesting and Survival in a Population of Florida Scrub Jays.

Zahavi, A. (197) : Cooperative Nesting in Eurasian Birds, Proc. XVI. Inernation Organisation Congress (Canberra Australia).

INDEX